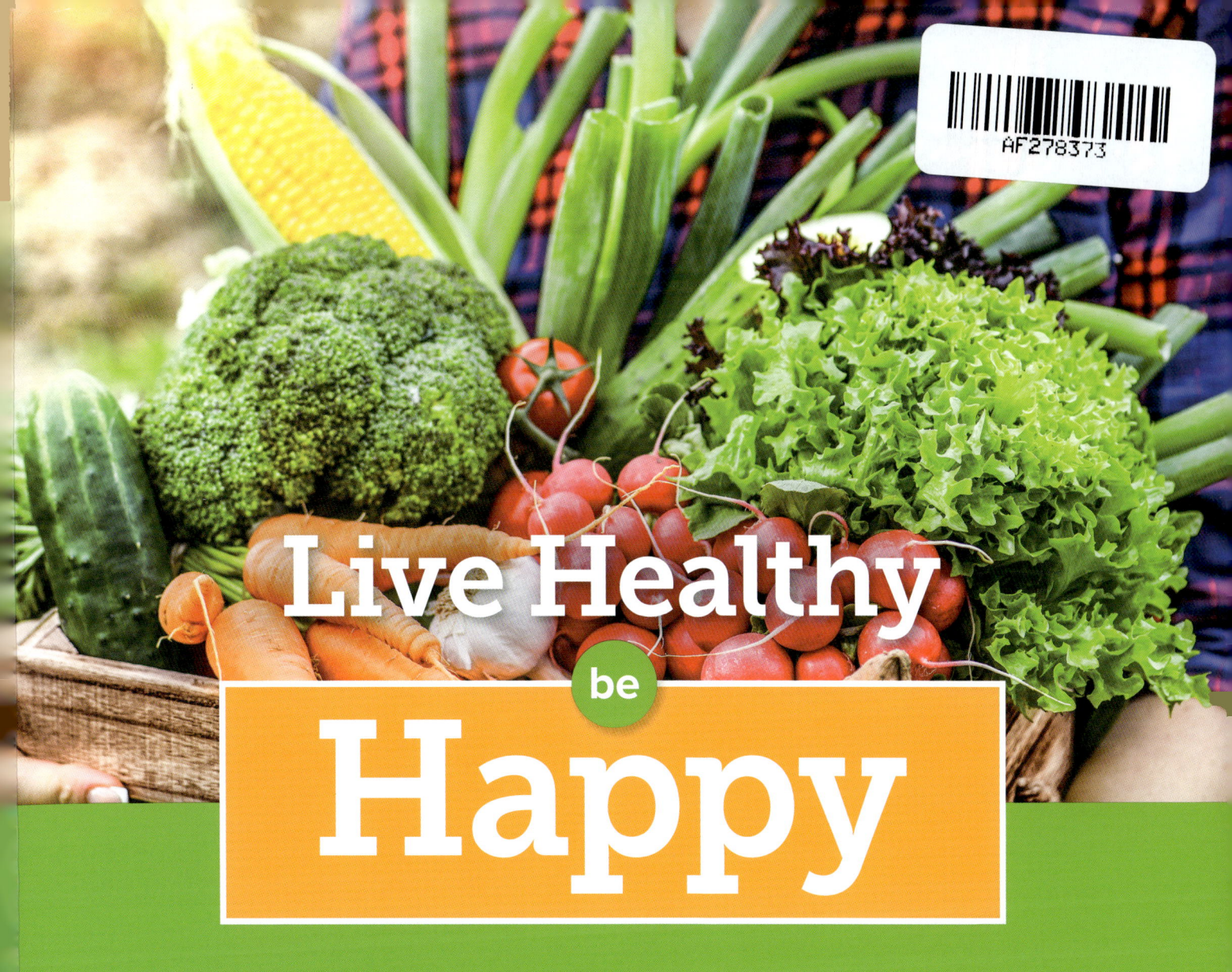

Live Healthy

be

Happy

CREATION Life

Guide For Students

Publisher and Editor in Chief	Robyn Edgerton, AdventHealth
Author	Jonathan Hickey
Production	Merita Ross, AdventHealth
Design and Layout	Carter Design, Inc., Denver, CO
Copy Editors	Matthew Janetzko, AdventHealth Katie Palacios, AdventHealth Jaclyn King, AdventHealth
Research	Heather Neal

Education Leadership
Jim Ingersoll, Associate Director, Secondary Education, Southern Union Conference
Keith D. Waters, Associate Director, Secondary Education, North Pacific Union Conference
Dennis Plubell, Associate Director, Secondary/Accreditation, North American Division

Review Committee
Burney Cullpepper, Bass Memorial Academy; Matthew Lee, Skagit Adventist Academy
Sandy Miller, Madison Academy; Tamara Ritterskamp, Forest Lake Academy
Andy Wade, Highland Academy; Chadd Watkins, Highland Academy

This book has been converted to an iBook format thanks to the following people:
Cameron Hathaway, Senior Interactive Designer
Stanley Pomianowski, Senior Videographer
John Boggs, Videographer
Olivia Crawford, Project Management
Camber Creative, Orlando FL

Published by AdventHealth | 833-854-8324

CONTENTS

INTRODUCTION   1

CHOICE   11

REST   33

ENVIRONMENT   61

ACTIVITY   89

TRUST IN GOD   113

INTERPERSONAL RELATIONSHIPS   135

OUTLOOK   165

NUTRITION   187

INTRODUCTION

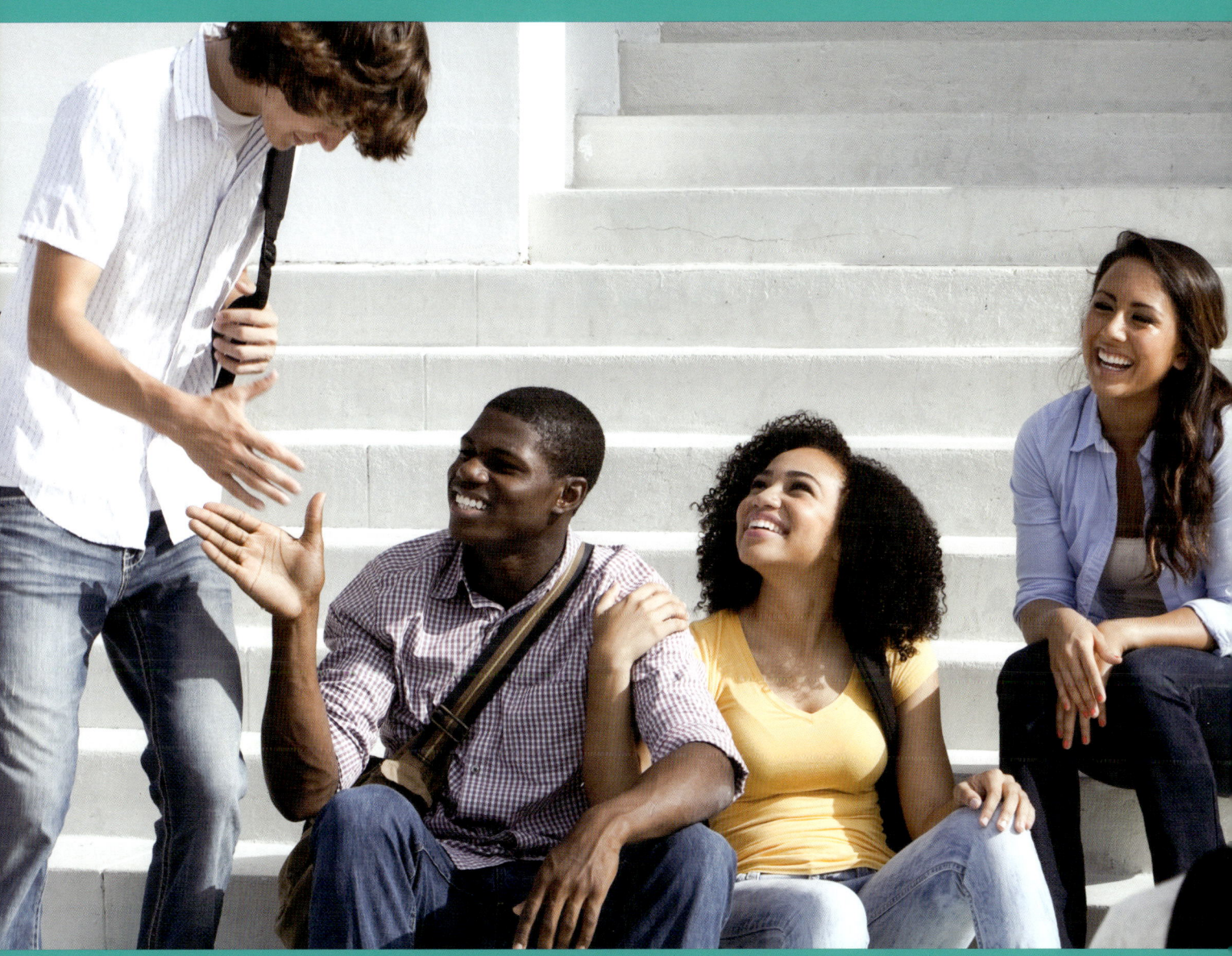

WELCOME

Right now you are young and bright, with a world of possibilities just waiting for you. Maybe you spend a lot of time thinking about living healthy or maybe you don't. Maybe you're a lot like Joe...

When Joe was your age, he didn't give much thought to making healthy choices. While he didn't make a lot of bad choices, he certainly didn't make a lot of good ones, either. Joe's biggest weakness was fast food. If it wasn't served at a drive-thru, then Joe didn't eat it. The only way he would touch a vegetable is if it was dipped in batter, fried and served G.B.D. (that's golden, brown and delicious). Joe didn't think his steady diet of grilled cheese, potato chips and deep-dish pizza was bad for him because he stayed relatively thin, but his choices eventually caught up with him. Once Joe got to college, he noticed he had gained some weight. It was something his classmates called "The Freshman Fifteen." Joe shrugged it off and kept eating junk food. Upon graduating, Joe's first job was working for a company where he spent the majority of his day at a desk. Joe never changed his diet to fit his less-than-active lifestyle, and he still ordered every meal through a loudspeaker. Then one day, Joe saw himself in the bathroom mirror. He couldn't believe his eyes. *When did I gain so much weight?*

Or maybe you're more like Katie. In high school, Katie was obsessed with her looks. She worked out every morning before school and was determined to stay slender. She typically ate very small portions or drank meal replacement shakes. On the rare occasion that she did overeat, she would punish herself by skipping meals later. Soon Katie's interest in diet and exercise took over her life. She stopped hanging around her friends after school because they always wanted to go out for ice cream. She was constantly comparing her looks to the beautiful women who graced the covers of magazines. *I'll never look like them*, she thought.

High school is full of people like Joe and Katie. They are trying to find satisfaction and happiness.

What does this have to do with CREATION Life? Everything. CREATION Life is about living your best life now. It's about living an abundant life. That means living the life God created you to live. It means not only can you be healthy, you can also be happy. You can start living the life God has in mind for you right now.

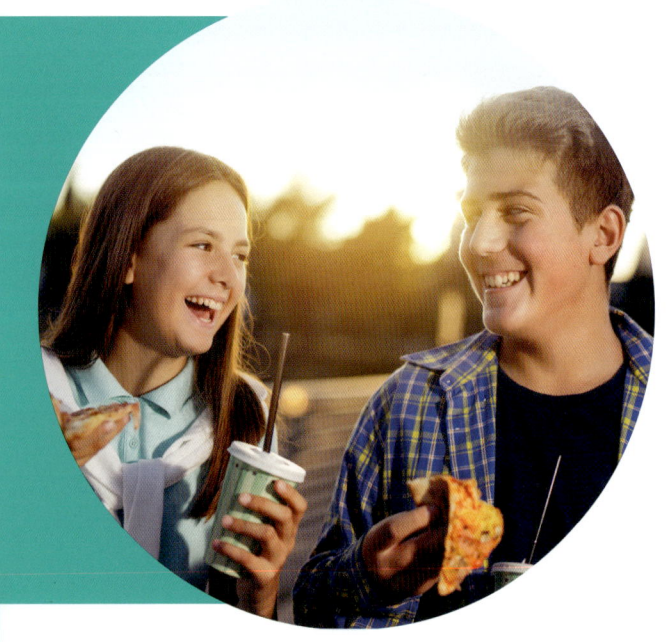

A WAY OF LIFE

CREATION Life isn't another program or diet, but a proven lifestyle that really works. The principles of CREATION may be as old as God's creation but are just as relevant and powerful today as they have ever been.

THE BEGINNING

If you want to know where CREATION Life began, you need to set your time machine for the mid-1800s. That is when James White, the first president of the Seventh-day Adventist church, was troubled by a series of mini-strokes. James' illness made it impossible for him to function from day to day, so he sought medical help. In those days, your options for treatment were fairly limited and in some cases even downright terrifying. Your doctor might have started by prescribing a small dose of arsenic, which is a lot like swallowing poison because... well, it is poison. Or your doctor might have suggested you try bloodletting, which is an even more peculiar practice. Many people believed the reason they got sick was because they had "bad blood" coursing through their veins. Naturally, the only way to get better was to let all that "bad blood" out. Veins were opened and patients would... well, *bleed*. Disturbing, isn't it? What's even more disturbing is that in its day, this chilling procedure was as common as taking an aspirin is today.

As you can imagine, these treatment options didn't appeal to James or his wife, Ellen, at all. They thought there had to be a better option out there somewhere. Since they were both believers in God, they turned to the Bible for answers. Inside its covers, they were surprised to discover many Scriptures written about how to live a healthy life, including some amazing concepts in the story of creation. They saw how God had placed the first humans, Adam and Eve, in the beautiful Garden of Eden. This made them wonder if the first step toward James' recovery might be as simple as relocating to a more "Eden-like" environment. So, James left his post, and the two of them moved to the country. James spent 18 months surrounded by nature, with plenty of fresh air, sunlight, water and exercise. He also worked hard physically, ate a vegetarian diet and got plenty of rest. At the end of the 18 months, his health was completely restored. James was able to return home with a renewed body, mind and spirit.

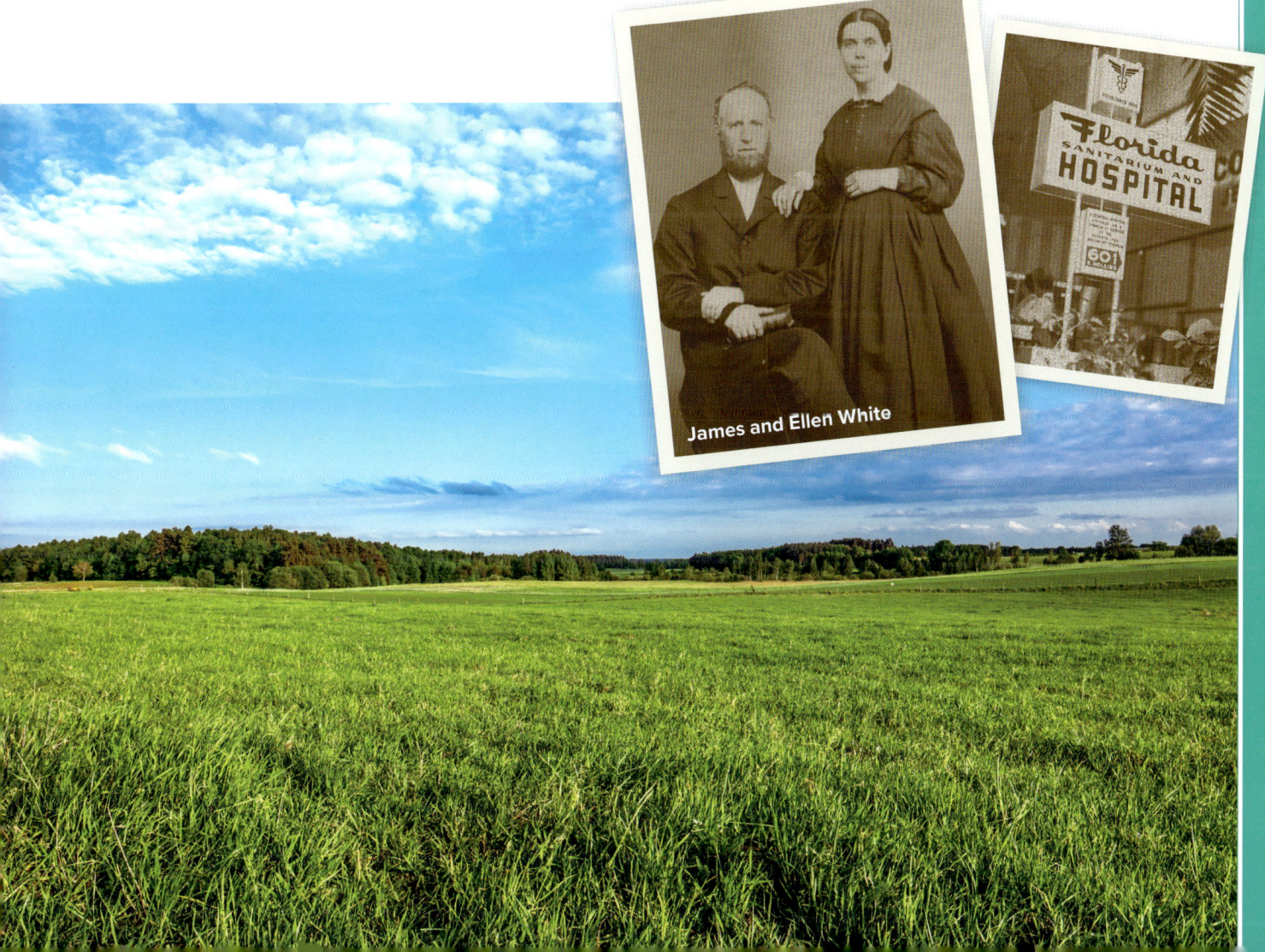

James and Ellen White

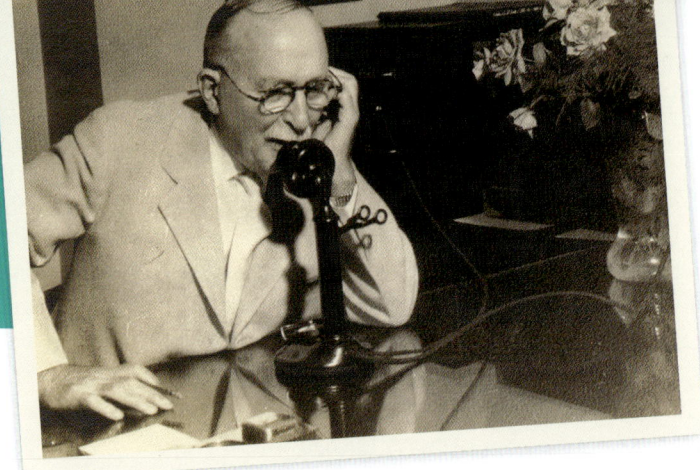

Dr. Kellogg making the first trans-Atlantic medical consultation in 1932.

After James' recovery the Whites noticed that many of their friends and coworkers were also experiencing a decline in their health and the devastating effects of disease. They knew if people followed the guidelines of Scripture, they would not only get better, they would stay better, so James and Ellen White decided to spread God's message of health and wellness to the world. In order to do this, they started a sanitarium in Battle Creek, Michigan. This was a special place where people could go not only to get well but to learn how to stay well. They also sent five young students to medical school — three men and two women, who all became doctors. One was John Harvey Kellogg. If you've ever enjoyed a bowl of Corn Flakes, you have John Harvey Kellogg to thank for it, but in those days Kellogg was known for much more than cereal. The prestigious *Journal of the American Medical Association* had this to say about the man:

Kellogg was without question one of the most famous physicians in the United States.... During his influential career, hundreds of thousands of persons with serious illnesses ranging from cancer and cardiac disease to gastric ulcers and debilitating digestive disorders demanded Kellogg's treatments, which combined modern medicine, surgery and bacteriology with an eclectic blend of hydropathy, vegetarianism, exercise and spiritual uplift. Those seeking treatment included such luminaries as John D. Rockefeller Jr., Thomas Edison and Henry Ford, whenever they were in need of a tune-up or recharge from the stresses of industrial gigantism; Amelia Earhart, before her important flights; Warren G. Harding, before embarking on his presidential run; and Booker T. Washington and Sojourner Truth, nursing wounds fresh from fighting the war against racism.... A vegetarian long before the term was coined, Kellogg developed his dietetic theories in protest against that era's standard fare of fatty, salted meats and fried foods. One of Kellogg's most popular books, *Tobaccoism or How Tobacco Kills*, was published in 1922 and is considered by many medical historians to be the first popular text alerting Americans to the dangers of tobacco smoking.... In his day Kellogg was the industrial king of wellness.[1]

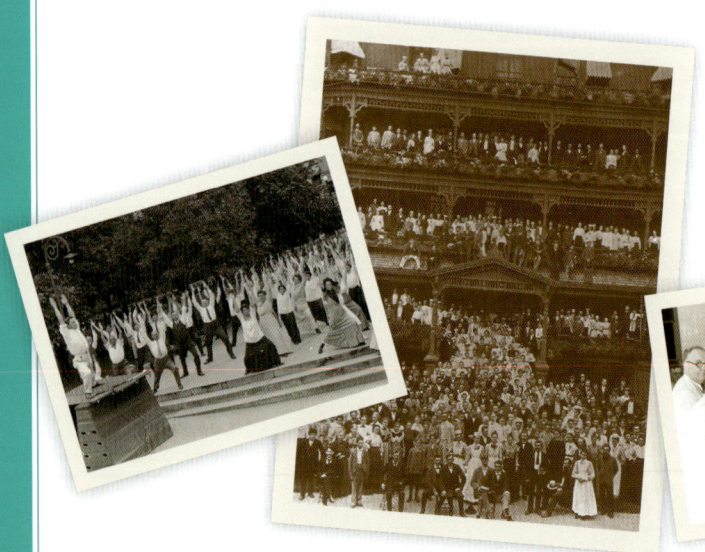

Kellogg became director of the Battle Creek Sanitarium in 1876, when he was only 24 years old. Under his guidance and leadership, the "San" (as it was affectionately called) became the first truly whole-person health center in the world, emphasizing that health involves the body, mind and spirit. Kellogg never ceased to make this connection for his many patients. As he once wrote, "Belief in God is the basis of all health."

Kellogg, who has been called "the father of natural health," was a prolific writer of over 50 health books and editor of the most popular health magazine of his day. When many of his patients suffered from life-threatening digestive and cardiac diseases, Kellogg correctly ascertained these illnesses were related to unhealthy eating habits, especially the typical high-fat American breakfast of his time. It was this understanding that led to Kellogg's ground-breaking invention — breakfast cereal — though in those early days, the only way you could have a bowl was with a doctor's prescription. Still, this healthy, nutritious breakfast soon launched a whole new industry promoting cereal as the foundation of a good breakfast. Kellogg's brother, W.K. Kellogg, had the vision and business sense to popularize the Kellogg's cereal brand around the world.

The health breakthroughs didn't stop with cereal. Peanut butter, soy milk and meat substitutes were quickly added as healthy diet choices. They extended beyond nutrition to exercise equipment, including the rowing machine, stationary bicycle, weight machines and the dynamometer — a machine designed to measure muscle strength that proved so valuable, it was adopted by the military. The program advanced to include aerobics and became, in conjunction with Columbia Records, the first exercise program set to music. The sanitarium also offered a variety of services, including massage therapy, weight loss and over 200 forms of baths. In fact, they had a lot in common with the modern specialty spas of today.

Kellogg's movement had such an impact that Battle Creek became known as "Health City." The thousands of physicians and nurses trained at the Sanitarium launched a health movement that today includes more than 550 Seventh-day Adventist hospitals and clinics around the world — all seeking to heal through renewing the body, mind and spirit.

"Physical fitness is not only one of the most important keys to a healthy body, it is the basis of dynamic and creative intellectual activity."

JOHN F. KENNEDY

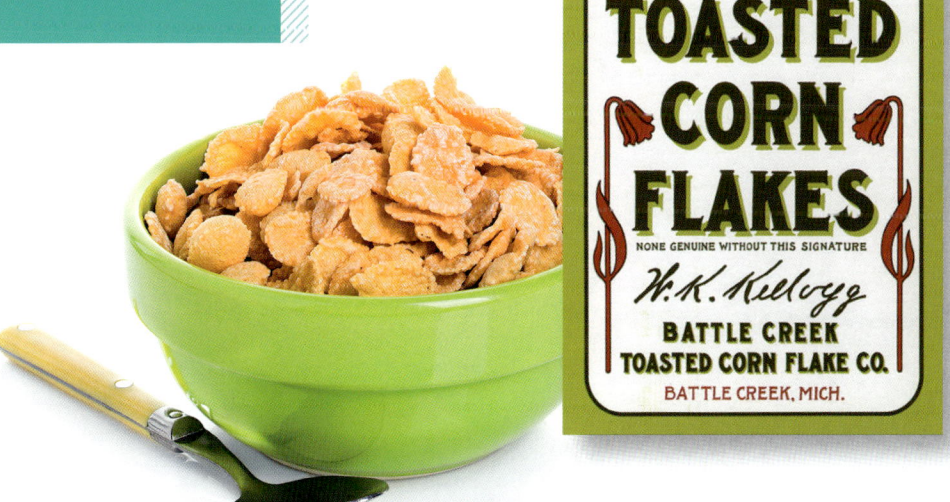

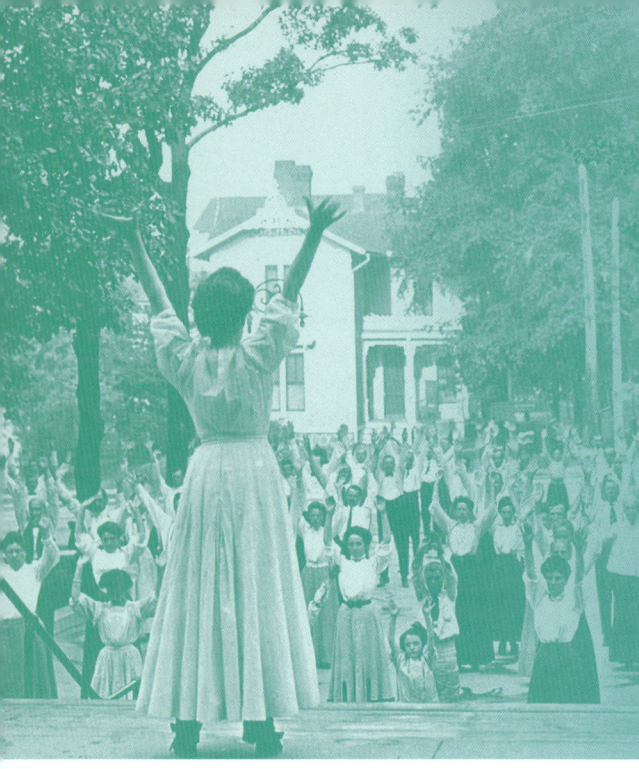

A DIFFERENT KIND OF HEALTH CARE

More than 150 years ago the first sanitarium doors opened in Battle Creek, Michigan through the effort of a small group of Seventh-day Adventist church pioneers who believed in a new way to live healthy and whole. This unique approach was grounded in caring for the body, mind and spirit, and today is seen in clinics and hospitals throughout the world.

To learn more about this incredible legacy, take a look at these short videos.

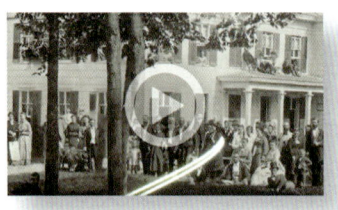

THE STORY OF WHOLE PERSON HEALTH

The first Adventist health care center opened in 1866, a time when most people, including Adventists, suffered from poor health. Medical practices were atrocious by today's standards. Doctors prescribed generous doses of opium, strychnine and other dangerous substances. The wisdom of the day dictated that water should be withheld from those with a raging fever. Hospitals functioned as a staging area for those at the end of life.

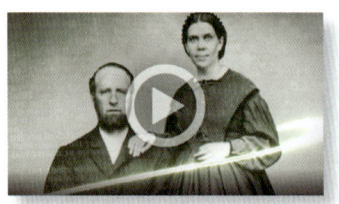

ELLEN AND JAMES WHITE

Ellen and James White were instrumental in forming the Seventh-day Adventist Church. They realized from their study of Scripture that Jesus devoted a great deal of His time on Earth to healing the sick and helping those in need. In fact, He seemingly sought out people experiencing hardships, offering them a new and better life. The members of the young church wanted to pattern a first-class institution after these principles — caring for the whole person: body, mind and spirit. In 1866, the first Adventist health care facility, named the Western Health Reform Institute, opened in Battle Creek, Michigan.

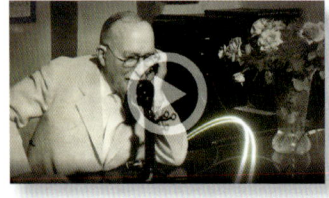

DR. JOHN HARVEY KELLOGG

Adventists see themselves as called by God to share with the world a message of wholeness for the body, mind and spirit. This model is the healing ministry of Christ, "who went about doing good" (Acts 10:38). This vision included a conviction that the health message should be shared. Thus they set out to share this healthier lifestyle. Dr. John Harvey Kellogg, the first medical director of the Battle Creek Sanitarium, researched new and better ways to help his patients stay healthy, and in the process created a more nutritious breakfast option, Corn Flakes.

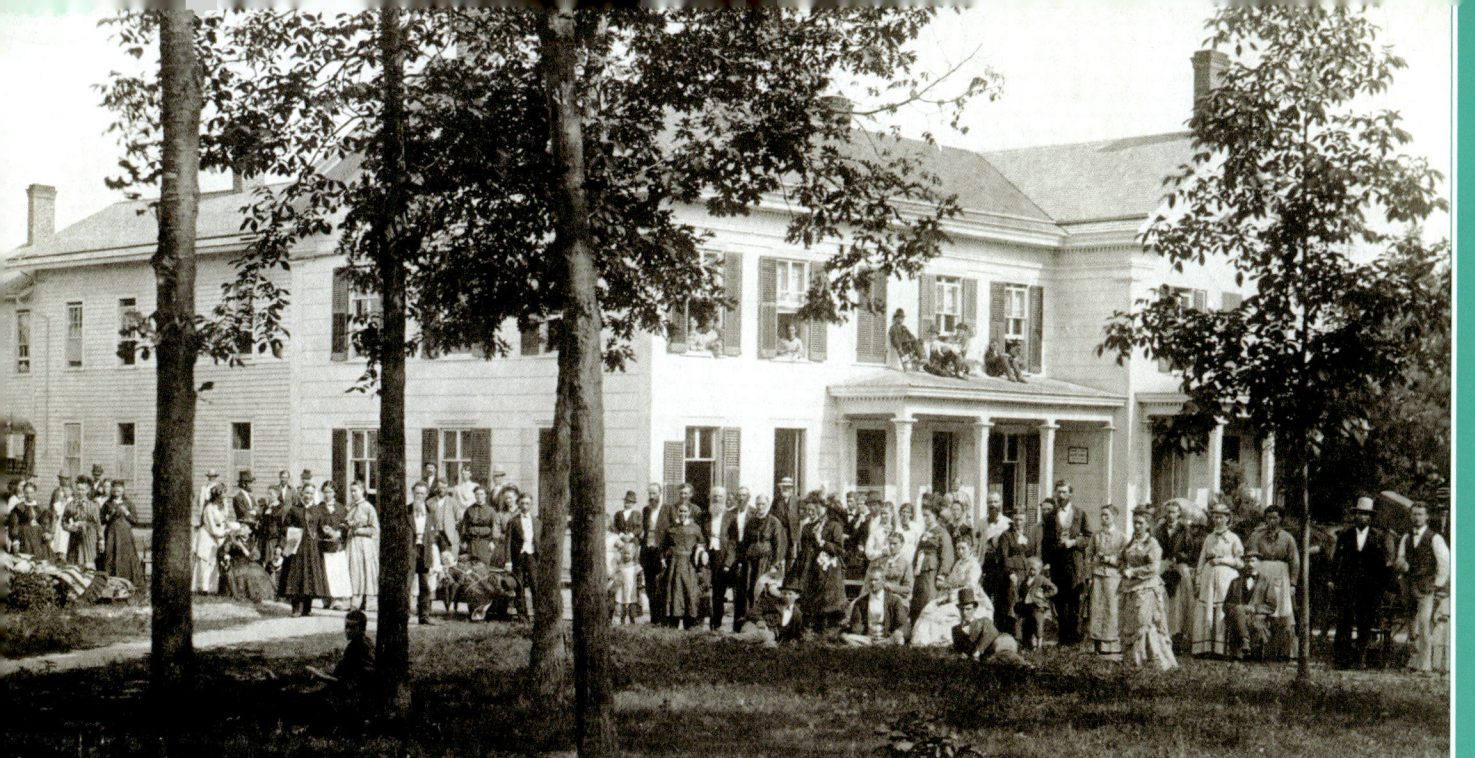

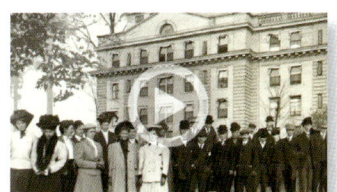 

GROWTH OF SANITARIUMS

The success of the unique health center in Battle Creek — and a widespread craving for the healing therapies found there — launched an Adventist health care movement that soon extended throughout the world. Today, more than 550 Adventist hospitals, clinics and other medical facilities care for people around the world.

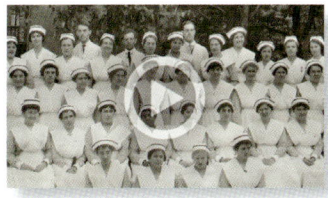 

A PLACE FOR LEARNING

The whole person principles of the Seventh-day Adventist Church are grounded in the biblical view of how God created us—an inseparable integration of body, mind and spirit. Pioneering Adventists realized from the beginning that education was the ideal way to nurture this concept. They created the Battle Creek Sanitarium as a place for people to learn how to stay well.

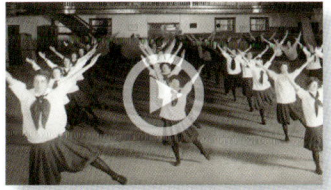 

NATURAL REMEDIES

Adventists founded the health care institutions based on the Bible's principles of health outlined in the Bible's story of creation. Unlike the common thought of the day, they believed health care should treat the disease rather than just the symptoms. Adventists began to advocate the benefits of diet, water, exercise, adequate rest and trust in God. This makes sense to us today, but more than 150 years ago it was a radical new approach.

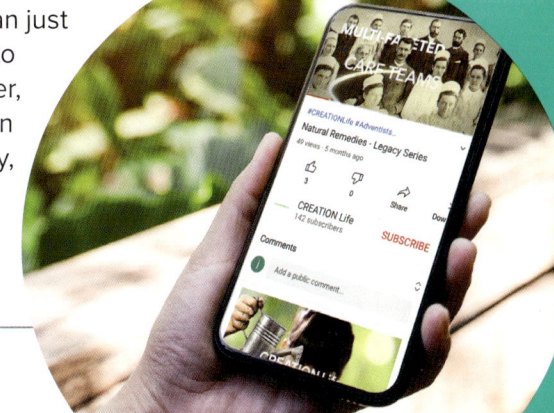

THE TRUE FOUNTAIN OF YOUTH

You may be familiar with NBA all-stars like Stephen Curry, LeBron James and Russell Westbrook, but did you know there's another group of all-stars in California identified by author Dan Buettner as the "All-Stars of Longevity?" In a special edition of *National Geographic* entitled "The Secrets of Living Longer," Buettner highlighted five major lifestyles: (1) Okinawans in Japan, (2) Sardinians in Italy, (3) Adventists in Loma Linda, California, (4) Icaria, Greece and (5) Nicoya, Costa Rica. While all five groups demonstrate remarkable longevity, the Adventist lifestyle is unique because it is the most universally transferable of the five:

- It has been reproduced in populations around the world.

- It is not dependent upon genetics and can transfer across races and ethnic groups.

- It has produced more people who have reached one hundred years of age than any other lifestyle in America — a remarkable achievement in a culture moving in the opposite health direction today.

Over time, these health principles based on the Bible's story of creation, have proven true beyond any doubt and the media has been paying special attention to the research. For example, a *U.S. News & World Report* article stated, "Americans who define themselves as Seventh-day Adventists have an average life expectancy of 89, about a decade longer than the average American. One of the basic tenets of the religion is that it's important to cherish the body that's on loan from God, which means no smoking, alcohol abuse or overindulging in sweets. Followers typically stick to a vegetarian diet based on fruits, vegetables, beans and nuts, and get plenty of exercise. They're also very focused on family and community."

Buettner's research later produced a best-selling book, *The Blue Zones*, which analyzed the data even further, citing scientific evidence collected over more than 50 years in a variety of Adventist Health Studies. The most current of which has over 96,000 participants in the U.S. and Canada. The study's preliminary results confirmed earlier findings that the way of life followed by these Adventists produces better overall health and a significant increase in longevity compared to people who do not practice this way of living.

All of the principles of this healthy lifestyle can now be found in a modern, innovative wellness philosophy known as CREATION Life. So, what is CREATION Life and where did it come from? It all started in Orlando, Florida, home to one of the world's most popular tourist destinations, Walt Disney World.

CREATION LIFE

In the early 1990s, the Disney Company had a plan to create a dream town where families could live and work in an ideal environment. From this dream came the city of Celebration, a storybook-like village where community was celebrated, neighbors were welcomed and the front porch was the most important part of the house. When Celebration needed a hospital, the people at Disney turned to many different health care providers. They were looking for the best care available.

As part of the approval process, each provider was asked to share its health care philosophy. One of the providers was then called Florida Hospital, a member of AdventHealth — a Seventh-day Adventist healthcare system.

The people at the hospital knew they couldn't talk about their philosophy without getting back to what they truly believed in. Whole-person health was at the center of everything they did because when Christ healed, He healed the whole person. While they took the opportunity to draw upon the principles of Adventists pioneers, including James and Ellen White and Dr. John Harvey Kellogg, they understood that the real foundation for these principles is in the creation story in Genesis. This led the team to come up with eight principles, which they expressed in an acronym that spells the word CREATION.

CREATION Life is about making good choices. For example, different colors of food on your plate means different nutrients are present. So, color your diet. Make it a goal to eat more than five colorful fruits and vegetables a day.

C CHOICE is the power to control your life. Consistently making wise decisions is key to becoming the person you were created to be.

R REST is the restoration of your body, mind and spirit. Your best rest includes a good night's sleep and making time to relax daily, weekly and yearly.

E ENVIRONMENT is what lies outside your body and affects what takes place inside you. What you perceive through your senses impacts your well-being.

A ACTIVITY is the movement of your body and the development of your mind. Exercising can keep you both alert and energized.

T TRUST IN GOD is knowing that God loves you unconditionally. This trusting relationship brings peace during tough times and gives hope for the future.

I INTERPERSONAL RELATIONSHIPS are the social connections you have with others. Healthy relationships bring happiness and make life better.

O OUTLOOK is the way you view your world. A positive attitude shapes your choices and how you interact with others.

N NUTRITION is nourishment for the body and energy for the mind. Understanding your relationship with food can lead to better choices and improved wellness.

Can you imagine what those early Adventist pioneers, such as the Whites and Dr. Kellogg, would have thought if they could have seen the results of their modest work, planted over a century ago? AdventHealth has grown to become the largest not-for-profit Protestant healthcare provider in the nation with each facility united in one mission — to extend the healing ministry of Christ.

This is your legacy, and it's worth getting excited about. In a world suffering from sickness and disease, you can be the all-star that brings these principles of health and healing to the ones who need it most.

START NOW.

The principles of CREATION Life come from the Maker Himself. This means they are universally applicable to *everyone*. Anyone can follow God's instructions for healthy living. Anyone can experience CREATION Life.

Before you begin, ask yourself this question: What is my vision for living?

Do you want to be like so many others who never reach their full potential, who know how to live a healthy, vibrant life but never apply their knowledge?

Or do you want to be well and live well so you can serve your Maker for as long as He leaves you here — to be able to live with such energy, enthusiasm and passion that it makes others want to know Him, too?

Should you choose the second option, here's one more question: When do you think would be a good time to begin? How about right now? Start living life to the fullest today through the principles of CREATION Life.

1. Markel, Howard. "John Harvey Kellogg and the Pursuit of Wellness." *Journal of America Medical Association* 305, no. 17 (2011): 1814-1815.

2. Buettner, Dan. "Secrets of Long Life." *National Geographic*, November 2005. https://www.bluezones. com/wp-content/uploads/2015/01/ Nat_Geo_LongevityF.pdf.

3. Kotz, Deborah. "11 Health Habits That Will Help You Live to 100." *U.S. News and World Report*, February 20, 2009. https://health.usnews.com/ health-news/family-health/living-well/ articles/2009/02/20/10-health-habits- that-will-help-you-live-to-100.

THE GIFT OF CHOICE

The Lord God commanded the man, saying, "From any tree of the garden you may eat freely; but from the tree of the knowledge of good and evil you shall not eat, for in the day that you eat from it you will surely die."

GENESIS 2:16–17

From the very beginning, God has been there to help us make the best choices. After all, He is the One who gave us the ability to choose in the first place. The gift of choice was first given to Adam and Eve in the Garden of Eden. It can be seen in the presence of the tree of the knowledge of good and evil. God gave humanity the freedom to choose between obedience and disobedience — between life and death — but Adam and Eve chose to disobey their Creator and listen to another voice. Of course, God could have stopped them from eating from the tree, but He did not interfere. He allowed His creations to make their choice freely. The power of choice comes with one serious stipulation — regardless of what you choose, you must always face the consequences of your actions. Adam and Eve's choice had serious consequences. They were separated from God, removed from the Garden of Eden and unable to eat from the Tree of Life. Their choice to sin and disobey God brought death and pain into the world.

Through Adam and Eve, God gave humanity the freedom to choose between life and death, good and evil. Adam and Eve were unwilling to keep God's commands. Humanity has suffered the consequences for their actions ever since. In John 14:15, Jesus tells His followers, *"If you love Me, you will keep My commandments."* When you make the choice to disobey God's commandments, you are actually choosing to love yourself more than Him. You are turning your back on His offer of abundant life.

> *"Happiness, like unhappiness, is a proactive choice."*
>
> STEPHEN R. COVEY

You have the God-given gift to make your own choices without coercion from others. Ultimately, you are only accountable to one being — God. This book is not intended to give you a list of what you should or should not do. Instead, it offers information that will allow you to make informed decisions for yourself. It is important to realize the responsibility for making those choices. The consequences that follow, good or bad, are uniquely and exclusively yours. Remember, not choosing is also a choice.

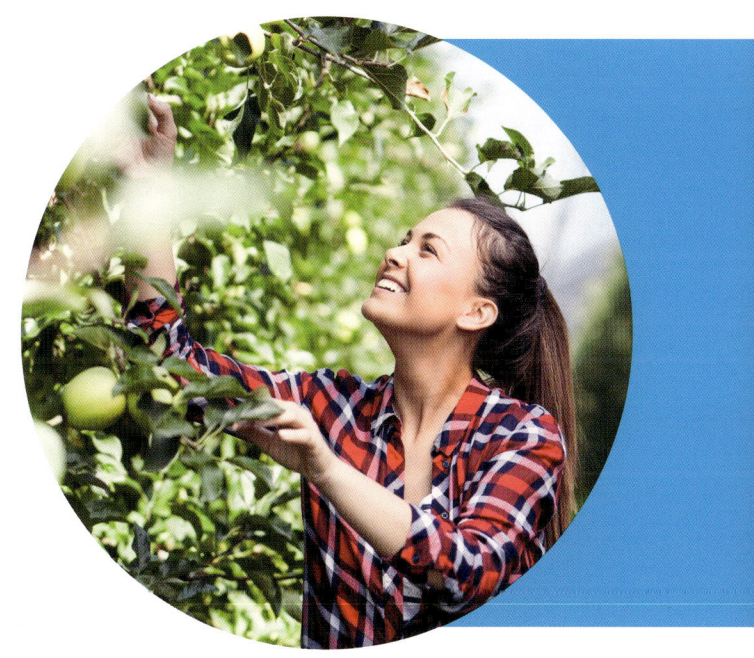

THE FRONTAL LOBE

So, from where does your power to choose come? Look no further than the grey matter inside your head. Like the circuits in a computer, God has hardwired choice right into your brain — into its frontal lobe to be exact. This is the unique area that gives you the power to choose. Just how unique is it? Well, let's compare brain sizes among the species:

- In a cat's brain, the frontal lobe makes up a mere 3.5 percent.

- In a dog's brain, it's double that at 7 percent (sorry, cat lovers).

- In a chimpanzee's brain, it's a little more at 17 percent.

- But in your magnificent brain, the frontal lobe is a whopping 33 to 38 percent.

You possess a natural ability to reason and plan that is much more complex than any other species in the entire world. You are distinct in all of creation, and it's all thanks to your frontal lobe. It's the seat of your judgment and reasoning. It's also where social norms are stored and long-term planning takes place. When these factors work together, you are able to make healthy, life-giving choices. In short, the power to choose is what makes you human.

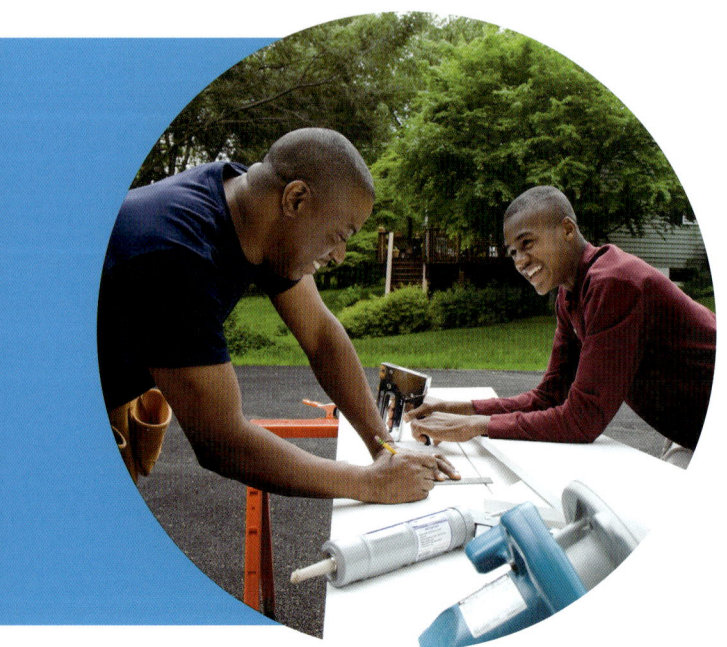

THE TRUE STORY OF PHINEAS GAGE

Just how important is the frontal lobe to your decision-making process? Consider the true, tragic story of Phineas Gage:

Phineas Gage was a railroad foreman who lived in the 1800s. One day, Gage was tapping blasting powder into a hole with a 13-pound iron bar. Suddenly the powder exploded, launching the iron bar like a missile straight through his head. The bar entered below his lower cheekbone and exited through the top of his skull, landing 25 to 30 yards behind him.

Amazingly, Gage survived the accident. He was even alert and talking on the ride into town. But in the days that followed, it became clear he was not the same. Before the accident, Gage had been known for his moral behavior. As a railroad foreman, his record was exemplary. But now he was often angry and overly emotional. He soon lost interest in spirituality. He began to swear and show little regard for social customs.

Even though Gage survived the accident, the iron bar caused severe brain damage, specifically to his frontal lobe. His doctor, John Harlow, shared how the accident destroyed Gage's "equilibrium or balance, so to speak, between his intellectual faculty and his animal propensities." In other words, Gage could no longer control or choose between his intellectual side and his more primitive animal side. Gage's traumatic frontal lobotomy cost him his personality, his moral standards and his commitment to family, church and loved ones.[2-3]

The story of Phineas Gage shows how damage to the frontal lobe can actually change your personality. At first, these changes may only be minimal, but over time they can build up until they significantly alter your life. Your health, happiness and even your future could all be at stake.

Message received, you may be thinking, *so I won't apply for any jobs working on the railroad.* But don't miss the real point. Many things can affect your frontal lobe, and the most common of them all come from your lifestyle habits — the foods you eat, the media you watch and the exercise you do or don't do. As a matter of fact, everything you choose will affect you for better or for worse.

BRAIN DRAIN

Keep your frontal lobe healthy and at optimal performance by avoiding these types of damaging behaviors:

- Large amounts of media can be numbing to your brain, so monitor your input. Take regular breaks from the Internet, social media and phones.

- A diet high in fat, sugar or alcohol can inhibit normal, healthy blood flow and have other deteriorating effects on your frontal lobe. So, eat a healthy, balanced diet of whole grains, fruits and vegetables.

- Cut the coffee. Avoid caffeinated drinks, with their highs and lows. Just drinking water is a much healthier choice.

- Illicit drugs and even legal medications can also be detrimental to frontal lobe function.

Making wise choices about what you eat, drink, hear or see can provide your frontal lobe with the good input it needs for a lifetime.

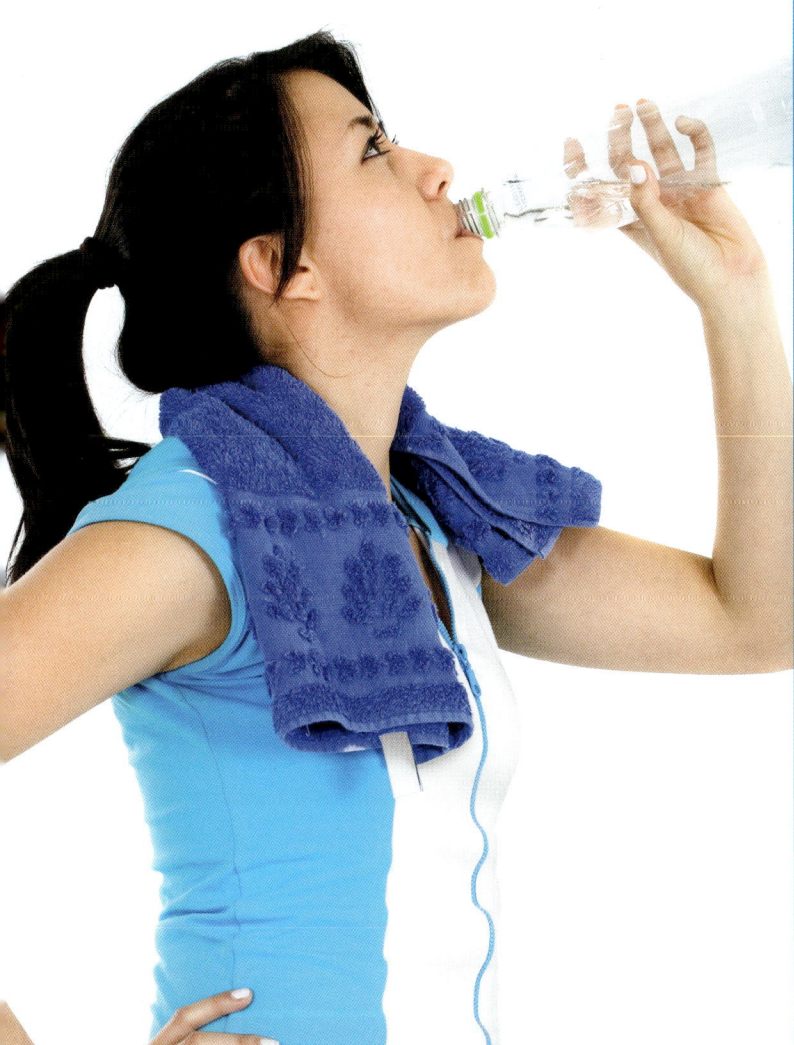

MAKING GOOD DECISIONS

Follow these four key steps for making good decisions:

1. **Focus.** Don't allow yourself to get distracted by the chaos in your life. Lack of sleep, demands from others or stress at home or school are just some of the factors that can lead you to make a poor decision. Keep focused on the real issues and the choices before you.

2. **Evaluate.** Look carefully at the risks and rewards of your decision. Examine the costs and benefits to you and the ones you love. Are things leaning in your favor, or will the decision put you in danger? Remember, not all rewards are beneficial and not all risks are dangerous.

3. **Consult.** Get input from others, who often see things from a different perspective. This could prove very helpful in your decision-making process. Seek out wise counsel from a parent, teacher or mentor.

4. **Decide.** Don't overanalyze a situation to the point where you are incapable of making a decision. While it's important to get all the data, don't let it keep you from being decisive. If you have an opportunity, then learn to make the most of it. Some opportunities will disappear if you wait too long to seize them. The good news is the more you make decisions, the more confidence you will build for making them in the future.

AN EXPERIMENT IN CHOICE

A now-famous study explored the benefits of letting people exercise choice and control in their lives. It was conducted in a nursing home called Shady Grove. Researchers divided the nursing home by floors. On the first floor, the director gave the residents a speech: "I'd like you to know about all the things you can do for yourself here at Shady Grove. There are omelets and scrambled eggs for breakfast, but you have to choose which you want the night before. There are movies on Wednesday or Thursday night, but you must sign up in advance before going. Here are some plants; pick one out and take it to your room, but you have to water it yourself."

But on the second floor, the director gave the residents a very different speech: "I want you to know about what we can do for you here at Shady Grove. There are omelets or scrambled eggs for breakfast. We make omelets on Monday, Wednesday and Friday, and scrambled eggs on the other days. There are movies on Wednesday and Thursday night. Thursday nights, residents from the left quarter go, and on Wednesday nights residents from the right quarter go. Here are some plants for your rooms. The nurse will choose one for you and take care of it."

Everyone at Shady Grove had access to the very same things, but only those on the first floor had choices. So, what happened?

The researchers found that the patients on the first floor did very well and even thrived at Shady Grove. Incredibly, 18 months later fewer people on the first floor had died when compared with the people on the second floor.[4-6] Could it be that having a choice and exercising a measure of control can actually save lives?

When someone has the ability to choose, it increases his or her sense of control and motivation. On the other hand, when choice is taken away, a person feels as if they have no control whatsoever. This has a variety of detrimental effects on their motivation, life satisfaction and personal well-being.[7-8]

POWER TOOLS

As anyone who's ever tried to hammer a nail with a block of cheese knows, having the right tool for the job can make all the difference in the world. In addition to the power of choice, you have many other tools at your disposal. These will help you make even better decisions and avoid choices that can harm you. Let's get to know them.

The first tool you should acquaint yourself with is knowledge. Think of the pursuit of knowledge as a way of life. You should always be learning something new. Don't expect to coast through life on intellectual autopilot. Learn to engage your intellect by reading or listening to books, watching informative programs and using the Internet wisely. Life should always be a pursuit of knowledge. Find ways to grow in knowledge, and as a result, you will be better equipped to make wise choices in the future.

Of course, you can't always know everything about every particular situation. Some information is going to be outside your reach (even if you own a smart phone). This is why you desperately need the next tool — reason. In order to make a good and reasonable decision, start by using the knowledge you have about the situation, applying the principles you live by, the rules you have to keep, the laws you are bound to follow and a good amount of common sense. All these factors taken as a whole will help you make good choices.

You can increase your ability to reason just as you can increase your knowledge. Consider reading books or taking classes on logic, philosophy or debate. Engage in stimulating discussions with your friends and practice your critical thinking skills. Soon you will be able to make good choices regardless of how much information you have available to you.

> *"Either you run the day or the day runs you."*
>
> JIM ROHN

STRESS TEST

Even though you have the power to choose, as well as the tools of knowledge and reason at your disposal, one thing can still affect your ability to make good decisions. We call it stress. When you find yourself in a stressful situation, you may feel your choices are limited or, worse, that you have no choice at all. That is because stress hurts your ability to think clearly. It gets worse. If you are in a situation where you feel you have little or no control, you may even begin to feel helpless. This may cause you to make one bad decision after another, all because your mind perceives it has no other options.

As these feelings continue, over time they become more permanent. Scientists call this behavior "learned helplessness." It occurs in nature as a response by animals when confronted with a persistent adversity, as was shown in a series of experiments conducted by Martin P. Seligman. Seligman placed dogs in pens where a series of electrical shocks were sent through the floor. At first, the dogs tried frantically to escape the pens, but after realizing there was no escape, they stopped trying. They decided there was no other choice except to endure the shocks. But then Seligman did something remarkable. He removed the barriers in the pens. Now the dogs were no longer prisoners; they had an escape. All they had to do was walk out of the pen, away from the rigged floor and they would be free. But amazingly, when Seligman resumed the shocks, the dogs did nothing. They didn't even try to escape. What happened?

The dogs believed they were helpless, and nothing could change that fact. Even though their circumstances had changed, the dogs remained in their pitiful, helpless state.[9-10] They no longer felt they were in control of their own destiny. They believed their surroundings, not their own options, determined their fate.

Is that how you feel? Have you experienced so many rainy days that you think the sun will never shine again? You don't have to settle for a life of helplessness. Determine right now to always exercise your power to choose. Regardless of how great the adversity in your life, remember you always have a choice.

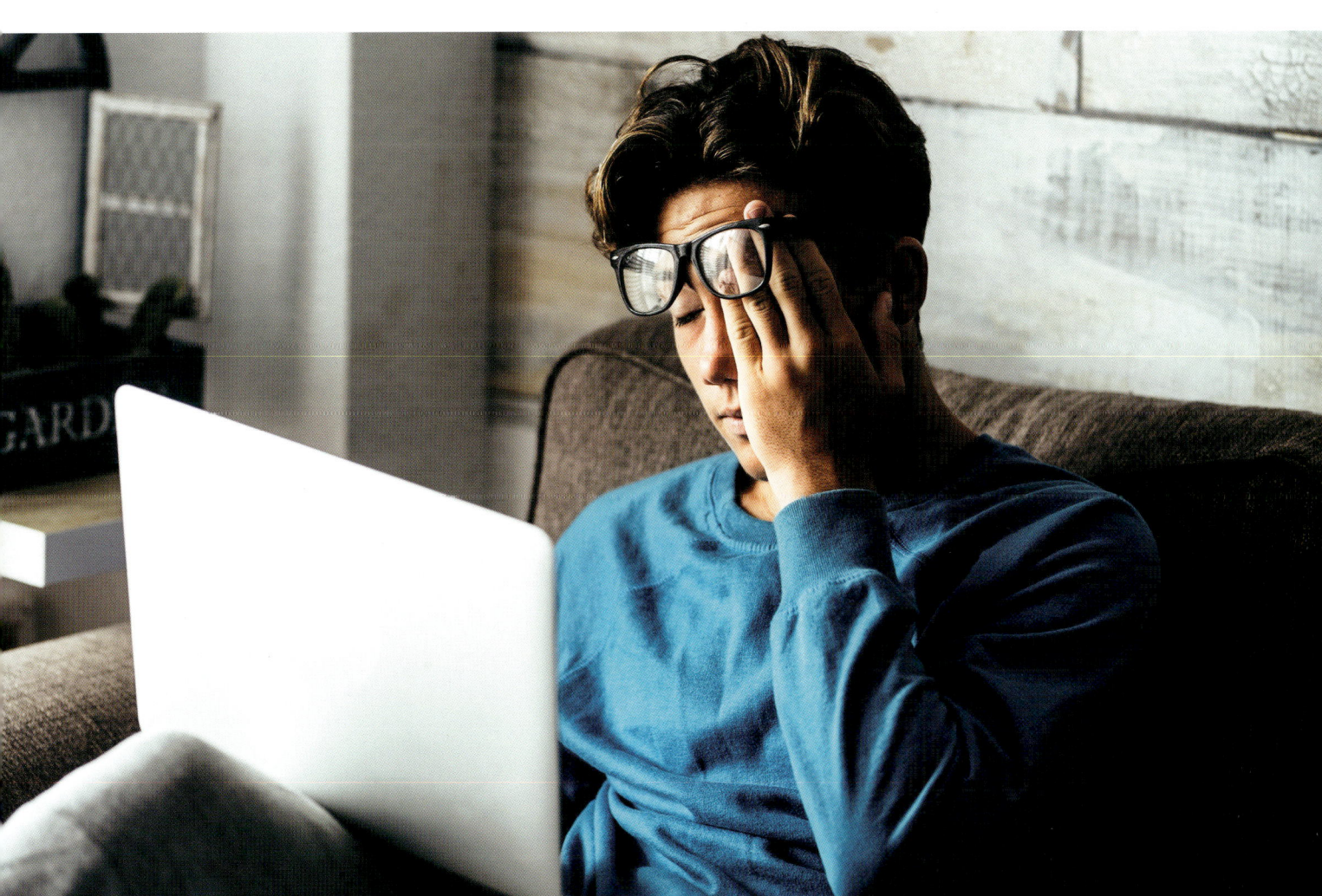

BALANCING ACT

Do you remember when you first learned to ride a bike? You were probably wobblier than a jellyfish on roller skates. Of course, over time you got better. All it took was a little practice and pretty soon you found your center of gravity. The next thing you knew you were popping wheelies and taking your bike off on sweet jumps. You just had to get everything in balance.

Learning to make healthy choices is a lot like riding your first bicycle. You have to balance things if you're going to get anywhere. This means you learn to choose good things in a positive, moderate way while avoiding things that are harmful for you. At first, you're bound to make some bad choices, but over time you'll find a way to keep everything where it needs to be. You will find your balance.

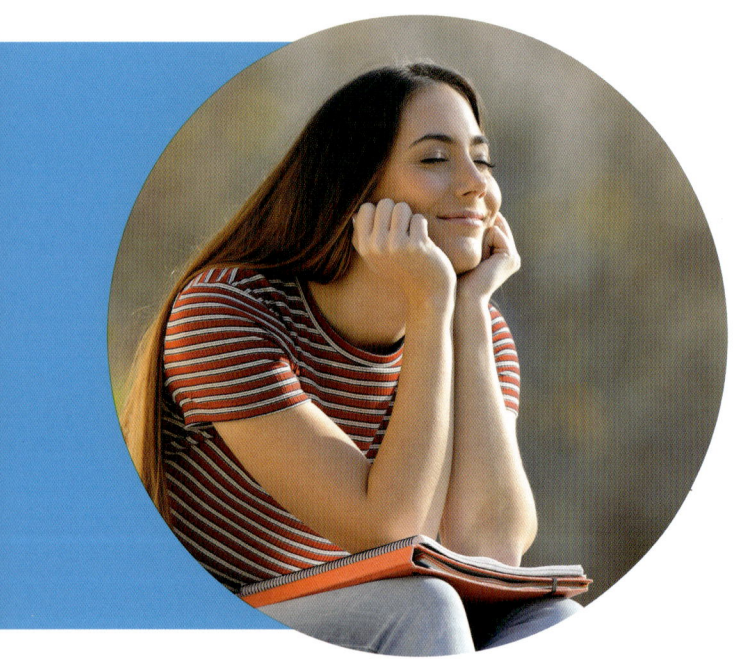

Think about how you adjust the equalizer on your car sound system. All the frequencies of a song need to be in just the right balance in order to produce the best sound. Too much treble and your favorite artist will sound like they're playing in a tin can. Too much bass and you'll melt your eardrums. The power of choice should be used to equalize your life. The goal is to avoid the extremes on both ends of the spectrum and aim for that all-important sweet spot — the place where everything is experienced as the Maker intended.

Without balance, your life will never reach its full potential. Even a good choice can be overdone. Think about people who are so obsessed with exercise they injure themselves from overdoing it. Think about people so consumed with weight loss that they end up with an eating disorder to achieve what they think is the perfect body. Make no mistake; exercise and weight loss may be good things, but when done to excess they can cause grievous harm with disastrous results. They must be balanced with proper nutrition and rest. This is the only way to achieve a balanced lifestyle.

You also can't use one good choice to cancel out all the bad ones. Maybe you've heard about the person who ordered a double cheeseburger and fries for lunch and then decided to cut their calories by having a diet soda. It doesn't work that way. Each choice has an impact on your life. Choosing to eat foods that are high in fat and cholesterol will eventually catch up with you, even if you always have a bowl of oatmeal for breakfast.

By using the power of choice to balance your life, you'll make wiser, healthier decisions. You'll feel better and have more energy to do all the things you want. You'll even add rewarding days to your life for years to come. The key is to find your balance.

THE HARD CHOICE

Dr. Martin Luther King Jr. knew there was a problem. Unjust laws promoting racial segregation and discrimination gave African Americans an inferior status. Just using the wrong water fountain or sitting in the front seat of a bus could mean serious repercussions. Dr. King knew that in the face of such injustice the only discourse was civil disobedience. Nonviolent protests erupted in the South as many blacks and whites staged sit-ins, peace marches and prayer vigils. The results were horrifying. Protesters were sprayed with fire hoses and jailed by policemen. A church in Birmingham was bombed in a shameful act of terrorism. Four girls lost their lives in the blast, none of them over the age of 14. People on both sides of the argument begged for the protests to stop, but King refused. It was a hard choice to make, but he knew that to stop would mean things would never change. He continued his efforts while encouraging his people to remain strong.

In 1964, King and the protestors' hard work and patience finally paid off when President Lyndon Johnson signed the Civil Rights Act into law. At last, segregation was overturned in the South. Dr. King was a victor, but victory came with a price. Four years later, King was assassinated in Memphis, Tennessee. He became a martyr for the cause of equality and freedom for all people everywhere.

Not every choice you make will be an easy one. Sometimes you may encounter great injustices or wrongs in the world. Sometimes you, like Dr. King, may be asked to make the hard choice —

to do what others believe is wrong in order to accomplish a greater good. Before you make such a choice, be sure that your desire to act does not come from within yourself. Dr. King was guided by something stronger than his own desires or sense of morality. He relied upon his faith in God to show him the truth and to strengthen him in the hard times. When his fellow clergymen accused his methods of being extremist, Dr. King answered their critiques in his now-famous letter from the Birmingham City Jail:

So, the question is not whether we will be extremists, but what kind of extremists we will be. Will we be extremists for hate or for love? Will we be extremists for the preservation of injustice or for the extension of justice? In that dramatic scene on Calvary's hill three men were crucified. We must never forget that all three were crucified for the same crime — the crime of extremism. Two were extremists for immorality, and thus fell below their environment. The other, Jesus Christ, was an extremist for love, truth and goodness, and thereby rose above His environment. Perhaps the South, the nation and the world are in dire need of creative extremists.

Hard choices often have serious repercussions. They might mean losing a treasured relationship, putting you at odds with your family or forcing you to endure difficult circumstances. They could even bring great injury or death. Determine now what you stand for and prepare yourself in advance. If that day comes and you are asked to make the hard choice, you'll be ready.

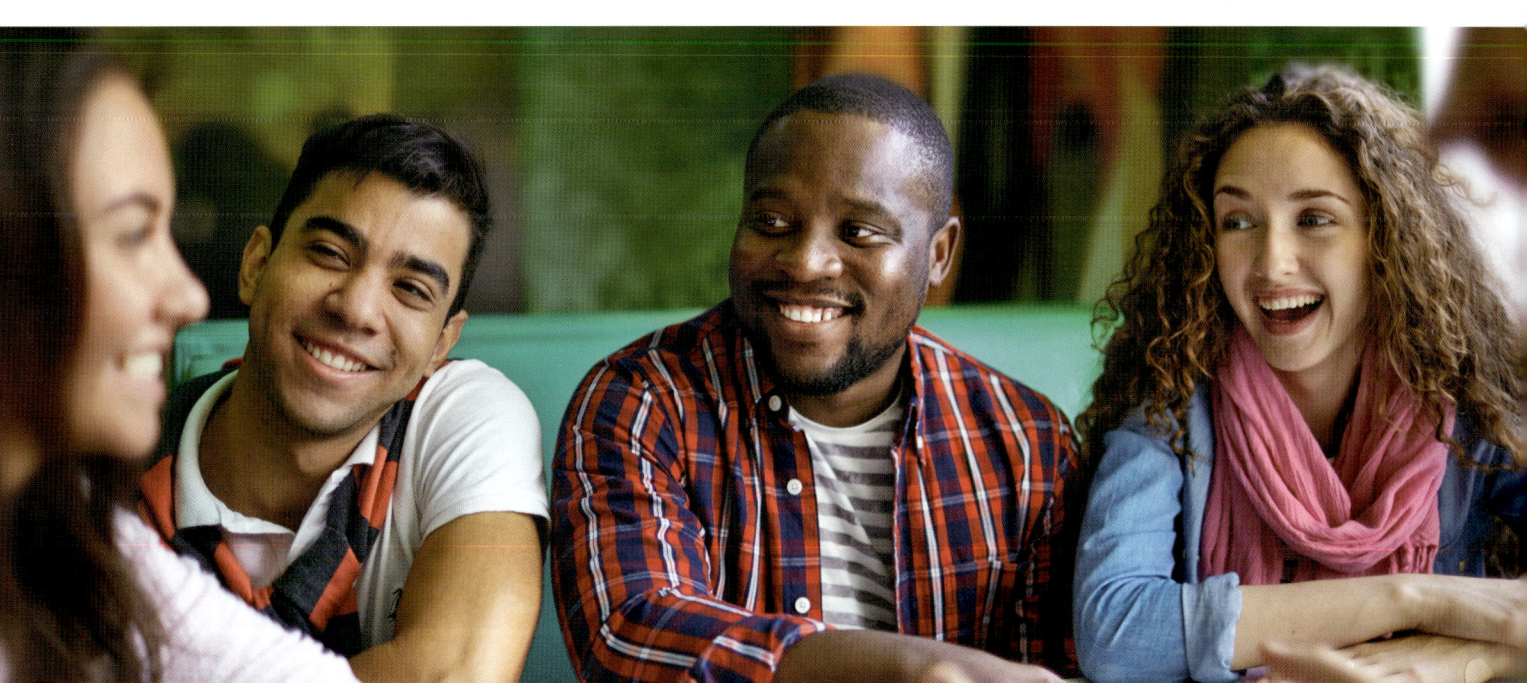

FREE TO CHOOSE

As a young child you probably didn't exercise much choice. Someone else chose for you — what clothes you wore, what foods you ate, what time you went to bed at night. But now as you are getting older, you are making more decisions for yourself. It's a great feeling, though there are still things about which you have little or no say. You have to go to school and you have to follow the rules. If you don't, there are consequences. So, even though you are free to make choices, you are not completely self-governed. Even if you were to pack up and move to another country you would still have to follow the laws of that land. Failure to do so would result in your losing much of your personal freedom.

Right now, you may be itching to leave school or home. Maybe you can't wait to be on your own. But hastily made choices can have long-lasting ill effects. Don't let a moment of frustration lead you to do something you may later regret. Remember, even though you are free to choose, the best choices are the ones that take into account as many pieces of information available. By using all the tools and resources God has given, you will be able to make the best choices.

FAMILY TIME

If you have a positive relationship with your parents, you are less likely to make harmful choices now and in the future. For example, children who have parents who talk with their teens regularly about drugs are 42 percent less likely to use drugs than those who don't. Unfortunately, only a quarter of teens report actually having these conversations.[12] Your parents may struggle or feel embarrassed talking about topics like drugs, alcohol or sexuality with you, but conversations like these are very important. They show you how much your parents care about you and how they want the best for your life. According to Angela Diaz, pediatrician and Director of the Mount Sinai Adolescent Health Center, "A child's well-being is every parent's priority, and one of the easiest ways to make sure your child is thriving is by keeping the lines of communication open."[13] If your parents are struggling with talking to you about a difficult topic, there is a way you can help. Consider reaching out to them. You don't have to wait for them to start a conversation in your home. With Choice, you have the power to take the first step.

If you do not have a good connection with your parents, seek help in repairing your relationship. A trusted pastor or counselor can help you find God's strength to forgive past wrongs and mend your relationships. But what if you have lost your parents through unfortunate circumstances? You may be hurting inside, unsure of how to handle difficult situations. The good news is you can also seek out support by finding a mentor. A mentor may be an extended family member, a pastor, coach, neighbor or someone from a formal mentoring program. Research has found that just like talking to a parent, having a mentor is also associated with decreased substance abuse.[14] But there are many other benefits to having a mentor. You are more likely to finish high school and attend college if you have a mentor in your life. Mentors are also associated with adolescents who have higher self-esteem, life satisfaction and increased health.[15]

God has made the family one of the most vital components in our society. Even if you are without your natural family, you can still experience all the benefits by choosing to create strong relationships with others.

"Man has a choice, and it's a choice that makes him a man." JOHN STEINBECK

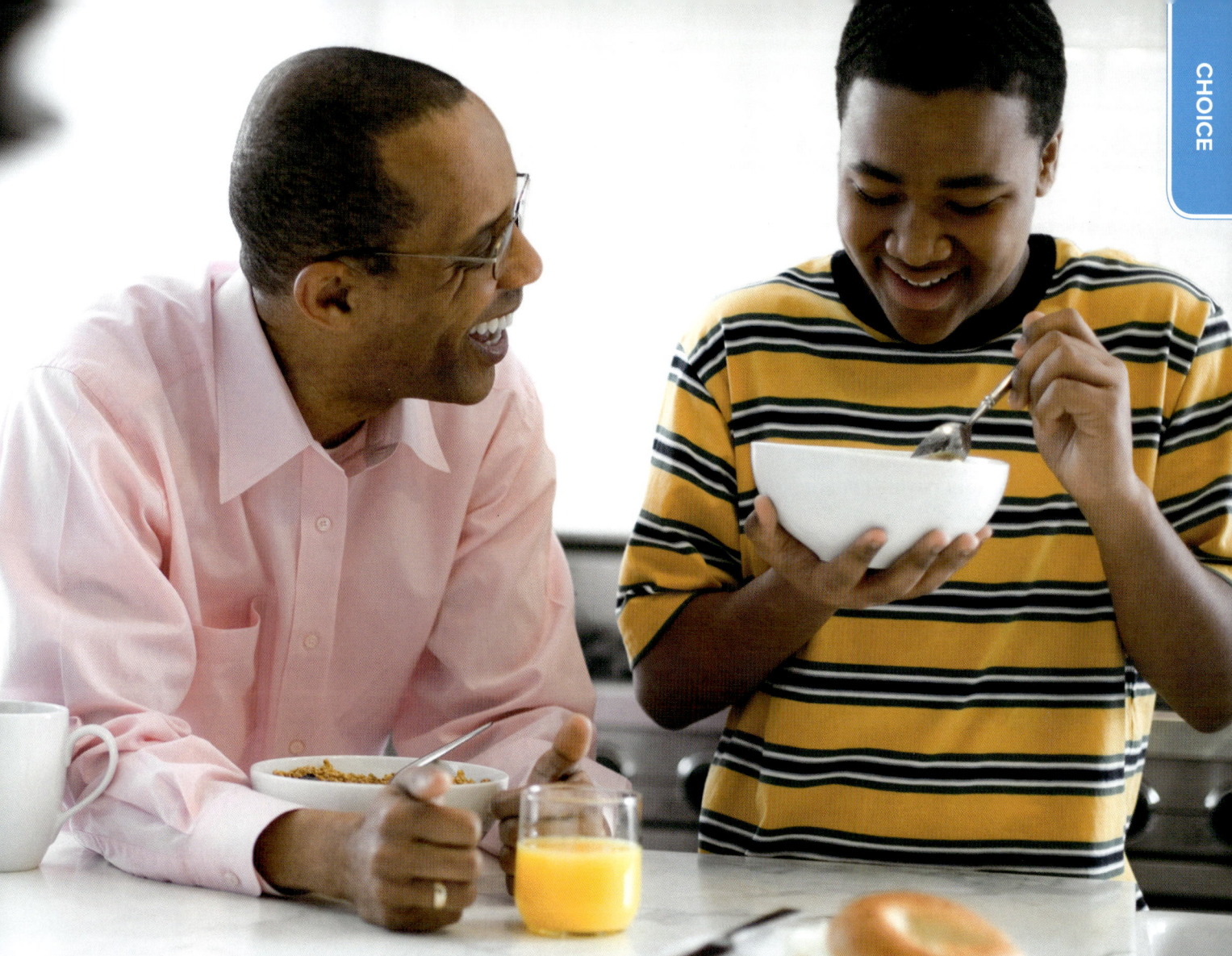

THREE WAYS TO TALK TO YOUR PARENTS

In *The 7 Habits of Highly Effective Teens*, author, speaker and executive Sean Covey gives some great ideas for improving communication between you and your parents:

1. **Listen.** Do you catch yourself telling your parents, "You just don't understand me?" Well, ask yourself one question: have you ever stopped to take the time to understand them? By first listening to what they have to say, you show your parents that you are at least trying to understand. Covey says, "If you want to improve your relationship with mom or dad... try listening to them just like you would a friend."

2. **Go First.** Start by asking them some questions. Covey asks, "When is the last time you asked your mom or dad, 'How was your day today?' or 'Tell me what you like and don't like about your job?' or 'Is there anything I could do to help around the house?'" These are great and easy ways to get the conversation going.

3. **Remember This.** "Hey, parents are people too. They laugh, they cry, they get their feelings hurt and they don't always have their act together, just like me and you."[16]

CHECK IT OUT

Did you know that feeling a strong sense of control over one's life has been associated with many amazing benefits, such as an increased ability to stop smoking[17], lose weight[18], stick to a medical regimen[19] and to perform better academically?[20]

SCHOOL RULES

Okay, be honest: In all your years attending school, have you ever skipped out on class? For some kids it's a "rite of passage." In reality, attending your classes is an important part of having a successful school experience. In fact, research has found what common sense has long told us — skipping class does impact your grades.

In one particular study, researchers measured a student's time commitments to a variety of activities to see how they impacted class performance. By far, the most valuable time commitment a student could make was their time spent in class. Nothing else was more important in determining how well the student would perform.[21]

Another study showed that missing classes was significant in explaining why a student earned a D in a class rather than an A, B or C. It found that students with regular class attendance significantly minimized their chances of getting a D or an F. This study also found that each absence from class lowered a student's grade point average by 0.06 in a 4.0 grading system. Being absent 10 times in a given term would be the difference between a C+ and a B.[22]

But skipping classes will cost you more than just good grades. If your performance in a class suffers too much, you might end up having to take that subject over. Miss several classes and you might not even graduate. Skipping class could also cause you problems in the future. Teachers are a lot less likely to give students a good recommendation when they know they're intentionally cutting class. A strong teacher recommendation is a plus when you're applying to get into college.

So, think twice the next time a friend wants you to bail on pre-calculus. The best choice is for you to make the most of the time you have in school. Attending and staying focused in your classes will help you to succeed.

Your school has its own unique code of conduct, which you are expected to obey. This may include guidelines on everything from class conduct to following the proper dress code or even abiding by certain food restrictions. Occasionally you may get so annoyed or upset by having to follow these guidelines that you begin to rebel against them. However, realize the rules are there first and foremost to protect you.

Staying compliant now to the guidelines of your school may also have a positive outcome for you in the future, especially as you enter the workplace. One article on student compliance and conduct put it this way, "Job dismissals rarely result from a lack of intellectual capacity. More often, they result from a failure in social or emotional skills, leading to dysfunctional relationships in the workplace."[23] Schools aren't the only places with rules and guidelines you must follow. It's highly probable your first job will also require proper attendance and a dress code. By keeping the rules now, you will be more likely to abide by your employer's guidelines in the future.

Every person is to be in subjection to the governing authorities. For there is no authority except from God, and those which exist are established by God. ROMANS 13:1

When God gave the Ten Commandments to the nation of Israel, it wasn't to keep them from having fun or enjoying life. It was to show them that His way was the best way. By abiding by the rules and guidelines of your institution, you are following the biblical command to "be subject to the governing authorities." You are living a life in humble obedience to God.

PROCRASTINATION

Procrastination is a challenge for many teens, especially in school. Maybe you think that project or research paper won't take a lot of time. Or maybe you're such a perfectionist that you don't want to start until you can do everything just right. Whatever your reason, you end up waiting until the night before, and then you're panicked, up late working until the last minute. This creates a ton of additional stress, which works against the finished product and you. One study revealed that students who procrastinated had higher stress levels and received lower grades on all assignments compared to students who completed things in a timely manner. The fact is, when you procrastinate you're never giving your best.

But the stress from procrastination affects you in other ways as well. It can actually make you sick. In the same study, it was found that those who were procrastinators reported greater illness late in the term. Overall, they were much sicker compared to the other students who did not procrastinate.[24]

In another large study, procrastinators were found to have less money and less happiness than those who did not procrastinate. Think about it. How can you be happy when you are anxious about the quality of your work or whether you'll be able to get the job done? And the financial impact of procrastination can be seen every April around tax time. Many people delay in filing their taxes, which costs each individual an average of $400 a year.[25]

There are so many distractions to get you off task: surfing the Internet, social media, playing video games, checking text messages, voicemail and email. Temptation is everywhere.

You may not believe it, but one of the best ways you can counter procrastination is by choosing to change your schedule. By following the body's natural rhythm of going to bed and getting up at an earlier time, you will get better results from all that you do. Research has found that those who stay up later at night are more likely to be procrastinators.[26-29] By choosing to get to bed at a decent hour, you'll be able to make better decisions about managing the time you have while you're awake. You'll be on the road to stop procrastination dead in its tracks.

> *"You cannot escape the responsibility of tomorrow by evading it today."*
> ABRAHAM LINCOLN

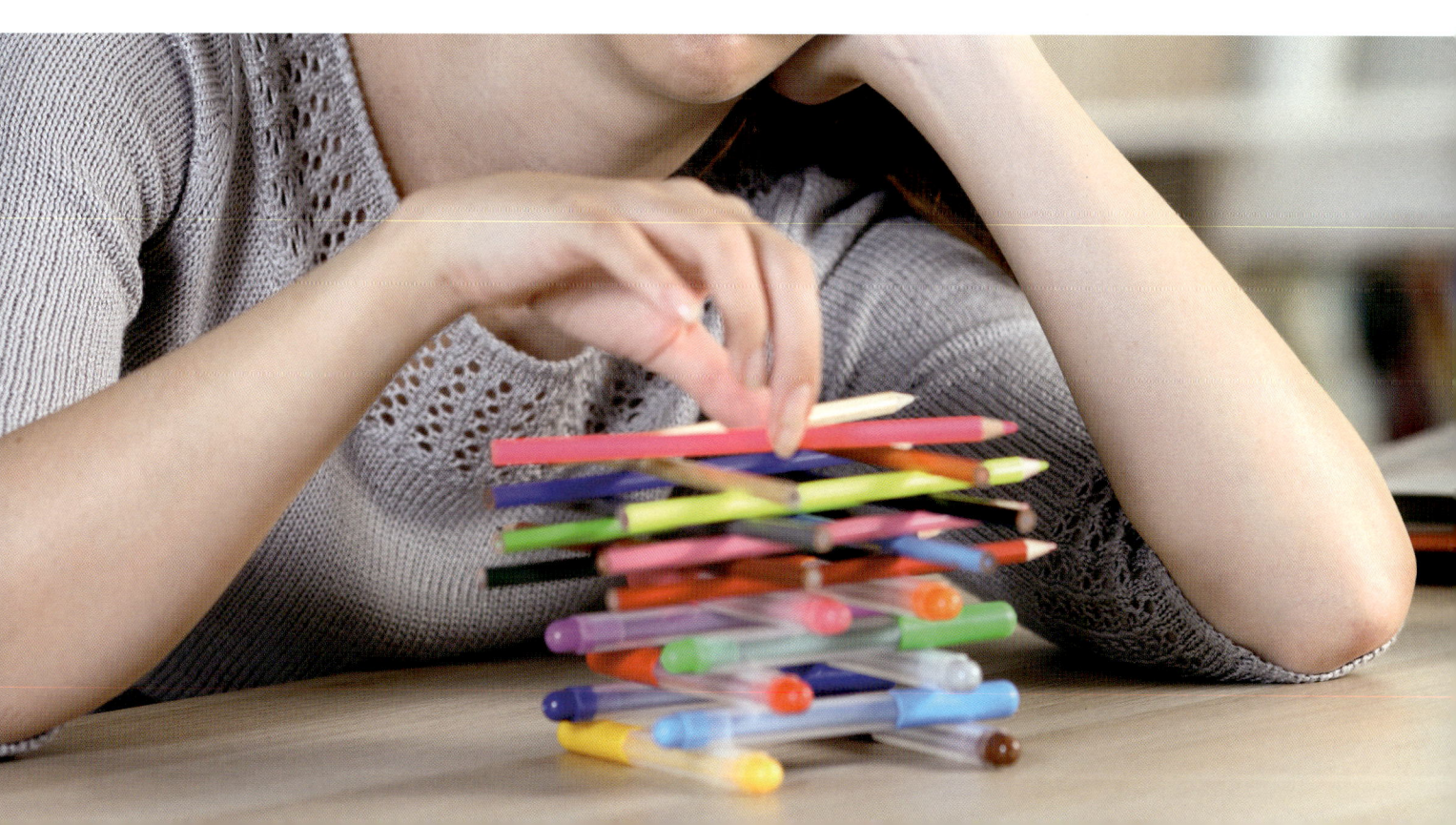

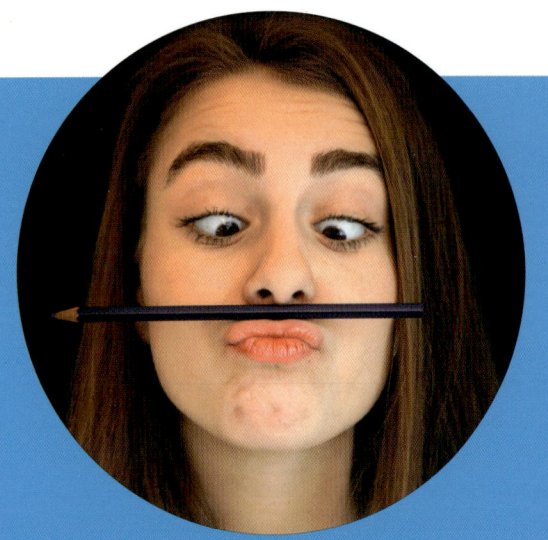

THREE WAYS TO STOP PROCRASTINATING... NOW

In the article "Why You Procrastinate — and How to Stop," Jennifer Nelson offers helpful ways to stop procrastination and get back to work. Nelson says, "It's not a time-management issue. For the vast majority of us, it's usually about doing a task we'd rather put off."

1. **Break it up.** If it's a big project, research paper or assignment — pace yourself. Break the task up into small chunks and then get started. Once you get started, you'll find your feelings about the task will change. If you have a 40-page report to write, start with a page. If you can't do that, start with a paragraph. Can't do that? Start with a sentence.

2. **Treat yourself.** Reward yourself for not procrastinating. "If I work for two hours, I can check social media for 10 minutes. If I exercise now, I'll talk to my friends later."

3. **Practice.** Willpower is like a muscle. It can be strengthened to help you beat procrastination, no matter your personality. Remind yourself that you will really benefit from working, seeing the doctor, finishing your research paper on time or studying before every class, not just for the exam.[30]

COLLEGE AND BEYOND

Is the choice to get a college degree a good financial investment for yourself? Absolutely. The typical Bachelor's degree recipient can expect to earn about 66 percent more over a 40-year working life than the typical high school graduate earns over the same period.[31] Although the college graduates may not see returns on their education dollars for at least four to six years, think of it as a long-term investment. College grads can also earn advanced degrees, which give even more payback. In 2018, those graduates who earned Master's degrees earned almost twice as much, and those with professional degrees earned over three times as much money per year as high school graduates. On average, this was $100,000 a year.

There are many more benefits to earning a degree than just making money. College grads are also able to get jobs more easily and hold onto them longer. They are also more likely to get jobs that have health insurance and other benefits.

Researchers have also found that college grads lead healthier lives overall. They have lower smoking rates and more positive perceptions of personal health than those who do not graduate from college. Higher levels of education are correlated with higher levels of participation in civic activities, which include volunteer work, blood donation and voting.[32]

With all these benefits, going to college sounds like a no-brainer, right? But there's just one problem — how are you going to pay for it?

STUDENT LOANS

You may decide to seek financial aid to help pay for your college degree. Student loans can definitely make it easier to pay for college, but make no mistake, once you graduate you could owe some serious money. It's called debt, and you must pay back what you borrowed plus the interest you owe on the loan.

In the article *What Does the Bible Say About Student Loans?*, author Palmer Muntz states that, "Loans, including student loans, are not inherently wrong. If you are committed to acting with integrity and to practicing good stewardship, loans could be a legitimate device for paying for college. Be sure to ask the right questions — even though they aren't easy ones — before deciding for yourself."

IMPORTANT QUESTIONS TO ASK BEFORE YOU BORROW MONEY:

"Is it God's will for my life to borrow this money?"

"How do I plan to repay it?"

"How long will it take me to repay it?"

"What is a reasonable amount to borrow?"

"Will I be able to pay this much back with the earnings that I make from my chosen profession?"

Did you know the Bible includes more than 2,000 verses concerning money and property? Many of these deal directly with the subject of borrowing money and going into debt. While the Bible does not prohibit borrowing in general, it does present important principles to consider. Muntz goes on to discuss why it is important to approach student loans with the principles of integrity and stewardship. You should always intend to pay your loans back and make every effort to do so. If you fail at this, your integrity will be damaged. It is also important to remember before you go to college that you are to follow God's will by being a trustworthy steward, and to develop the talents He has given you.

Muntz also states that when thinking about student loans, a key word to focus on is "reasonable." "First, it is important to exhaust all other options. Second, a student should borrow only *if* necessary and only *what* is necessary. It is altogether too easy to take out student loans these days and many students find themselves borrowing more than they really need. Often, they don't even truly realize that they are borrowing. It's only when they make the first of what may be 10 years' worth of monthly payments that they realize they really could have been a bit more frugal while in college and borrowed less."[33]

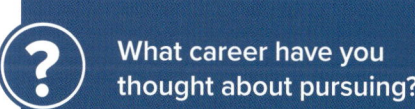

? What career have you thought about pursuing?

OTHER CHOICES

Remember that student loans aren't the only ways to pay for your college degree. Parental assistance, personal savings, scholarships, grants and work study employment can all help you get to school without breaking the bank. So, before you fill out that loan application, be sure to consider all the options you have available to you.

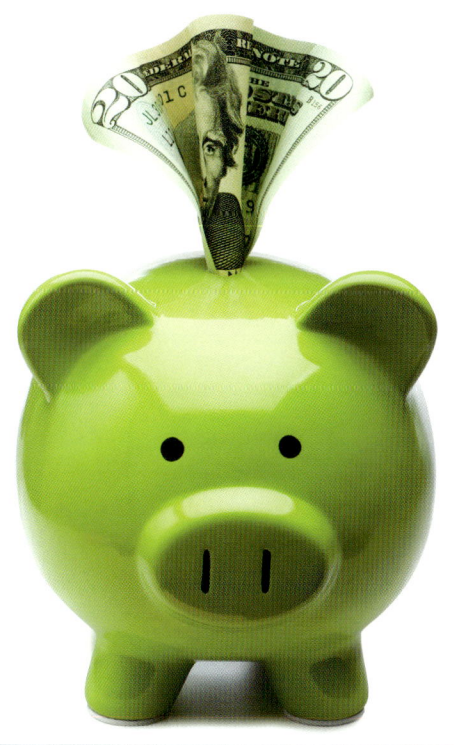

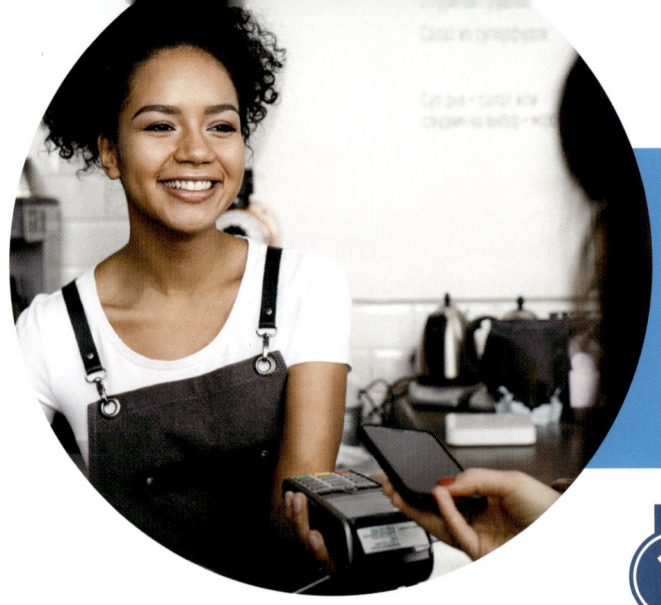

Research has found that part-time work is linked with higher grades, better self-image and increased independence and social opportunities.

? What will you enjoy and what will challenge you about your career choice?

MONEY TALKS

Right now you might be more broke than a glass baseball bat, but at some point you will need to learn how to make good decisions with money. Let's see how the power of choice can help you find the right solution to the problem.

For example, if you do want to make more money, choosing to take a part-time job is a good idea. In fact, it may benefit you in more ways than just an increase in cash flow. Some people think that when students take on jobs they end up neglecting their schoolwork. However, research has found that part-time work is linked with higher grades, better self-image and increased independence and social opportunities. Even when those who worked part-time studied less than those who did not, they had more efficient use of their time and more effective study habits.[34]

When you do make money, it's important to remember to give back to God.

"Bring the whole tithe into the storehouse, so that there may be food in My house, and test Me now in this," says the Lord of hosts, "if I will not open for you the windows of heaven and pour out for you a blessing until it overflows." MALACHI 3:10

The truth is, any money you make belongs to God first. You are not its owner; you are only a steward. God wants you to give back to Him through tithes and offerings.

The word tithe means "a tenth" and is usually expressed by giving God 10 percent of your regular income through your local church. Offerings are gifts, which go above and beyond your regular tithe giving. Whatever you decide to give, remember these words from the apostle Paul, *"Each one must do just as he has purposed in his heart, not grudgingly or under compulsion, for God loves a cheerful giver,"* (2 Corinthians 9:7, NASB). Your giving reveals what you are like on the inside. Yes, God wants you to give, but not out of obligation or for selfish reasons. He wants you to give because you love Him.

The amazing thing is that your giving has a huge impact on your personal happiness. In one study, a team of Harvard researchers surveyed people about their spending and their happiness. They made an interesting discovery — contrary to popular belief, spending money on oneself does *not* boost happiness. However, spending money on others does. In fact it's as important to a person's happiness as the total amount of money they make.[35]

The generous man will be prosperous, and he who waters will himself be watered.

PROVERBS 11:25

God created you to give. He wants you to help and serve others, and He promises to bless you when you do. It's only natural that doing what God desires actually helps you to be happier. By being generous with your giving, you are helping others, but you are also helping yourself.

MORE BANG FOR YOUR BUCK

Another way you can boost your happiness and get the most out of your money is by experiential purchases rather than material ones. Experiential purchases, such as going out to dinner or saving up for a vacation, not only increase your life-satisfaction but also the satisfaction of others. When you invest in experiences, you have something to look forward to and can reflect on the memory for years to come. Sharing these experiences also helps you to connect with others.[36-37]

When researchers looked at why these experiential purchases made people happier, they found a couple factors. First, you are less likely to regret experiential purchases as opposed to material ones. This increases your satisfaction when you make these purchases over time. Second, people tend to examine material purchases more and make comparisons to other options available. This comparison shopping often undermines the ultimate choice because they can't stop thinking about the other possibilities they've passed up.[38]

Another way you can make the most of your money is by avoiding purchases when you feel discouraged or depressed. Why do so many people think a shopping spree is just the thing to improve their mood? They head to the mall to stock up on items they don't want or even need just because they think it will help them to feel better. However, in the end it does just the opposite. In fact, feelings of sadness may

influence you to spend more than you can afford. This was seen in a study of several shoppers who were asked to watch certain videos before shopping. One group watched a neutral, middle-of-the-road video, while another group was shown a video designed to induce sadness. When the groups were later given the opportunity to shop, the second group of shoppers offered to pay nearly four times as much for their products compared to the first group. In spite of this major difference, the viewers of the sad video still insisted that the content did not influence their decision. They were unaware of how much their emotions were controlling their shopping habits.[39]

Don't let your emotions wreak havoc on your bank account. Recognize when you are feeling down, and don't try to spend your way out of depression.

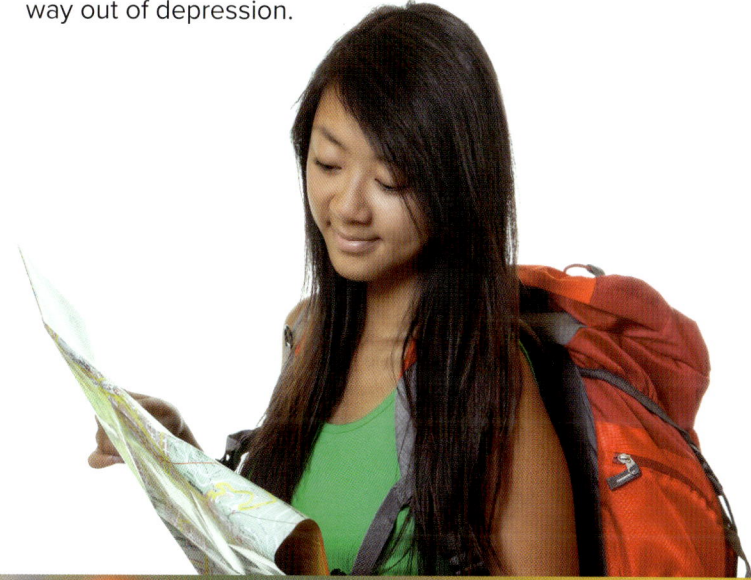

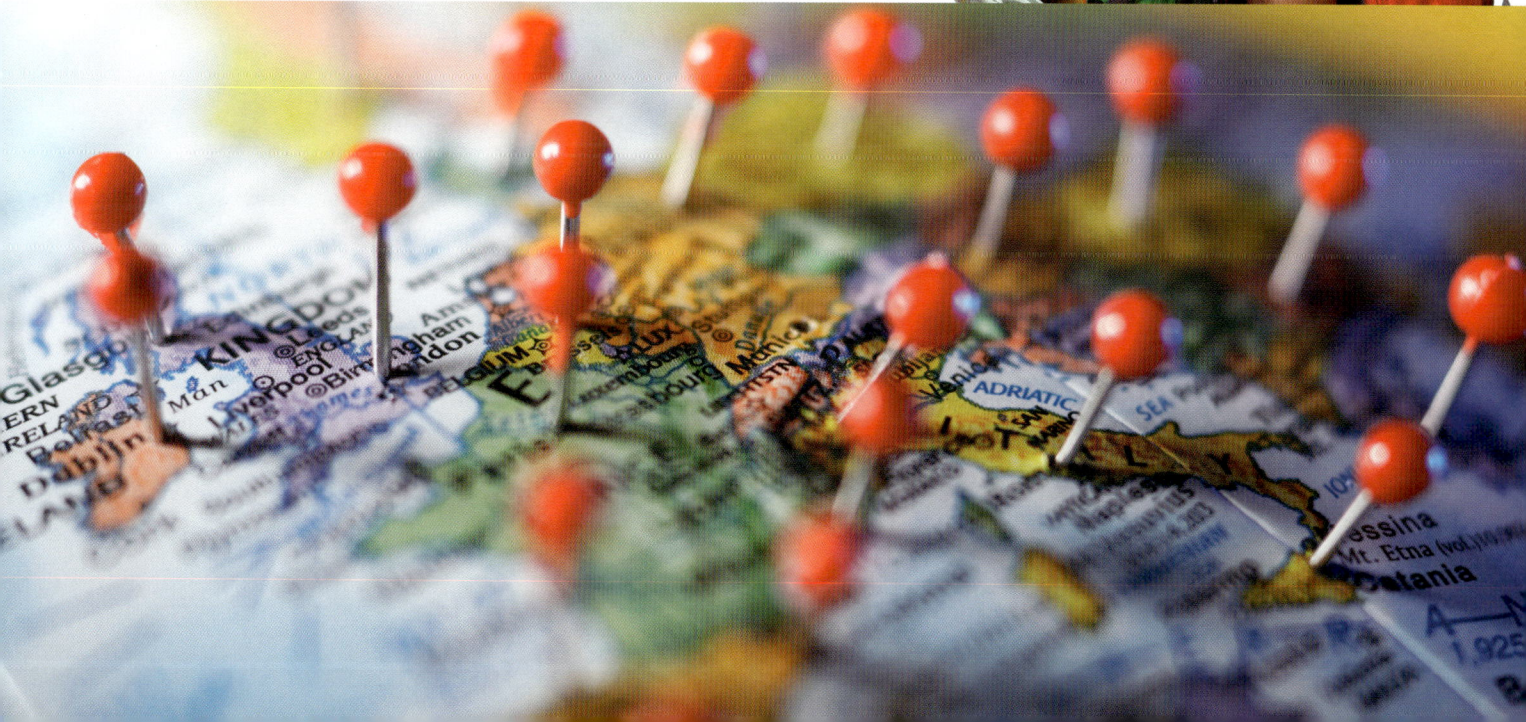

THE TRUTH ABOUT CREDIT CARDS

At some point, you're going to leave home and be on your own. You'll be excited to get your own place with a succulent plant, DYI book shelf and mix-and-match towels. Money will be so tight you'll have to find a roommate who won't do the dishes but will eat your food. You'll long for the days when someone else bought the groceries and did your laundry, but hey, at least you'll be on your own. One day you'll pick up your mail. You'll be surprised to find an envelope. It will be from a major credit card company and inside will be an offer. They will want to give you thousands of dollars in credit with "Zero-percent APR till February." "Thank-you points." and "Cash-back bonuses." You're not sure what all that means (and it would take an electron microscope to read the fine print), but you figure your place could really use a new TV... and a waffle maker, some food in the fridge, gas in your car and a few other things you haven't been able to afford. A minute ago you were eating ramen noodles straight out of the bag and suddenly you have it all! Awesome, right?

Not exactly. Remember that "credit" is just a fancy word for borrowing money, and every dollar you borrow must be paid back with interest. Some of these interest rates can be deceptively low at first, but they jump to astronomical heights after just a short trial period. If you're not careful, you can rack up a huge amount of debt in no time. Credit cards can bring other problems besides debt. One study that looked at the impact of credit card debt on college students revealed that students who had greater debt reported greater stress and decreased financial well-being. The research found that the amount of debt a person had was related to their age, their lack of financial knowledge, the number of credit cards they had, how well they could delay gratification and their attitude toward credit card use.[40]

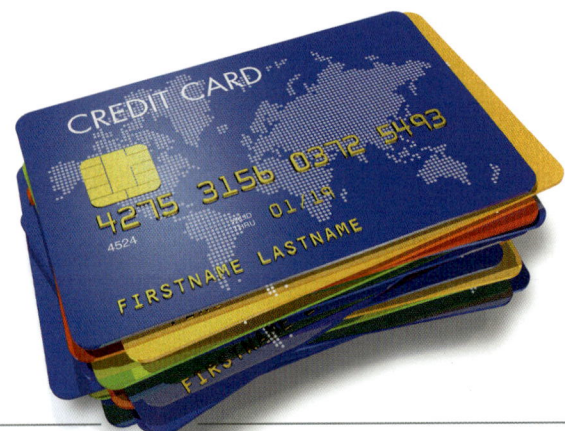

Researchers have also found that students with a tendency toward compulsive buying are more likely to have credit card debt. This is because carrying a credit card in your wallet is a huge temptation to live beyond your means, or spend more than what you can afford. Peer pressure or an attempt to alleviate negative feelings such as difficulty, anxiety or frustration in your life can also lead you to make compulsive or impulsive purchases. You can escape the dangers of debt by educating yourself on strategies to use a credit card wisely. Start by talking to your parents or a financial counselor about how you can best move forward.[41]

"WHAT DO YOU WANT TO BE WHEN YOU GROW UP?"

Whatever you do, do your work heartily, as for the Lord rather than for men, knowing that from the Lord you will receive the reward of the inheritance. It is the Lord Christ whom you serve. COLOSSIANS 3:23–24

So, what do you want to do for the rest of your life? This is a basic question many people have trouble answering. But figuring it out can help you decide upon a career and its importance to your life.

In one Gallup poll, several workers were asked, "Do you like what you do each day?" Sadly, only 20 percent of the workers surveyed answered with a strong "Yes." This is a clear indication that something is wrong. The majority of people in this country are not happy in their work.

Why is it that when people first meet, the first question they ask each other is, "So, what do you do?" This is because what you spend your time doing each and every day shapes who you are. It becomes your identity. The fact is, after you have finished high school and college, you will spend the majority of your waking hours doing something. You might call it a career, an occupation or just a job, but research shows that if you actually like what you do, it's because you have found something fulfilling and meaningful. You will have a strong sense of "Career Well-being."

? What are your personal strengths and how will these help you in your career?

Career Well-being is important because it impacts your health and wellness. Gallup researchers also found that if you do not have high Career Well-being, the odds of you having high well-being in other areas is diminished. People who have high Career Well-being are more than *twice* as likely to be thriving in other areas of their lives overall. "Imagine that you have great social relationships, financial security and good physical health — but you don't like what you do every day. Chances are, much of your social time is spent worrying or complaining about your lousy job. And this causes stress, taking a toll on your physical health. If your Career Well-being is low, it's easy to see how it can cause deterioration in other areas over time."[42]

"Each morning when I open my eyes I say to myself: I, not events, have the power to make me happy or unhappy today. I can choose which it shall be. Yesterday is dead, tomorrow hasn't arrived yet. I have just one day, today, and I'm going to be happy in it."

GROUCHO MARX

To really appreciate how much our careers shape our identity and well-being, consider what happens when someone loses a job and remains unemployed for a full year. In a landmark study, researchers found that unemployment might be the only major life event from which people do not fully recover within five years. The researchers followed 130,000 people for several decades, which allowed them to assess how major life events such as marriage, divorce, birth of a child or death of a spouse affected life satisfaction over time. On an encouraging note, the researchers found that after one of the most tragic life events, like the death of a spouse, people did recover to the same level of well-being they had before the spouse passed away. This was not the case for those who were unemployed for a prolonged period of time, and this number was even more significant among men. Amazingly, according to this research, our well-being actually recovers more rapidly from the death of a spouse than it does from a sustained period of unemployment.[43]

? What steps do you need to take to find out what career path fits you best?

THE MOST IMPORTANT CHOICE

You have one choice to make that is far more important than all the others. In fact, it's the most important choice you can possibly make in life, more important than any decision regarding your future, your career or your deepest dreams and desires. That choice is this: *"... choose for yourselves today whom you will serve... but as for me and my house, we will serve the Lord"* (Joshua 24:15). Choosing to serve God, to have Him as your personal Friend, Counselor, Helper, Guide and Savior is the most important choice you can make today, tomorrow and every day. This choice has the power to impact every other choice you will make for every moment of your life.

Why has God given you the power of choice? It's so you can choose Him on a daily basis. *"... I have set before you life and death, the blessing and the curse. So, choose life in order that you may live, you and your descendants, by loving the Lord your God, by obeying His voice, and by holding fast to Him; for this is your life... "* (Deuteronomy 30:19–20). The best path to choose is God's way of living. Instead, most people so often choose another path, one that provides them with immediate pleasure. This pleasure lasts only for a short time. Like an addict coming off a drug, they're soon looking for another hit. By choosing God's way, you will not only receive blessings in this life, but also in the life to come. God has promised to give the ultimate blessing of eternal life to those who have chosen to place their trust in Him. The choice for God is truly the choice for life — now and forevermore.

CHOOSE LIFE

Today you are on the brink of something big. You have the opportunity to change your life. All it takes is one choice, but no one can make it for you. You alone have to decide to change. Will you make that choice today?

In John 10:10, Jesus says, "I have come in order that you might have life." The Greek word for life is "zoe." This isn't just any ordinary life Jesus is talking about. This is life as God has it. Imagine sharing and enjoying that kind of life. How does it compare to the life you have now?

Wherever you are today, understand this: you are just one choice away from a new beginning. Through the power of God, you can become a new creation. You can have a new life just as God intended it. It's a life that's available to you right now through the power of CREATION Life.

> *"God always gives His best to those who leave the choice with Him."*
>
> JIM ELLIOT

God wants to give you eternal life.

What does that mean to you personally? What is your response to God's gift?

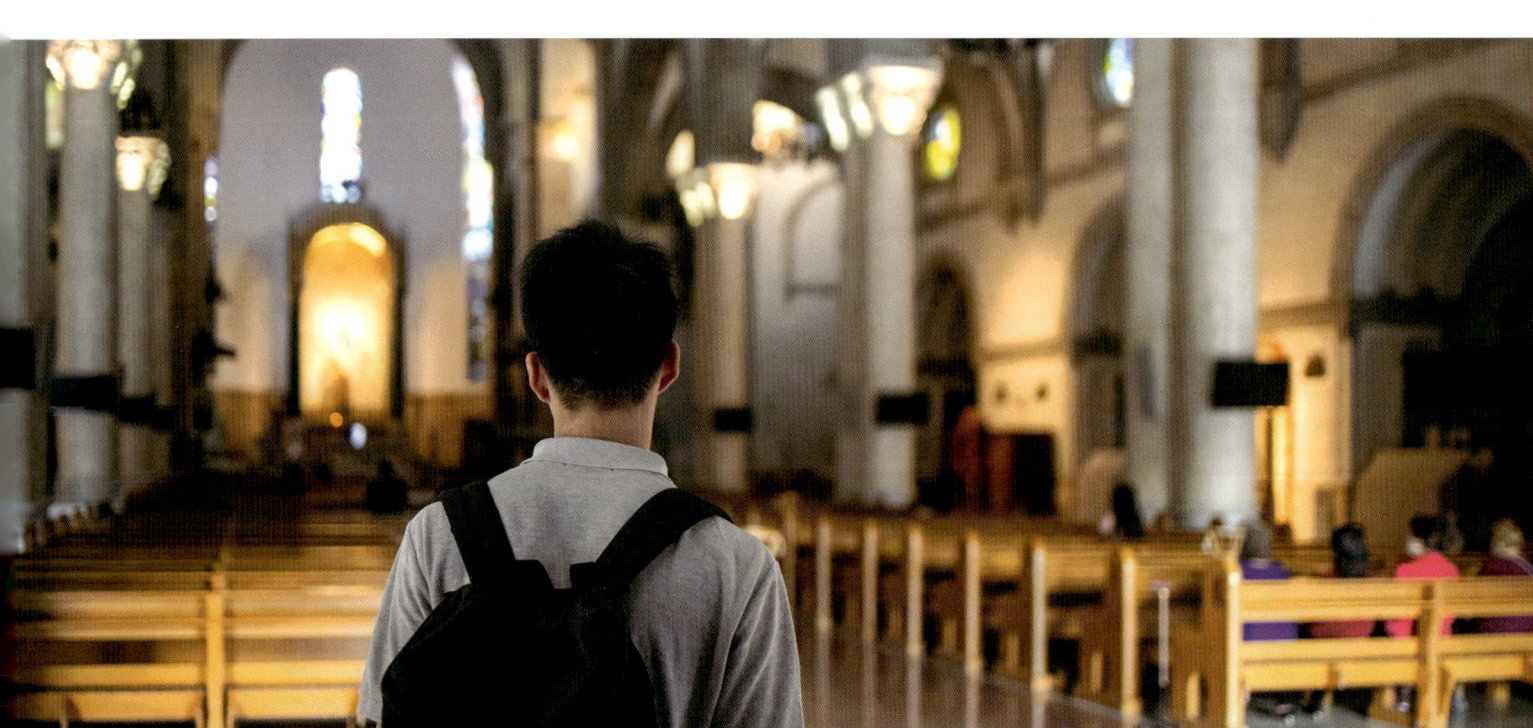

REFERENCES

1. Fuster, Joaquin M. *The Prefrontal Cortex: Anatomy, Physiology, and Neuropsychology of the Frontal Lobe*. New York: Raven Press, 1989. 3-9, 125.

2. Damasio, Hanna, Thomas Grabowski, Randall Frank, Albert M. Galaburda, and Antonio R. Damasio. "The Return of Phineas Gage: Clues about the Brain From the Skull of a Famous Patient." *Science* 264, no. 5162 (1994): 1102-1105. https://doi.org/10.1126/science.8178168.

3. Baldwin, Bernell E. and Marjorie V. Baldwin. "Frontal Lobes and Character." *Ministry Magazine*, February 1976: 26-29. https://gcmin-rnr.s3.amazonaws.com/cdn/ministrymagazine.org/issues/1976/issues/MIN1976-02.pdf.

4. Langer, Ellen J., Judith Rodin, and John T. Lanzetta. "The Effects of Choice and Enhanced Personal Responsibility for the Aged: A Field Experiment in an Institutional Setting." *Journal of Personality and Social Psychology* 34, no. 2 (1976): 191-99. http://dx.doi.org/10.1037/0022-3514.34.2.191.

5. Rodin, Judith and Ellen J. Langer. "Long-term Effects of a Control-relevant Intervention with the Institutionalized Aged." *Journal of Personality and Social Psychology* 35, no. 12 (1977): 897-902. http://dx.doi.org/10.1037/0022-3514.35.12.897.

6. Seligman, Martin E. P. *Learned Optimism: How to Change Your Mind and Your Life*. 1st Vintage Books ed. New York: Vintage Books, 2006.

7. Deci, Edward L, Nancy H. Spiegal, Richard M. Ryan, Richard Koestner, and Manette Kauffman. "Effects of Performance Standards on Teaching Styles: Behavior of Controlling Teachers." *Journal of Educational Psychology* 74, no. 6 (1982): 852-59. http://dx.doi.org/10.1037/0022-0663.74.6.852.

8. Schulz, Richard and Barbara H. Hanusa. "Long-term Effects of Control and Predictability-enhancing Interventions: Findings and Ethical Issues." *Journal of Personality and Social Psychology* 36, no. 11 (1978): 1194-201. http://dx.doi.org/10.1037/0022-3514.36.11.1194.

9. Garber, Judy and Martin E.P. Seligman. *Human Helplessness: Theory and Applications*. Academic Press, 1980.

10. Overmier, J. Bruce and Martin E. Seligman. "Effects of Inescapable Shock Upon Subsequent Escape and Avoidance Responding." *Journal of Comparative and Physiological Psychology* 63, no. 1 (1967): 28-33. http://dx.doi.org/10.1037/h0024166.

11. King Jr., Martin Luther. *Letter from a Birmingham Jail*. April 16, 1963. https://kinginstitute.stanford.edu/king-papers/documents/letter-birmingham-jail.

12. Johnston, Lloyd D. and Patrick M. O'Malley. "Why Do the Nation's Students Use Drugs and Alcohol? Self-Reported Reasons from Nine National Surveys." *Journal of Drug Issues* 16, no. 1 (1986): 29-66. https://doi.org/10.1177/002204268601600103.

13. Albert, Sarah. "Talk to Your Teens (It's Important.)." *Frederick News Post*, June 9, 2013. https://newspaperarchive.com/frederick-news-post-jun-09-2013-p-63/.

14. Yancey, Antronette K., Judith M. Siegel, and Kimberly L. McDaniel. "Role Models, Ethic Identity, and Health-Risk Behaviors in Urban Adolescents." *Archives of Pediatric & Adolescent Medicine* 156, no. 1 (2002): 55–61. https://doi.org/10.1001/archpedi.156.1.55.

15. Dubois, David L. and Naida Silverthorn. "Natural Mentoring Relationships and Adolescent Health: Evidence from a National Study." *American Journal of Public Health* 95, no. 3 (2005): 518-524. https://doi.org/10.2105/AJPH.2003.031476.

16. Covey, Sean. *The 7 Habits of Highly Effective Teens: The Ultimate Teenage Success Guide*. New York: [Great Britain]: Fireside, 1998. 176-177.

17. Coan, Richard W. "Personality Variables Associated with Cigarette Smoking." *Journal of Personality and Social Psychology* 26, no. 1 (1973): 86-104. http://dx.doi.org/10.1037/h0034213.

18. Balch, Phillip and A. William Ross. "Predicting Success in Weight Reduction as a Function of Locus of Control: A Unidimensional and Multidimensional Approach," *Journal of Consulting and Clinical Psychology* 43, no. 1 (1975): 119. http://dx.doi.org/10.1037/h0076495.

19. Lewis, Frances Marcus, Donald E. Morisky, and Brian S. Flynn. "A Test of Construct Validity of Health Locus of Control: Effects of Self-Reported Compliance for Hypertensive Patients," *Health Education Monographs* 6, no. 1 (1978): 138–148. https://doi.org/10.1177/109019817800600105.a

20. Findley, Maureen J. and Harris M. Cooper. "Locus of Control and Academic Achievement: A Literature Review." *Journal of Personality and Social Psychology* 44, no. 2 (1983): 419–427. http://dx.doi.org/10.1037/0022-3514.44.2.419.

21. Schmidt, Robert M. "Who Maximizes What? A Study in Student Time Allocation." *The American Economic Review* 73, no. 2 (1983): 23-28. http://www.jstor.org/stable/1816808.

22. Park, Kang H. and Peter M. Kerr. "Determinants of Academic Performance: A Multinomial Logic Approach." *The Journal of Economic Education* 21, no. 2 (1990): 101-11. https://doi.org/10.1080/00220485.1990.10844659.

23. Elias, Maurice J. and William H Trusheim. "Beyond Compliance: Rethinking Discipline and Codes of Conduct." Education Week. Last modified July 25, 2013. https://www.edweek.org/ew/articles/2013/07/25/37elias.h32.html?tkn=XS%20MFVIzoUtKkJIQxZWf%2FK3Ao3e4xElXyh3Bf&cmp=clp-edweek.

24. Tice, Dianne M. and Roy F. Baumeister. "Longitudinal Study of Procrastination, Performance, Stress, and Health: The Costs and Benefits of Dawdling." *Psychological Science* 8, no. 6 (1997): 454-58. https://doi.org/10.1111/j.1467-9280.1997.tb00460.x.

25. Steel, Piers. "The Nature of Procrastination: A Meta-Analytic and Theoretical Review of Quintessential Self-Regulatory Failure." *Psychological Bulletin* 133, no. 1 (2007): 65-94. https://doi.org/10.1037/0033-2909.133.1.65.

26. Díaz-Morales, Juan Francisco, Joseph R. Ferrari, and Joseph R. Cohen. "Indecision and Avoidant Procrastination: The Role of Morningness—Eveningness and Time Perspective in Chronic Delay Lifestyles." *The Journal of General Psychology* 135, no. 3 (2008): 228-240. https://doi.org/10.3200/GENP.135.3.228-240.

27. Ferrari, Joseph R., Jesse S. Harriott, Lucy Evans, Denise M. Lecik-Michna, and Jeremy M. Wenger. "Exploring the Time Preferences by Procrastinators: Night or Day, Which is the One?" *European Journal of Personality* 11, no. 3 (1997): 187-196. https://doi.org/10.1002/(SICI)1099-0984(199709)11:3<187::AID-PER287>3.0.CO;2-6.

28. Hess, Brian, Martin F. Sherman, and Mark Goodman. "Eveningness Predicts Academic Procrastination: The Mediating Role of Neuroticism." *Journal of Social Behavior and Personality* 15, no. 5 (2000): 61-74.

29. Digdon, Nancy L. and Andrew J. Howell. "College Students Who Have an Eveningness Preference Report Lower Self-Control and Greater Procrastination." *Chronobiology International* 25, no. 6: 1029–1046. https://doi.org/10.1080/07420520802553671.

30. Nelson, Jennifer. "Why You Procrastinate – and How to Stop." Today. Last modified April 15, 2011. https://www.today.com/news/why-you-procrastinate-how-stop-wbna42578065.

31. CollegeBoard. "Lifetime Earnings by Education Level." Accessed September 19, 2018. https://trends.collegeboard.org/education-pays/figures-tables/lifetime-earnings-education-level.

32. Baum, Sandy, Jennifer Ma, and Kathleen Payea, Education Pays 2013: *The Benefits of Higher Education for Individuals and Society.* CollegeBoard, 2013. https://trends.collegeboard.org/sites/default/files/education-pays-2013-full-report.pdf.

33. Muntz, Palmer. "What Does the Bible Say About Student Loans?" Accessed July 20, 2018. http://www.geneva.edu/student-financial-services/documents/What_does_the_Bible_about_loans.pdf.

34. Elling, Susan R. and Theodore W. Elling. "The Influence of Work on College Student Development." *NASPA Journal* 37, no. 2 (2000): 454-470. https://doi.org/10.2202/1949-6605.1108.

35. Dunn, Elizabeth W., Lara B. Aknin, and Michael I. Norton. "Spending Money on Others Promotes Happiness." *Science* 319, no. 5870 (2008): 1687-1688. https://doi.org/10.1126/science.1150952.

36. Rath, Tom and Jim Harter. *Wellbeing: The Five Essential Elements.* New York: Gallup Press, 2010. 55.

37. Carter, Travis J., Thomas Gilovich, and Laura King. "The Relative Relativity of Material and Experiential Purchases." *Journal of Personality and Social Psychology* 98, no. 1 (2010): 146-159. http://dx.doi.org/10.1037/a0017145.

38. Van Boven, Leaf and Thomas Gilovich. "To Do or to Have? That Is the Question." *Journal of Personality and Social Psychology* 85, no. 6 (2003): 1193-1202. http://dx.doi.org/10.1037/0022-3514.85.6.1193.

39. Cryder, Cynthia E., Jennifer S. Lerner, James J. Gross, and Ronald E. Dahl. "Misery Is Not Miserly." *Psychological Science* 19, no. 6. (2007): 525-530. http://journals.sagepub.com/doi/pdf/10.1111/j.1467-9280.2008.02118.x.

40. Norvilitis, Jill M., Michelle M. Merwin, Timothy M. Osberg, Patricia V. Roehling, Paul Young, and Michelle M. Kamas. "Personality Factors, Money Attitudes, Financial Knowledge, and Credit-Card Debt in College Students." *Journal of Applied Social Psychology* 36, no. 6 (2006): 1395-1413. https://doi.org/10.1111/j.0021-9029.2006.00065.x.

41. Wang, Jeff and Jing. J. Xiao. "Buying Behavior, Social Support and Credit Card Indebtedness of College Students." *International Journal of Consumer Studies* 33, no. 1 (2009): 2-10. https://doi.org/10.1111/j.1470-6431.2008.00719.x.

42. Rath, Tom and Jim Harter. *Wellbeing: The Five Essential Elements.* New York: Gallup Press, 2010.

43. Clark, Andrew E., Ed Diener, Yannis Georgellis, and Richard E. Lucas. "Lags and Leads in Life Satisfaction: A Test of the Baseline Hypothesis." *The Economic Journal* 118, no. 529 (2008). https://www.econstor.eu/bitstream/10419/150633/1/diw_sp0084.pdf.

REST

Refresh and restore

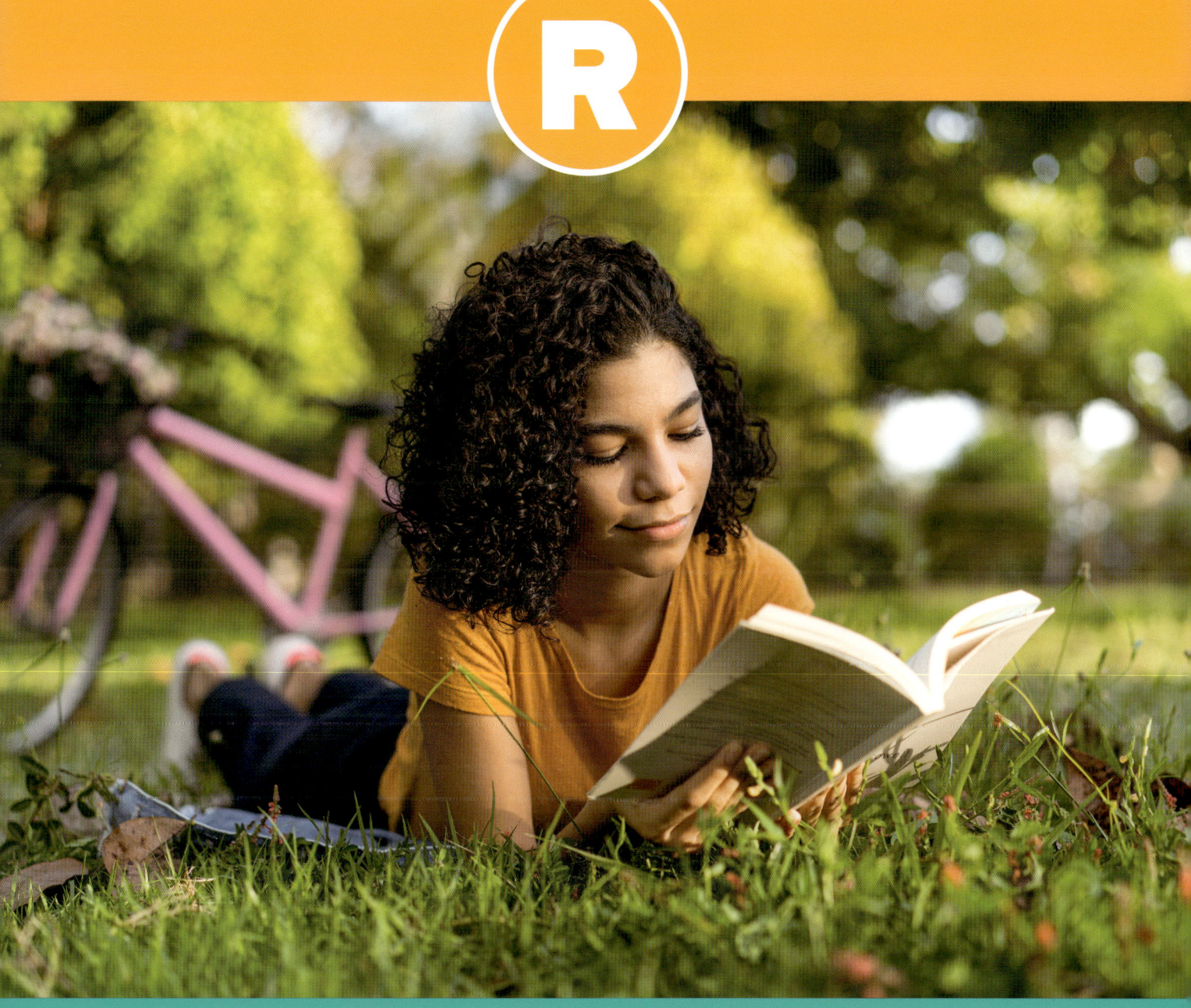

REST [rest] *verb* **1:** the restoration of your body, mind and spirit. Your best rest includes a good night's sleep and making time to relax daily, weekly and yearly.

THE BIG PICTURE

Imagine, you're sitting in biology class and the teacher is droning on and on about the life cycles of protozoa. You know you should be taking notes because this will all be on the quiz, but you are too sleepy to care. You rub your eyes, yawn and regret staying up all night. It's too late to change things now because your eyelids are already at half-mast. The next thing you know you're out for the count, but hey, at least your mouth is still closed; otherwise you'd be drooling all over your homework.

Suddenly the teacher calls your name. You jump up in your seat as if you've been struck by lightning. The entire class is looking straight at you, snickering. You feel embarrassed, disoriented and worried. After all, it's only first period and you've got a long day to go.

You've probably experienced a similar scenario. And to think, this could have been avoided if you had just gotten enough rest. Rest does much more than keep you awake during boring lectures.

Rest is powerful. It refreshes, regenerates and rebuilds your body, mind and spirit. Rest allows you to function at your very best. Most students misunderstand or simply don't appreciate the true benefits of proper rest. They allow the stress of life and the pressures they face at home or school to build until they feel overwhelmed. At that point, it's almost impossible for them to get a good night's sleep. If they only knew that good and proper rest is life's first antidote to stress.

Why do so many students fall into this trap? Probably because they have been taught to build their lives around the concept of success. They are encouraged by friends, society or even family members to do whatever it takes to be the best they can be. Each day is filled with so many important and urgent responsibilities that getting rest becomes a low priority. Ironically, many students would be more likely to reach their goals of success if they gave themselves the right kind of rest at the right time. That's why this section is so important to living a CREATION Life. In order for you to be your best, you first have to get good rest.

In this chapter, you'll see how Rest, the second principle of CREATION Life, plays a vital role in your well-being. You'll learn how important sleep is to keeping you healthy, and you'll examine the benefits of taking regular periods of rest through naps, a weekly day of rest and vacations.

Rest includes a good night's sleep as well as taking time to relax and rejuvenate daily, weekly and annually.

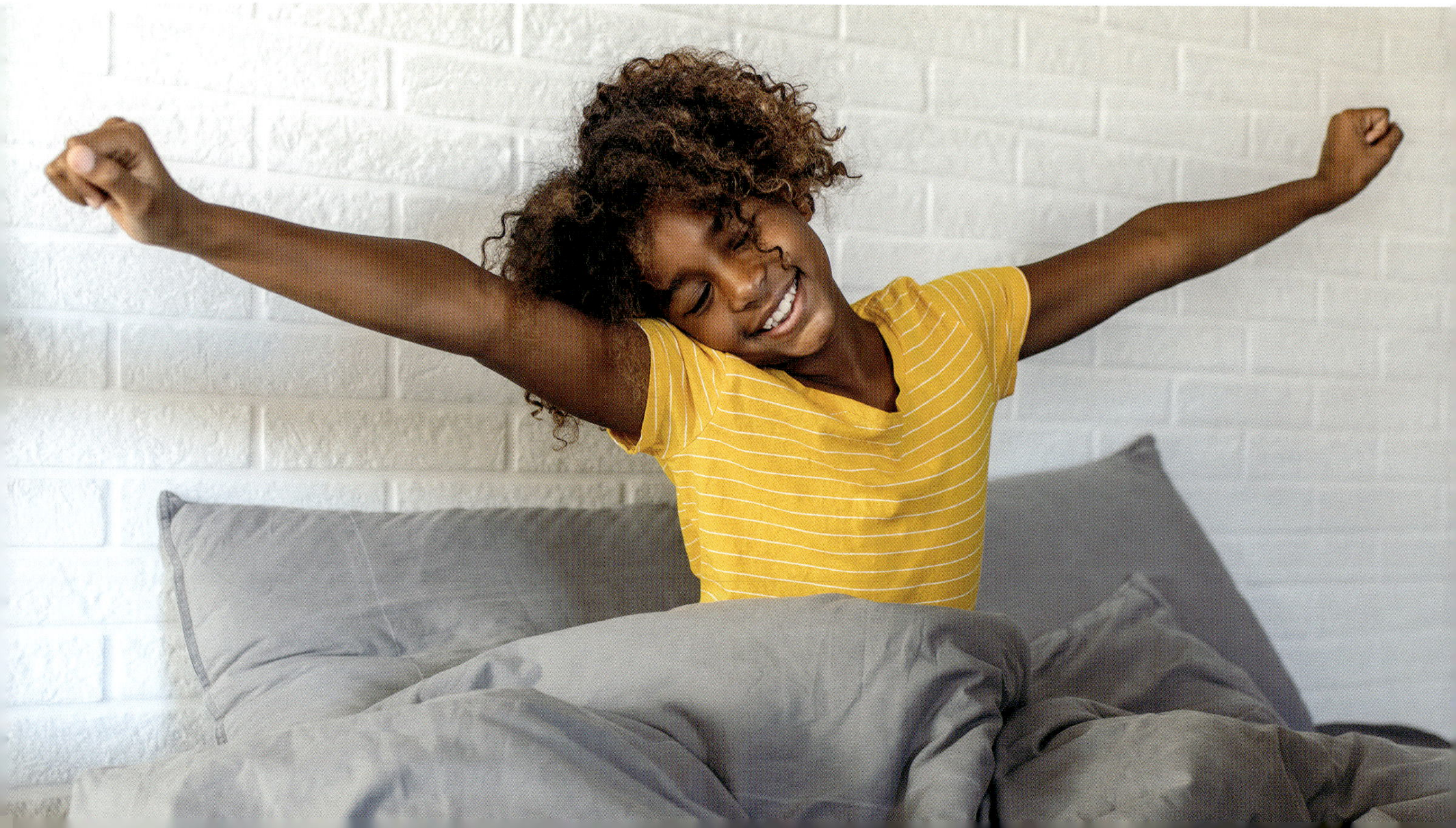

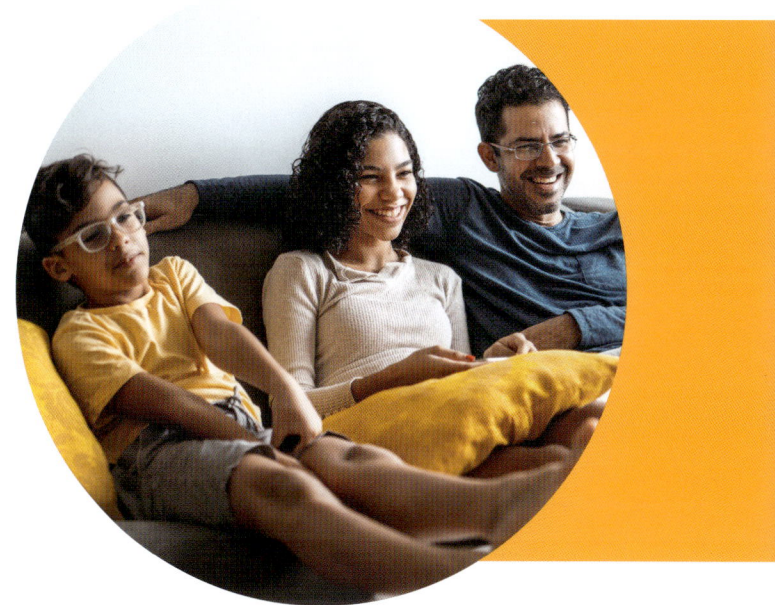

THE GIFT OF REST

Then God said, "Let there be light;" and there was light. And God saw the light, that it was good; and God divided the light from the darkness. God called the light Day, and the darkness He called Night. So the evening and the morning were the first day.

GENESIS 1:3–5

For His very first act of creation, God set in place a pattern of day and night. This cycle naturally gave birth to nightly rest. Though there are a few exceptions, most people still work or play during the day and sleep at night. As you will see, following this pattern of rest allows you to live an abundant and healthy life.

But God gave you another gift at creation. For His final act, God set apart a special time not just for rest, but also for reflection and communion with Him. God gave you the gift of the Sabbath. This special day of rest allows you to find strength from spending time with God Himself. It affords you a day when you can be free from the stress brought about by school, work, relationships or finances. God desires for you to have rest, not just at night, but also through communing with Him on a weekly basis. In this chapter, you will see there are numerous benefits from honoring God's commandment and taking this day of rest.

"To me, rest is the space within my life — space to step back and to reconnect with God, with my family, with my friends. Rest is time to recharge my batteries and restore my enthusiasm with life and people."

SCOTT BRADY, M.D.

SLEEPY TIME

Most everyone knows about the benefits of eating a healthy diet and getting regular exercise, but they overlook the important benefits of sleep. In an editorial in the journal *Archives of Internal Medicine*, two neurologists at Northwestern University said that sleep should be considered as "essential to a healthy lifestyle as exercise and nutrition."[1] Amazingly, you can make all the healthy changes you want — eating nothing but kale salad and quinoa while you run marathons till you're blue in the face — but if you don't improve your sleep at the same time (especially your nightly sleep), you will never get the maximum benefits from your diet and exercise.

Research has found that teenagers function best on eight and a half to more than nine hours of sleep each night.[2] But most likely, you're not getting anywhere near that amount. Typically, students your age voluntarily alter their sleeping habits in order to better manage their lives. One study found that more than 90 percent of teenagers reported sleeping less than the recommended time, with 10 percent sleeping less than six hours each night.[3] Since a lack of sleep affects your brain and body in many negative ways, this can lead to some serious problems.

For starters, it can make you more susceptible to sickness and disease. A study conducted at the University of Chicago found that chronic sleep deprivation could hasten the onset and increase the severity of diabetes, high blood pressure and obesity.[4] Lack of sleep is also linked to a significantly increased risk of coronary heart disease.[5] Another study revealed that losing just three hours of sleep on any given night could cut the effectiveness of your immune system in half.[6] That means staying up a few hours past your bedtime makes it a lot harder for your body to fight off infections.

Why is this the case? According to Dr. Lisa Shives, founder of Northshore Sleep Medicine in Chicago, sleep is when the body heals itself. "Sleep is a quiescent period where the cells are doing a lot of repairing. Your hormones act differently when you're asleep, and your immune system as well." Dr. Shives goes on to say that "if your immune system is out of whack, you can't fight off illness — and I would venture to say that you can't repair your cells very well, either."[7]

Lack of sleep also slows your brain function. How do you feel when you haven't had enough sleep — groggy, cranky, like your head is full of rice pudding? That's because you've decreased your ability to perform tasks controlled by the frontal lobe. This includes tasks such as planning, concentrating, motor performance and high-level intellectual skills.[8] Not getting enough sleep also decreases memory and your ability to learn.[9] This is why for optimal brain functioning, you must allow your mind to take advantage of the rejuvenating effects of regular sleep. As you saw in the previous chapter, the frontal lobe is the center of your ability to make wise and healthy choices. If your frontal lobe is impaired due to a lack of sleep, you will be less likely to do so.

A lack of sleep will also affect how well you perform in school. Not enough sleep can result in excessive daytime sleepiness and reduced neurocognitive function.[10] This makes staying awake in class a real challenge. Sleep restriction has also been shown to contribute to increased attention problems in schoolchildren.[11] This explains why it is so hard to stay focused in your classes when you've missed sleep. In one study of college-age students, sleep restriction negatively affected their academic measures in contrast to those who had better quality sleep.[12] Regardless of what grade you're in, the challenge with any sleep-deprived student is that they are often not aware that their academic challenges may be related to their lack of sleep.[13] These same students may even go so far as to wrongfully rate their cognitive performance as being better than that of students who have had a normal night's sleep. This would explain the comment so often heard in schools: "I don't understand why I did so badly. I studied for hours."[14-15] You can avoid the feelings of pity and confusion that accompany a poor performance in the classroom. By getting plenty of good rest, you will be free to achieve your best in high school and throughout your entire college career.

Do you want to know what's scary? If you are sleep deprived you may not even realize just how tired you really are. In one study, individuals who were sleep deprived for 14 days reported feeling only slightly sleepy. This means they were completely unaware of just how impaired they had become. Their lack of sleep seriously reduced their ability to pay attention and react during important activities such as driving or monitoring security at airports. It also affected their abilities to think quickly, avoid mistakes and multitask.[16]

What do large-scale disasters like the 1989 Exxon Valdez oil spill and the nuclear accidents at Three Mile Island and Chernobyl all have in common? Each of these devastating man-made tragedies occurred in the early predawn hours, and lack of sleep was a major factor in all three.[17] This is because sleep deprivation puts you at a greater risk for accidents. For example, you have probably heard about the dangers of drinking or texting while driving, but getting behind the wheel when you are sleepy can have severe consequences as well. A study published in the *British Medical Journal* found that moderate sleep deprivation produces impairments in cognitive and motor performance equivalent to legally prescribed levels of alcohol intoxication.[18] The American Academy of Sleep Medicine also reports that one in every five serious motor vehicle injuries is related to the driver being fatigued. 80,000 drivers fall asleep behind the wheel every day, and 250,000 accidents every year are related to sleepy drivers.[19] Younger drivers are even more at risk for having a crash. In fact, researchers found that drivers younger than 30 accounted for almost two-thirds of drowsy-driving crashes, in spite of the fact that they represent only about one-fourth of the licensed drivers. They were also four times more likely to have a crash due to sleepiness than were drivers 30 years of age or older.[20] With statistics like these, it's important that you take sleep deprivation seriously. If you are driving while drowsy, pull over at a rest stop or another convenient location. Better yet, get adequate sleep before you get on the road. Your life, and the lives of others, may depend on it.

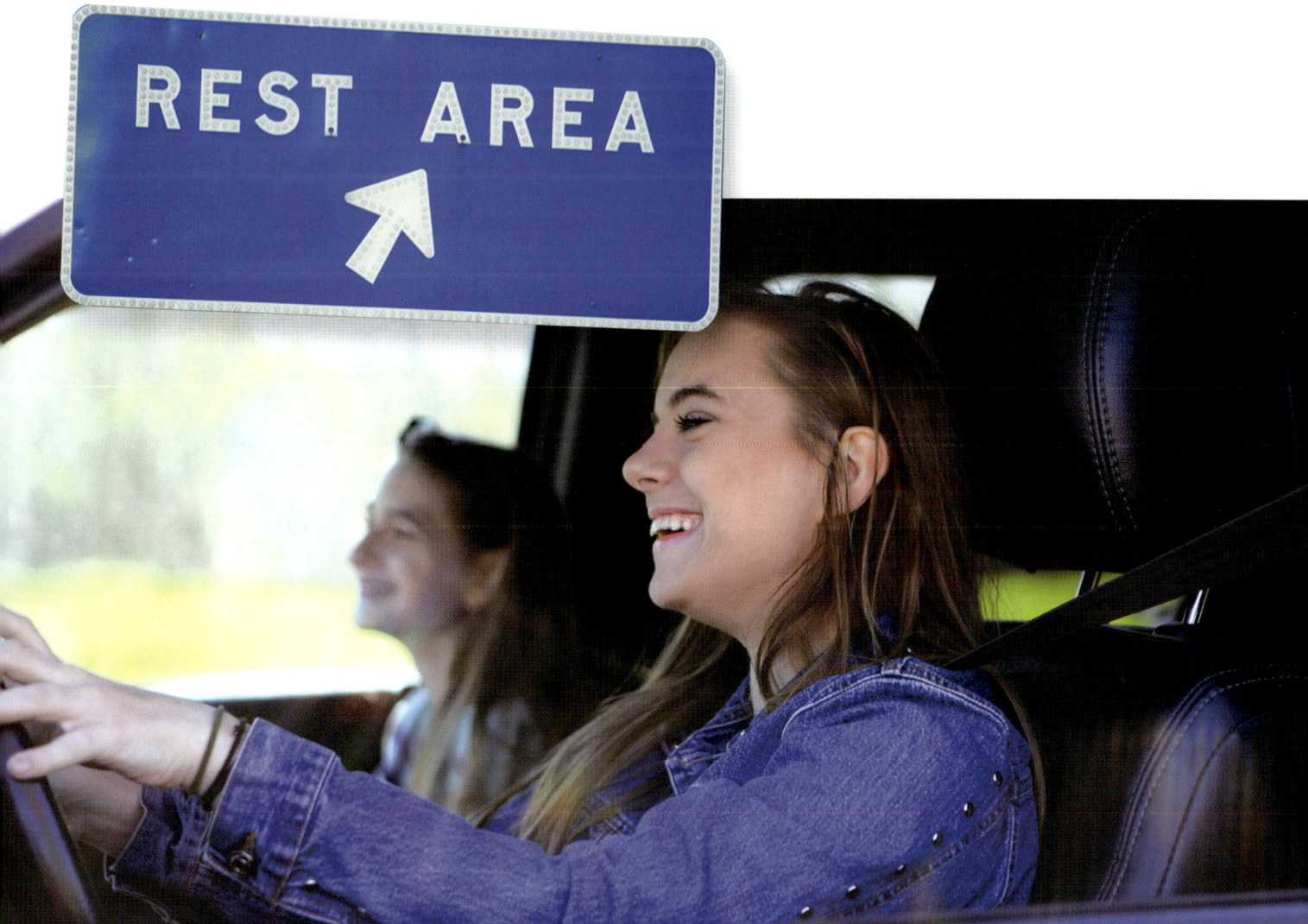

EARLY TO BED, EARLY TO RISE

Benjamin Franklin may have invented bifocals and posed for the picture on the one hundred dollar bill, but he is even more famous for his well-known saying:

Early to bed and early to rise, makes a man healthy, wealthy and wise.

New research indicates that Franklin wasn't just trying to come up with a catchy rhyme. His words actually contain a great deal of wisdom. For starters, those who go to bed early and get up early have lower rates of heart disease, diabetes and overall lower death rates than those who stay up late and get up late.[21] God created you and all human beings as diurnal creatures. That means you are made to function during the day. Your body is designed to work best when you get to sleep early in the evening and get up early in the morning. Dr. Timothy H. Monk, one of the foremost authorities on sleep, said, "Human beings are built to be daytime creatures. It's hard wired into our circuitry... when you deliberately try to shift the sleep/wake cycle, it's like having a symphony with two conductors, each one beating out a different time... your delicate internal rhythms go haywire... you need to treat sleep as a precious and fragile thing."[22] Monk has found that morning people, or larks as they are often known, are more likely than night owls to stick to healthy routines and have better sleep. Larks wake up, eat meals, exercise and get to bed at pretty much the same time each day. Night owls, on the other hand, are not so consistent with healthy daily practices.[23]

Developing regular patterns in your life is worth getting out of bed. For example, getting up early means you're more likely to eat breakfast and to exercise. This will naturally improve your physical and mental performance at school and throughout the rest of the day.

BUT I'M NOT A MORNING PERSON.

Do you dread when the alarm goes off every morning? Do you stay in bed till the last possible minute? When you finally do get up, do you have all the friendliness of a Bengal tiger with a hangnail? A lot of people have excused themselves from early rising with what they think is a rock-solid, ironclad excuse: *I'm just not a morning person.* People have heard it so many times they start to believe it's true... but is it? Is being a morning person in your genes?

Genetics may play a role in keeping some people bright eyed and bushy tailed in the morning, but this only applies to a small amount of people. Doctors feel that for 80 percent of the population it comes down to one thing — lifestyle. Everything — from the people you hang out with to the activities you participate in to how you spend your free time — all affect you.[24]

In 2005, the National Sleep Foundation conducted a national poll of adults that provides insight into why being a morning person is so beneficial. Twenty-seven percent of the respondents to the survey were categorized by the foundation as *Healthy, Lively Larks*. Members of this group were the least likely to have problems sleeping and were the most likely to enjoy a good night's sleep. As morning people, they began their day early and fell asleep quickly at night without the use of sleep aids. They were also the least likely of all those who responded to the survey to have any medical conditions. In addition, they were also the most likely to say that during their time awake they never or rarely felt tired, fatigued or less than par. Compared to average sleepers, *Healthy, Lively Larks* are much less likely to have missed work or events and/or made errors at work at least once in the past three months because of being too sleepy.[25]

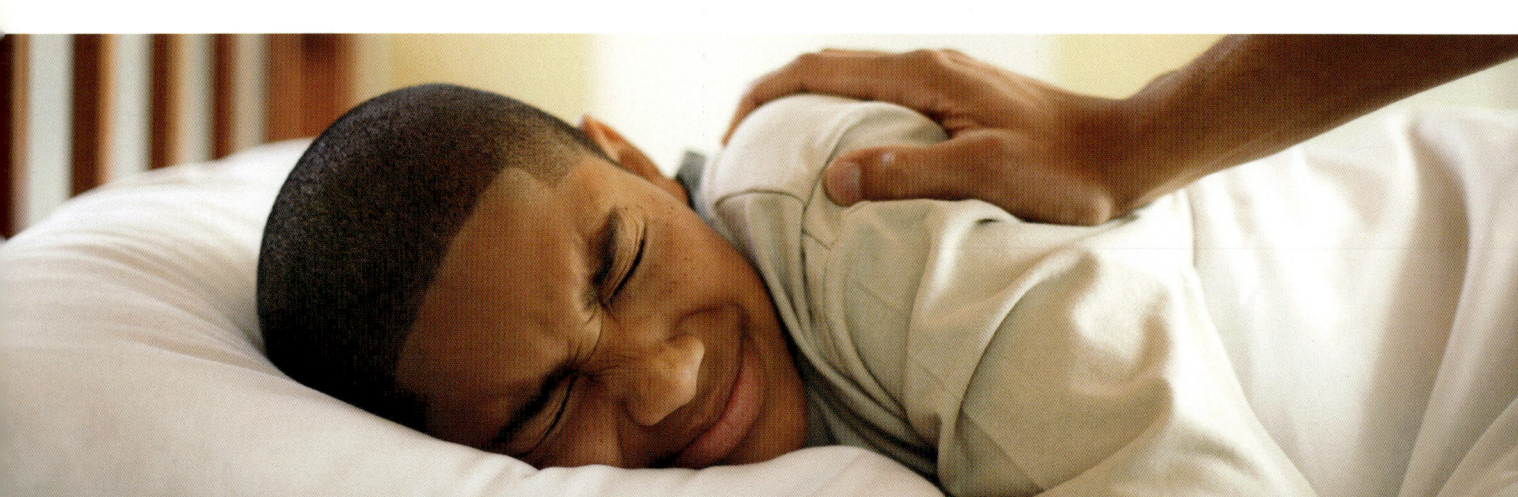

Many years of research and hundreds of well-conducted studies show that our bodies were created to follow the day and night pattern — to work when it is light and go to sleep when it gets dark. Following this pattern now can maximize your health, but what if you're a night owl? Are you destined to forever be a victim of your poor sleeping habits?

The good news is you can change. Becoming a morning person is not only doable, it comes with tremendous rewards for your health and wellness. Maybe you're thinking, *I've tried to go to bed earlier, but I can't do it.* Your sleep habits can become firmly ingrained over time, so making a change will require an intelligent and determined effort on your part. But, rest assured — you can.

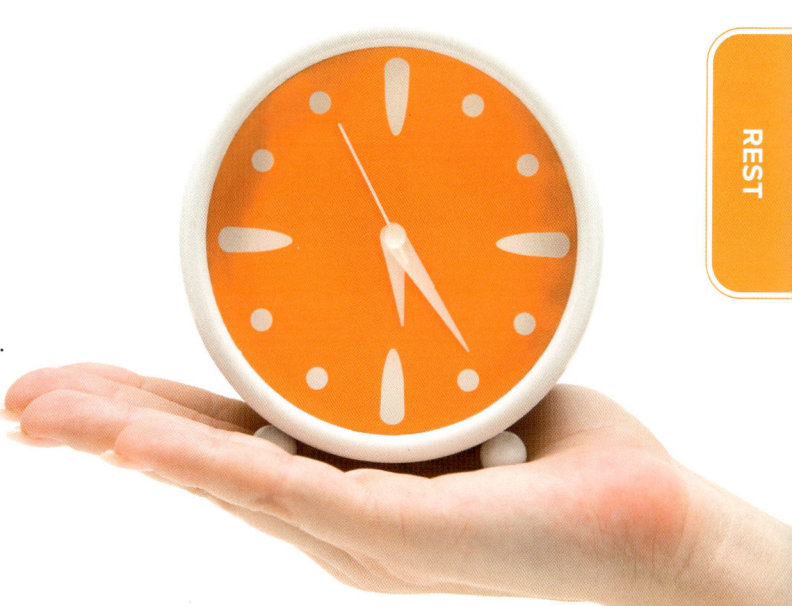

BECOME A BETTER MORNING PERSON

In an article for *Psychology Today,* Dr. Susan Krauss Whitbourne identifies five ways that night owls can reset their clocks and adopt the habits of a morning person:

1. **Find your hidden morning person.** A lot of teens may think going to bed early means missing out on valuable social opportunities with friends, but according to Dr. Whitbourne, "You may actually be more of a morning person than you think you are." Getting yourself to bed early will help you feel better in the long run, so don't feel pressured to stay up late if you don't want to. "When you're tired," Dr. Whitbourne says, "go to bed, even if your friends think you're being lame."

2. **Watch the noise.** A noisy environment can ruin your chances of getting a good night's sleep, so Dr. Whitbourne offers some solutions: "If you're stuck in a noisy environment that you can't control, get yourself a good set of ear protectors or headphones that play white noise."

3. **Get organized.** According to Dr. Whitbourne, staying up past your bedtime to get work done only makes things worse. "People who stay up past their preferred bedtime to finish the work they didn't get done during the day are only adding to their woes," she says. "The further behind they get at work, the more midnight oil they have to burn for more nights. Follow the principles of effective time management and you won't be so pressured and far behind."

4. **Don't give up.** Making any important change takes a lot of hard work and diligence, so stay with it and don't get discouraged. "You may have thought you were an evening person," Dr. Whitbourne points out, "but perhaps you've discovered here that you're not. If that's the case, then you can definitely adjust to a healthier sleep schedule."

5. **Make small adjustments.** Slowly begin to adjust your sleep patterns. Don't jump from getting up at nine o'clock every morning to getting up at five o'clock all at once. Make small, incremental changes over a period of weeks and months. "Don't rush through the steps," Dr. Whitbourne warns. "Give your body enough time to adjust so that the newer sleep and wake times will come more easily to you."[26]

THE ALL-NIGHTER

So, you put off studying for that 20-page calculus final to the last minute? No problem. You can always pull an all-nighter. Stay up all night studying, and by tomorrow morning you'll ace that test for sure, right?

While you might think pulling an all-nighter is a good way to get a large amount of work done in a short amount of time, research shows this is not true. Skipping rest means you're also skipping a very important step in the learning process. In fact, pulling an all-nighter does a lot more harm than good.

For starters, your memory will be negatively affected the next day. In one study, it was found that students who were sleep deprived for 24 hours were "not only increasing their feelings of sleepiness during the day, thus decreasing their ability to pay attention in class, but are also negatively affecting their ability to perform on exams."[27] What good is it to stay up all night studying if you're actually hurting your ability to take the exam in the process? In essence, all the good you do by studying is undone by your staying up late.

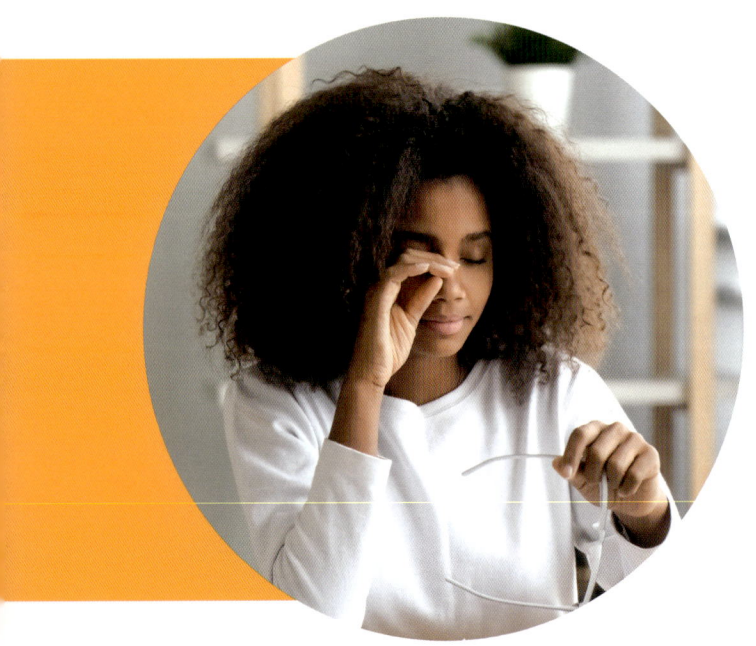

Another study found that your temporal memory is impaired after staying up 36 hours or more. Your temporal memory is your ability to remember how long ago something happened. In this study, young adults were given a simple memory test after staying up for 36 hours. The test consisted of pictures of unknown faces and had two parts: recognition memory and recency (knowing when a face had been previously presented). Recognition was unaffected by sleep deprivation, but for recency, those who did not sleep scored much worse compared to those who did. This study also revealed two interesting findings. First, when test subjects were given caffeine, it reduced their sleepiness, but it did not help them perform any better on the test. So, doubling that espresso shot isn't going to double your grade. Second, sleep deprivation increases a person's belief that they are correct, especially when they are wrong.[28] Think about how damaging this could be the next time you decide to pull an all-nighter and study. At test time, you might be writing down answers, confident that you are correct, only to find when your grade comes back just how wrong you were.

So, why does pulling an all-nighter work against you? Because sleep is when your brain turns the brand new knowledge you have learned into long-term memories you can recall later. Studies have shown a critical period for sleep and memory consolidation occurs soon after you learn the new information. Researchers examined a student's ability to remember vocabulary words and found that declarative memory is enhanced when sleep follows within a few hours of learning, independent of time of day.[29] So, if you're thinking of pulling an all-nighter, remember, this will prevent new information that you are studying from being consolidated in your mind. It will also prevent you from recalling it when you need it most come test time. It's much better to have a study plan so that you are prepared. Review things as you go along, and be sure to get a good night's sleep the night before the exam.

TIME MANAGEMENT

Learning to manage the time you do have will not only keep you from having to pull another all-nighter, it will also reduce your stress and make you better prepared to complete your work. Try following these steps to better time management.

1. **Plan for your day.** As anyone who's ever been behind on an assignment knows, teachers are very fond of saying, "Lack of preparation on your part does not constitute an emergency on mine." This is all the more reason to take time each day to plan. You'll actually get more done and feel a greater sense of accomplishment if you think in advance about what you have to do. Every morning before school take 15 to 20 minutes and run through your daily schedule. If you have tasks that require your attention, make a to-do list. Be sure to put your important tasks at the top.

2. **Learn to say, "No."** Let's face it; there are only so many hours in a day. If you're going to learn good time management skills then you've got to be able to say no to things that are robbing you of your time. You may find that too many extracurricular activities or afterschool practices are keeping you from doing what is essential such as schoolwork or spending time with friends or family. Even volunteering in your church can sometimes zap your time. But you also have to learn to say no to one other person — yourself. When it comes to time management, you are your own worst enemy. Think about how much time you spend each day on distractions like playing games on your phone or scrolling social media. Keep yourself disciplined and focused.

3. **Keep it short.** Pop quiz hotshot. You have a test tomorrow on European socialism. You've put off studying until the last minute, and if you don't do well you'll be grounded until the Browns win the Super Bowl. What do you do? Everyone has to face dreaded tasks more often than they would like. The secret is to work on the task for short intervals of time until you've completed it. For example, if you are dreading studying, force yourself to work for 10 minutes. Then take a break and return for another 10 minutes. Pretty soon you may be able to study longer. By following the 10-minute rule, you'll be able to tackle even the most dreaded of tasks.

4. **Get it right the first time.** Nothing is more discouraging than having to redo something you've already done. This means you should always put your best foot forward and try to get it right the first time. You've probably experienced that nagging voice in your head. It shows up when you know you're not doing your best work. Listen to it. Don't turn in something that you know is less than your best. Take the time you need to do a stellar job and you'll save yourself a lot of time in the future.

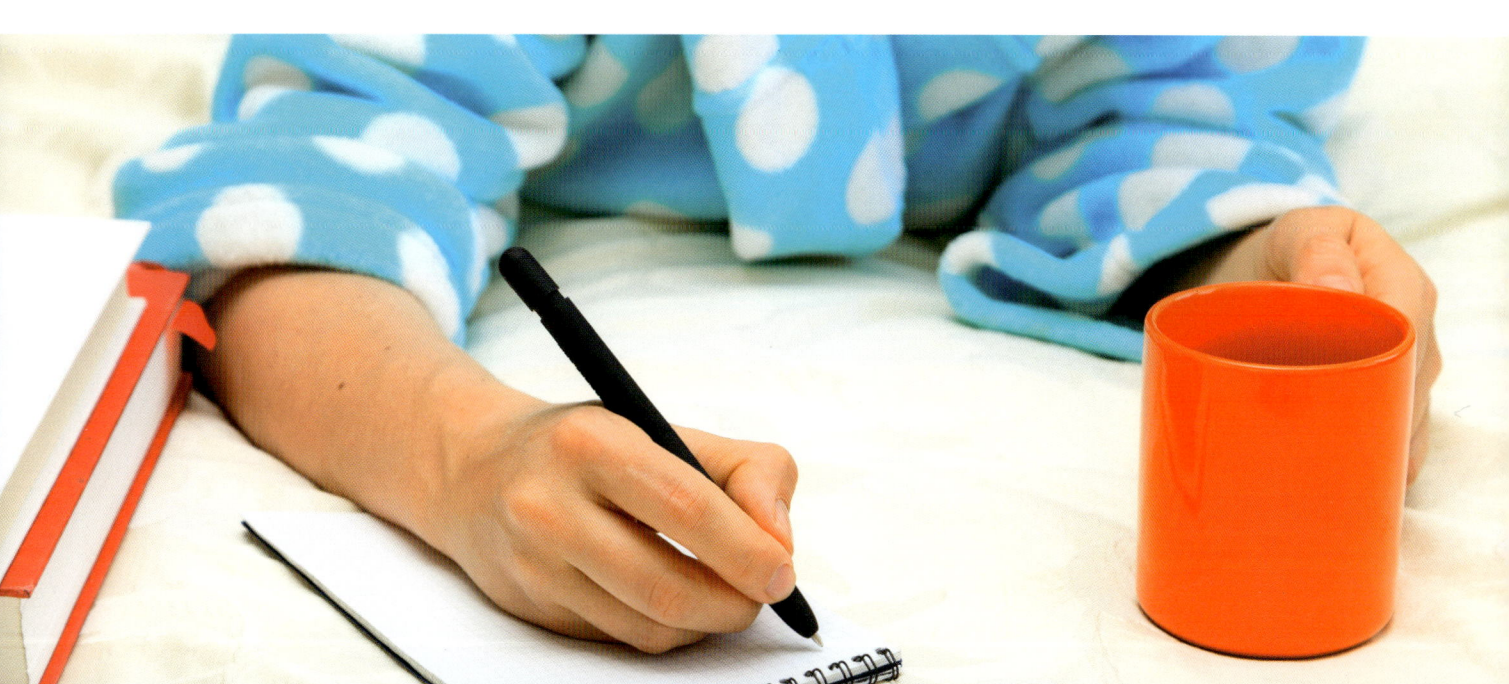

SLEEP AND MEMORY

Maybe it's true that an elephant never forgets, but you, on the other hand, have probably experienced a few memory slips along the way. The fact is you have two types of memory at your disposal — declarative and non-declarative.[30] Declarative memory gives you the ability to encode and recall facts, events and arbitrary associations.[31] This is the kind of memory you need to perform well in your classes at school. Non-declarative memory includes procedural memory, which gives you the ability to learn motor skills like playing the piano, shooting a basketball or typing up a report.[32] Sleep helps enhance and consolidate both kinds of memory. Research has found that if you are not getting enough sleep you are decreasing your ability to remember and learn new things.[33]

You may think your brain shuts off when you go to sleep, but your brain is active in incredible ways even when your body is not. German researchers illustrated this in a study where they taught people a specific method to complete a complicated math problem. Participants completed the problem three times and were then given an eight-hour break before completing the problem 10 more times. During the break some participants slept while others did not.

What the researchers did not tell the participants was that there was a much simpler way to solve the problem. Over time, many in the study discovered the shortcut on their own, but one thing helped them do it. That thing was sleep: 59.1 percent of the participants who slept found the shortcut, compared with only 22.7 percent of those who stayed awake between the sessions. "The study revealed how the sleeping brain was actually solving a problem — even though the person did not know there was a problem to solve."[34]

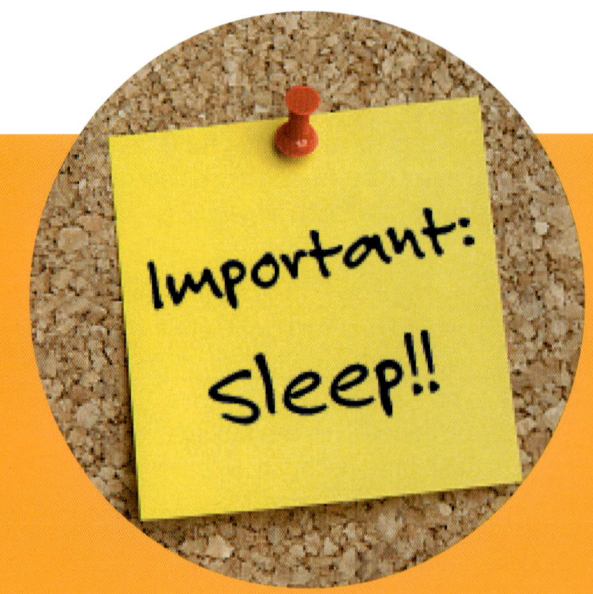

SLEEP TIPS:

- Make an effort to go to bed and wake up at the same time every day.

- Create a sleep-friendly environment in your room by darkening it, removing distractions and making sure it is a cool temperature.

- Sneak in a power nap here and there.

- Try and have a good laugh at least once every day. Laughing is a good way to reduce stress.

- Find a place that allows you to break away from life — somewhere you can be alone to take a break to relax and renew your spirit.

- Put sleep at the top of your priority list.

- Spend 20 to 30 minutes on a relaxing activity before bedtime.

A GOOD NIGHT'S SLEEP

You've seen how important it is to get a good night's sleep on a regular basis, but what exactly does that mean? How do you know if you're getting a good night's sleep, and is there such a thing as a "bad night's sleep?"

Actually, there is a way to measure how well you sleep at night. This is called your *sleep quality*, and it's determined by looking at several factors:

- Your sleep quantity or how long you sleep a night
- The length of time it takes you to fall asleep
- The number of times you wake up at night
- The length of time it takes you to fall back asleep after waking up
- The feelings of fatigue/restfulness upon awakening in the morning
- Your overall general satisfaction with your sleep[35]

Many factors contribute to poor sleep quality. The biggest is simply choosing to stay up later for whatever reason. This could include academic obligations, work requirements, extracurricular activities[36] or social interactions.[37] The use of stimulants such as caffeine or certain prescription drugs can also disturb your rest.[38-39]

The only way to get optimal sleep quality is by going to bed at the same time every night and getting up at the same time each day. Dr. Michael Brues, clinical psychologist and diplomat of the American Board of Sleep Medicine, says, "Remember everything you do, you do better with a good night's sleep."[40]

You've seen how restricted sleep is harmful to your health, but it is also possible to get too much of a good thing. Researchers have discovered that subjects who reported long periods of sleep (nine or more hours a night) shortened their lives by an average of nine years when compared with people who slept seven to eight hours per night.[41] Keep in mind that these numbers are for adults and should be adjusted for teenagers. You need anywhere between eight to 10 hours of sleep each night. Still, it's not a good idea to sleep longer than is necessary. Make sure you're following the recommended amounts so that you can achieve good sleep quality.

"You've gotta take time for yourself, to renew and to relax. If you don't, you'll lose your zest for life."

SEAN COVEY
The 7 Habits of Highly Effective Teens

REST

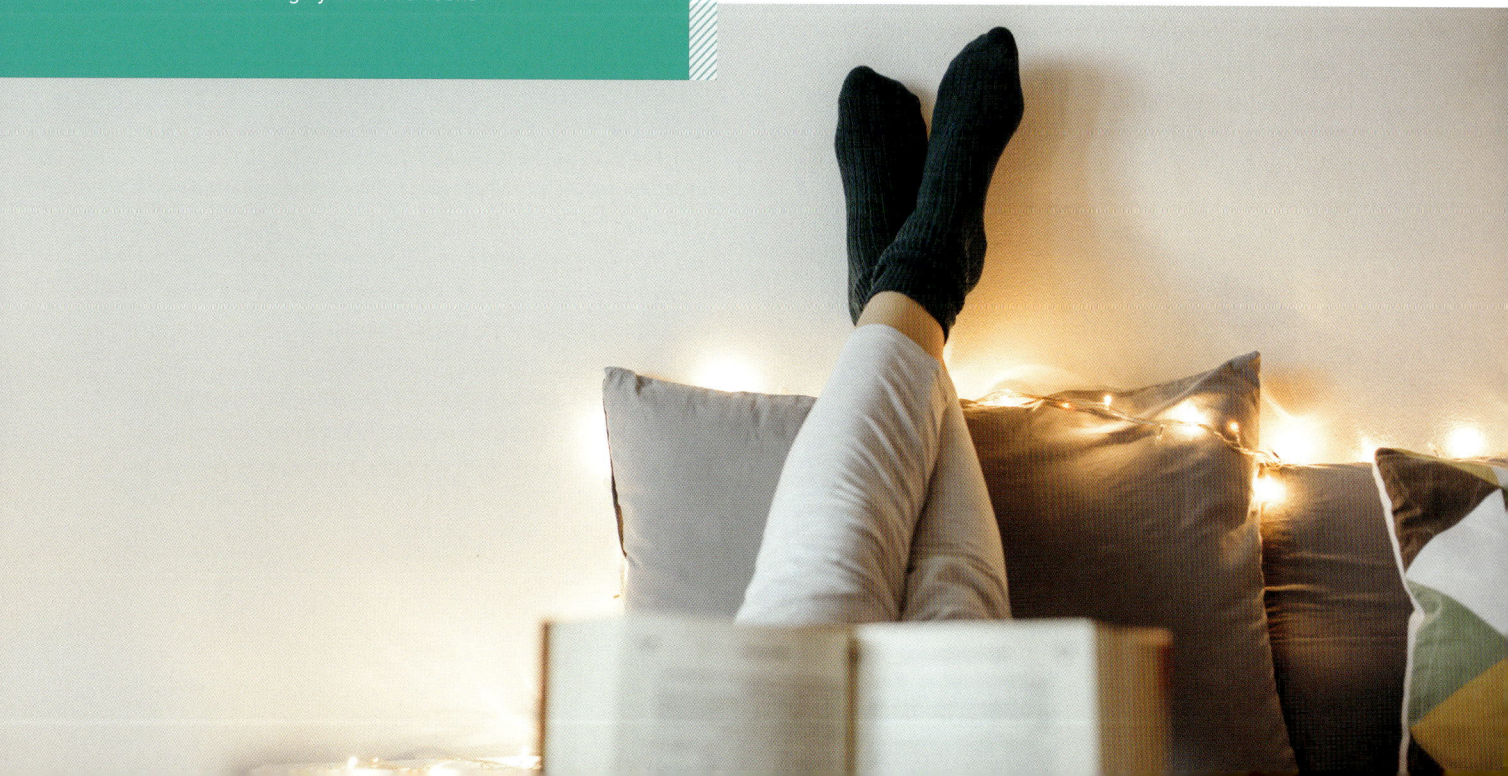

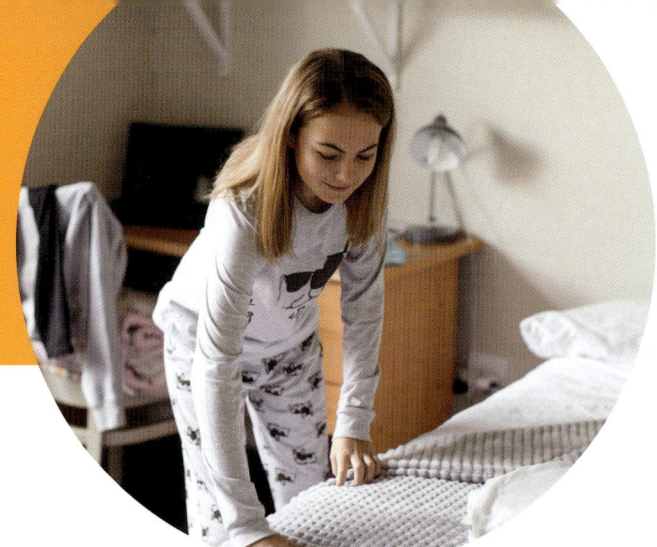

Create a sleep-friendly environment in your room by darkening it, removing distractions and making sure it has a cool temperature.

SLEEP CHEMISTRY

Every night when your head hits the pillow and your eyes close, amazing things are happening inside your body. Even before you start to get sleepy, your body begins to release a chemical called melatonin. This natural hormone is made by your body's pineal gland, which is located just above the middle of your brain. In the daytime this gland doesn't do much, but once the sun goes down and it gets dark, the pineal gland gets to work releasing melatonin into your bloodstream. You begin to feel less alert and sleep becomes more appealing. But melatonin does more than get you in the mood to put on your jammies. It stimulates immune function and is a potent antioxidant. Immune function is the state in which your body recognizes foreign materials and is able to neutralize them before they can do any harm. Antioxidants remove potentially damaging oxidizing agents from your body and are believed to play a big part in preventing cancer, heart disease, stroke and several other life-threatening illnesses.[42] This makes melatonin a big player in keeping you healthy, so make the most of it. Since melatonin release naturally increases in the late evening, arrange your schedule so that you can go to bed in sync with this natural disease fighter.

Two other hormones that are regulated by sleep and affect your health are ghrelin and leptin. Both play an important role in regulating your appetite.[43] Ghrelin is the hormone that makes you feel hungry while leptin makes you feel full. Research has found that missing sleep causes an increase in the level of ghrelin in your body and a decrease in the level of leptin. This means that being sleepy could also make you think you are a lot hungrier than you really are. You may be more likely to overeat. Some studies even show that not enough sleep could lead to obesity.[44-45] It is also possible that a lack of sleep is contributing to the increasing obesity rates in America.[46]

Researchers have also discovered that ghrelin plays an important role in metabolism, heart function and immune functions. It also promotes slow-wave sleep (see the "Five Stages of Sleep" chart for more information).[47]

According to the U.S. Department of Health and Human Services, sleep can also help you grow. "When you were young, your mother may have told you that you need to get enough sleep to grow strong and tall. She may have been right. Deep sleep triggers more release of growth hormone, which contributes to growth in children and boosts muscle mass and the repair of cells and tissues in children and adults."[48]

Your body may still be growing and developing up until you reach age 20. This makes it all the more imperative for you to get the best sleep now. The largest and most predictable release of growth hormone occurs about an hour after you fall asleep. This is because growth hormone is strongly associated with deep sleep.[49] Deep sleep takes place more in the early hours of night and diminishes as the morning approaches. So, if you want to maximize the health improvements that growth hormone and these other hormones provide, you must get to bed as early as possible in the evening.

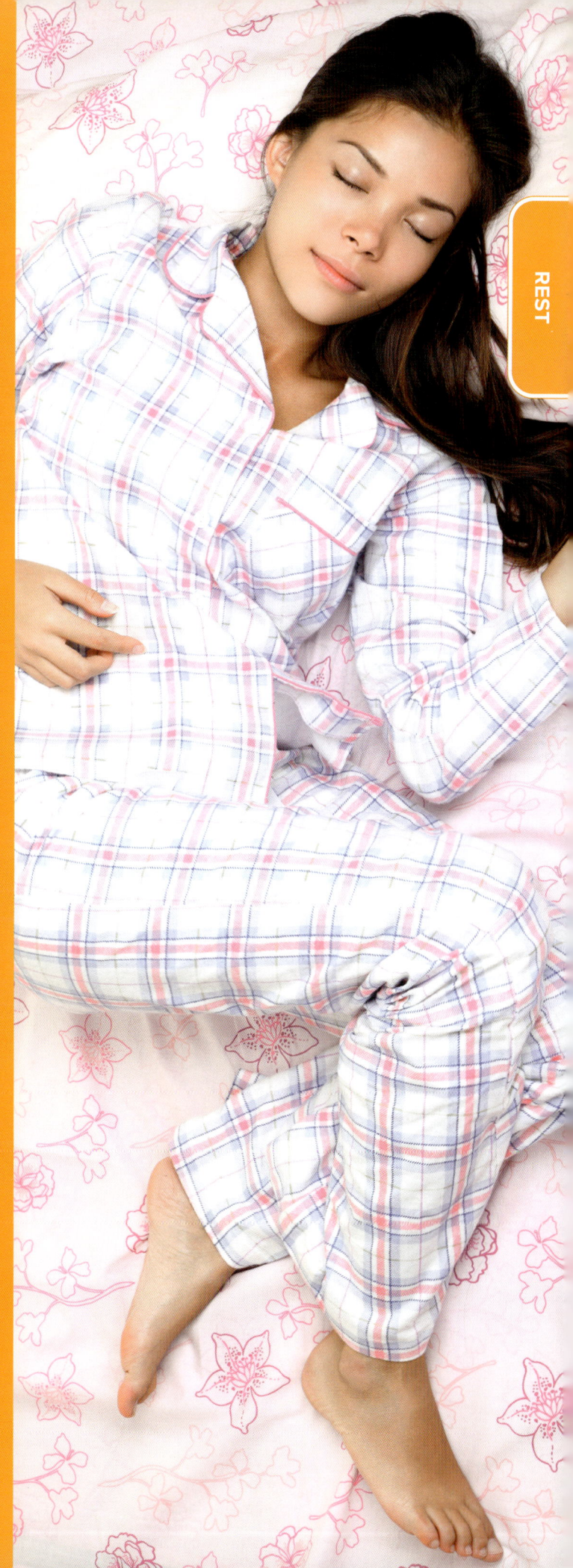

FIVE STAGES OF SLEEP[50]

Stage One Sleep is the lightest and comes as a person just dozes off. This is a light sleep where people drift in and out of sleep. The eyes move slowly, and muscle activity slows. A person can be awakened easily. Some may experience sudden muscle contractions after a sensation of falling.

Stage Two Sleep is when eye movement stops and brain waves become slower, although there will be an occasional burst of rapid brain waves.

Stage Three Sleep is when an EEG (Electroencephalogram) records very slow brain waves called delta waves that are interspersed with smaller, faster waves. This is the first stage of deep sleep and is also known as "Slow Wave Sleep" (SWS).

Stage Four Sleep is when most of the slow delta waves are seen. Stages three and four are called deep sleep. It is very difficult to awaken someone from these levels. There is no eye movement or muscle activity during these stages. Bed-wetting, sleepwalking or night terrors happen during this stage.

Stage Five Sleep is called REM or rapid eye movement sleep. Breathing is more rapid, irregular and shallow. The eyes jerk rapidly. The arm and leg muscles are temporarily paralyzed. The EEG brain waves during this stage are similar to levels experienced by an individual who is awake. The REM stage is when most dreams occur. Our circadian rhythms contribute to a variety of hormonal releases, and these in turn contribute to the production of an optimal sleeping environment that will facilitate the greatest possible restoration for our bodies.

The good news in all of this is that you can choose to synchronize yourself with these natural rhythms and reap the benefits. In order to do this, you should go to bed early on a regular basis.

CAFFEINE

When it comes to caffeine, many people think it's a miracle drug. Adults and teens alike turn to coffee concoctions, tea, sodas and energy drinks daily to help them feel more alert. However, they don't realize that caffeine could be the reason they're so sleepy in the first place. One review article summarized the effects of this so-called "miracle drug:" "Caffeine is one of the most widely consumed psychoactive substances, and it has profound effects on sleep and wake function. Laboratory studies have documented its sleep-disruptive effects.... Studies have shown that caffeine dependence develops at relatively low daily doses and after short periods of regular daily use."[51] This means you could develop a caffeine addiction even if you are only consuming small amounts and after a relatively short time. It's no secret that caffeine disturbs your sleep, but the younger you are, the less caffeine it takes for you to feel the effects. "Children and adolescents, while reporting lower daily, weight-corrected caffeine intake, similarly experience sleep disturbance and daytime sleepiness associated with their caffeine use. The risks to sleep and alertness of regular caffeine use are greatly underestimated by both the general population and physicians."[52] So, the next time you turn to that steaming cup of java to help you stay awake, just remember, you may be doing more harm than good since caffeine intake is actually associated with those feelings of daytime sleepiness.

A VICIOUS CYCLE

In the Bible story "Daniel and the Lion's Den," you see a clear picture of how stress and worry can negatively impact your sleeping habits. King Darius spends a sleepless night in his royal palace, tossing and turning as he worries about the fate of his servant, Daniel. In sharp contrast, Daniel finds peace amid the ravenous lions because he knows that God has everything under control. Nothing keeps you up at night more than a worried mind full of stress. Psychologist and author Sherrie Bourg Carter says, "Stress leads to a loss of sleep and a loss of sleep leads to an increase in stress, which can become a vicious cycle."[53] Picture it; you are stressed about something at school so you stay up all night worrying about it. Now your lack of sleep only adds to the stress you are already experiencing. You become more worried, more stressed and more exhausted. How can you break this cycle?

First, you need to understand what's happening inside your body. Not getting enough sleep affects the level of the stress hormone cortisol. Cortisol is the body's normal reaction to the stresses of life, but too much cortisol can have negative effects on your health. Research has found that sleep loss brings about an increase in your evening cortisol levels.[54] Normally at night your levels decrease and this allows you to relax and prepare for rest. However, research shows the rate of decrease is much slower in people who have had sleep restrictions.[55] This means that just by missing sleep you are already adding extra stress to your body.

Stress affects your sleep in many harmful ways. One study found that people with high stress reported shorter sleep times, poorer sleep quality, increased likelihood of sleep apnea, daytime sleepiness and fatigue.[56] Sleep apnea is a common disorder where your breathing stops momentarily or becomes shallow while sleeping. It's an ongoing condition that disrupts your sleep and keeps you from receiving the full benefits of rest. Sleep apnea can also have powerful negative effects on your physical, mental and emotional health. Depression, anxiety, decreased memory, hypertension, heart disease, type 2 diabetes and premature death have all been linked to this problem.[57-59]

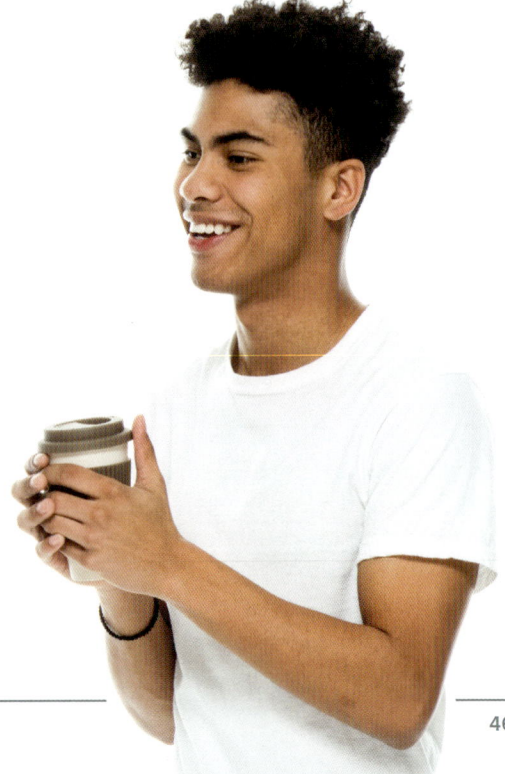

Research shows that students who experience good quality sleep also have the benefit of higher life satisfaction. That's compared with students who report poor sleep quality.[60] Over time, stress and worry can lead to feelings of depression. In the National Longitudinal Study of Adolescent Health, 15,000 teens were surveyed. It was discovered that teens whose parents required a 10 PM or sooner bedtime were 25 percent less likely to be depressed. They were also 20 percent less likely to have suicidal thoughts when compared to teens who went to bed at midnight or later.[61] The same study also found that teens who regularly slept five or fewer hours per night were 71 percent more likely to report feeling depressed.[62] Choosing to get good rest will improve your mood and help you feel more relaxed. This is the first step to breaking free from the cycle of stress and worry. Here are some more tips for kicking stress to the curb and getting your life back on track:

1. **Give Thanks.** Research has shown that people who regularly write down what they are grateful for have several qualities that help with stress management. These include higher levels of optimism, enthusiasm, determination, attentiveness and energy. They are also more likely to have a better duration and quality of sleep.[63] Make time to list the people and things for which you are thankful.

2. **Stay Positive.** Research also shows that being optimistic is a very powerful promoter of health and well-being.[64] Don't always assume the worst about every situation. Learn to focus on the positive things in your life.

3. **Get Support.** Sharing your concerns with a friend or family member will help alleviate the stress you are experiencing. Let them hear what's worrying you, and don't be afraid to ask for help.

God doesn't want stress and worry to rob you of rest. In his letter to the Philippians, Paul encourages you to *"Be anxious for nothing, but in everything by prayer and supplication with thanksgiving let your requests be made known to God"* (Philippians 4:6). This means prayer is also a vital part of good rest. Think of prayer as *"casting all your anxiety on Him, because He cares for you"* (1 Peter 5:7). You don't have to worry about bothering God or burdening Him with your requests, because He wants you to pray to Him. He also gives you an amazing promise that when you turn to Him in prayer, *"the peace of God, which surpasses all comprehension, will guard your hearts and your minds in Christ Jesus"* (Philippians 4:7). God wants you to have His peace. This is a peace that will not only provide you with wonderful, refreshing rest, but will also protect you from harm by guarding your heart and your mind. Turn to God and find His peace.

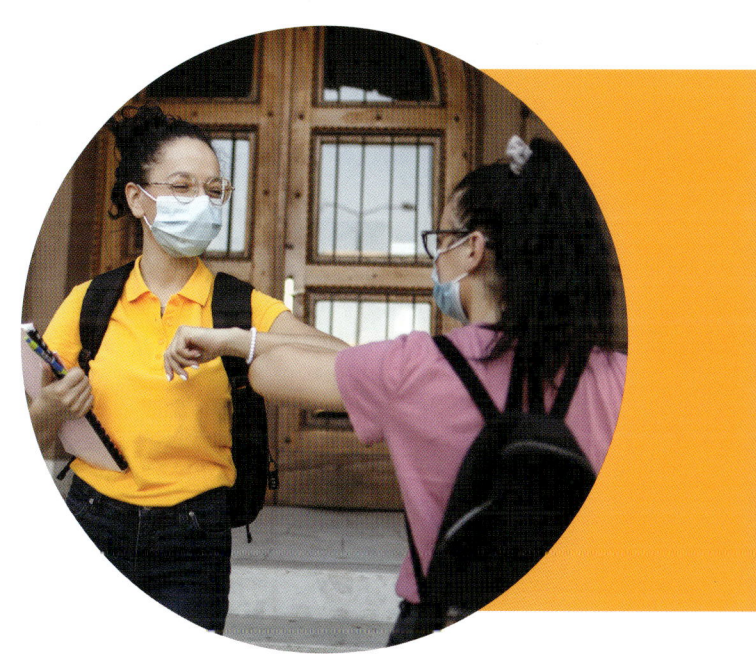

"The time to relax is when you don't have time for it."

ATTRIBUTED TO BOTH
JIM GOODWIN AND SYDNEY J. HARRIS

Is there a challenging situation that you are facing right now, either at home or school, that you could give to God? Pray and ask God for wisdom and His help to know how to proceed.

GO DEEPER

The Bible says, *"Be still, and know that I am God"* (Psalm 46:10). When was the last time you allowed yourself to slow down from your busy routine to be still and seek God's help through prayer?

DAILY REST

Another great way for you to deal with the pressures of stress is to take some time each day for personal relaxation. This relaxation could be anything from taking a walk outside to reading a favorite book or magazine. Keep in mind that many people feel that to relax they need to do something totally different from their normal routine. One really simple way to relax is to get some fresh air outdoors. Try this exercise the next time you have a moment between classes — go outside and take several deep breaths of fresh air. Fresh air taken deeply into the lungs is a wonderful, vitalizing force that can energize you for the rest of your day. Fresh air has many positive benefits. First of all, it's chemically different than the recirculated indoor air that most Americans

breathe on a daily basis.[65] Fresh air is electrified. It's negatively charged, or "negatively ionized," by the oxygen molecule — which actually has a positive result. There are over 5,000 published studies reporting on experiments with ionization. All of these studies support the conclusion that an overdose of positive ions is harmful to your health while extra negative ions, the good ones, are beneficial.[66] Negatively charged oxygen reportedly brings an improved sense of well-being, increases the rate and quality of growth in both plants and animals, improves function in your lung's protective cilia, decreases anxiety through a tranquilizing and relaxing effect, lowers your body temperature, lowers your resting heart rate, improves learning in mammals, decreases severity of stomach ulcers and decreases survival of bacteria and viruses in the air.[67-73] But even if you can't get outside into the fresh air, you can still enjoy the benefits of deep breathing. Long and slow abdominal breathing will reduce anxiety and improve the quality and quantity of your sleep.[74]

Another great relaxation method is to meditate on something positive and encouraging. For example, meditating on the personal meaning of a Bible promise can have powerful renewing and peace-promoting effects.

Daily relaxation can also come in the form of a daily vacation, "a piece of time when you wholeheartedly pursue something *you truly enjoy.*"[75] A daily vacation can be packed into as little as 10 or 15 minutes and is completely up to you. The idea is to find something that you have a passion for doing: reading, painting or mastering a musical instrument. It can be enjoyable, invigorating and relaxing.

What activities would you like to do as a part of your daily vacation?

STUDY BREAKS

As a high school student, you study… a lot. Sometimes your homework might start to feel like a bottomless pit of math problems and book reports. That's when short breaks can make a world of difference. If you notice you're starting to feel sleepy or your performance level is dropping, try one of these quick tips for getting over the slump and back on track:

1. **Short Breaks.** Psychology professor Alejandro Lleras led a study that looked at a participant's ability to focus on a repetitive computerized task for almost an hour. As the task went on, most of the participants' performances declined, but those who took two short breaks during the 50-minute experiment saw no drop in their performance.[76]

   Lleras said, "Our research suggests that, when faced with long tasks… it is best to impose brief breaks on yourself. Brief mental breaks will actually help you stay focused on your task."[77]

   One word of warning: be careful what kind of breaks you take. For example, taking a break to check out something online might turn into a very long break indeed.

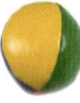

Laughing is a good way to reduce stress. Try and have a good laugh at least once every day.

2. **Exercise Breaks.** One of the best things you can do to overcome the feelings of fatigue is to get some physical activity. In a comprehensive analysis of more than 70 studies, it was found that doing physical activity is much more effective at eliminating fatigue than prescription drugs.[78]

   So, if you want to boost your morale and your ability to complete your study session, take a five-minute green exercise break. That means you do your exercise in a relatively natural environment. In a study, researchers looked at the best dose of nature and green exercise for improving mental health. It was found that the greatest improvements in mood and self-esteem came from as little as five minutes of green exercise.[79] You can certainly find five minutes to take a walk around the neighborhood or ride your bike. It's easy and fun to do. Plus, it will clear your mind and help you focus when you return.

3. **Power Naps.** Power naps are brief periods of sleep that stop before you reach stage three sleep. There are a lot of great benefits to grabbing a quick power nap, including higher perceived alertness,[80] improved declarative memory,[81] procedural memory,[82] alertness and performance,[83-84] mood,[85-87] physiological activation[88-89] and level of alertness.[90-91] Power naps have also been shown to help modulate or calm emotions.[92]

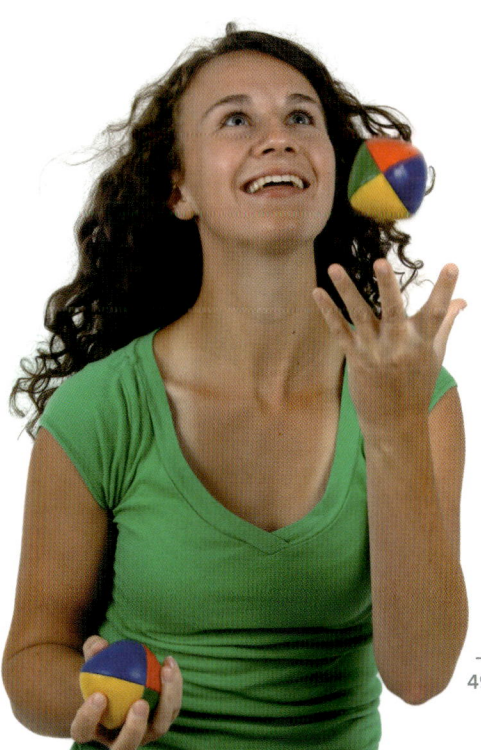

MAKING THE MOST OF YOUR NAP

Do you want to get the maximum benefits next time you take a nap? Check out these tips from Harvard psychologist and sleep expert, Dr. Sara C. Mednick:

1. **Cut yourself some slack.** Dr. Mednick says, above all, you should realize that "you're not being lazy; napping will make you more productive and more alert after you wake up." So, give yourself permission to put the work on hold and catch some Z's.

2. **Choose your nap time wisely.** Your body has a system of biological clocks that control your daily rhythm, also called your circadian rhythm. Because of this, Dr. Mednick says the best nap times are, "In the morning or just after lunch." Napping in the late afternoon means you are likely to fall into deep (slow-wave) sleep, which will leave you feeling groggy.

3. **Watch what you eat.** Large amounts of caffeine and foods that are heavy in fat and sugar will hinder your ability to fall asleep. "Instead, in the hour or two before your naptime, eat foods high in calcium and protein, which promote sleep."

4. **Find the perfect spot.** Seek out a quiet place, free of distractions, where you won't be disturbed.

5. **Get in the dark.** "Try to darken your nap zone, or wear an eyeshade," Dr. Mednick suggests. "Darkness stimulates melatonin, the sleep-inducing hormone."

6. **Set your alarm.** You don't want to nap too long or miss out on something important, so be sure you have an alarm to wake you up. To get the benefits of your power nap, don't go too long, either. Dr. Mednick says, "20 minutes is ideal."[93]

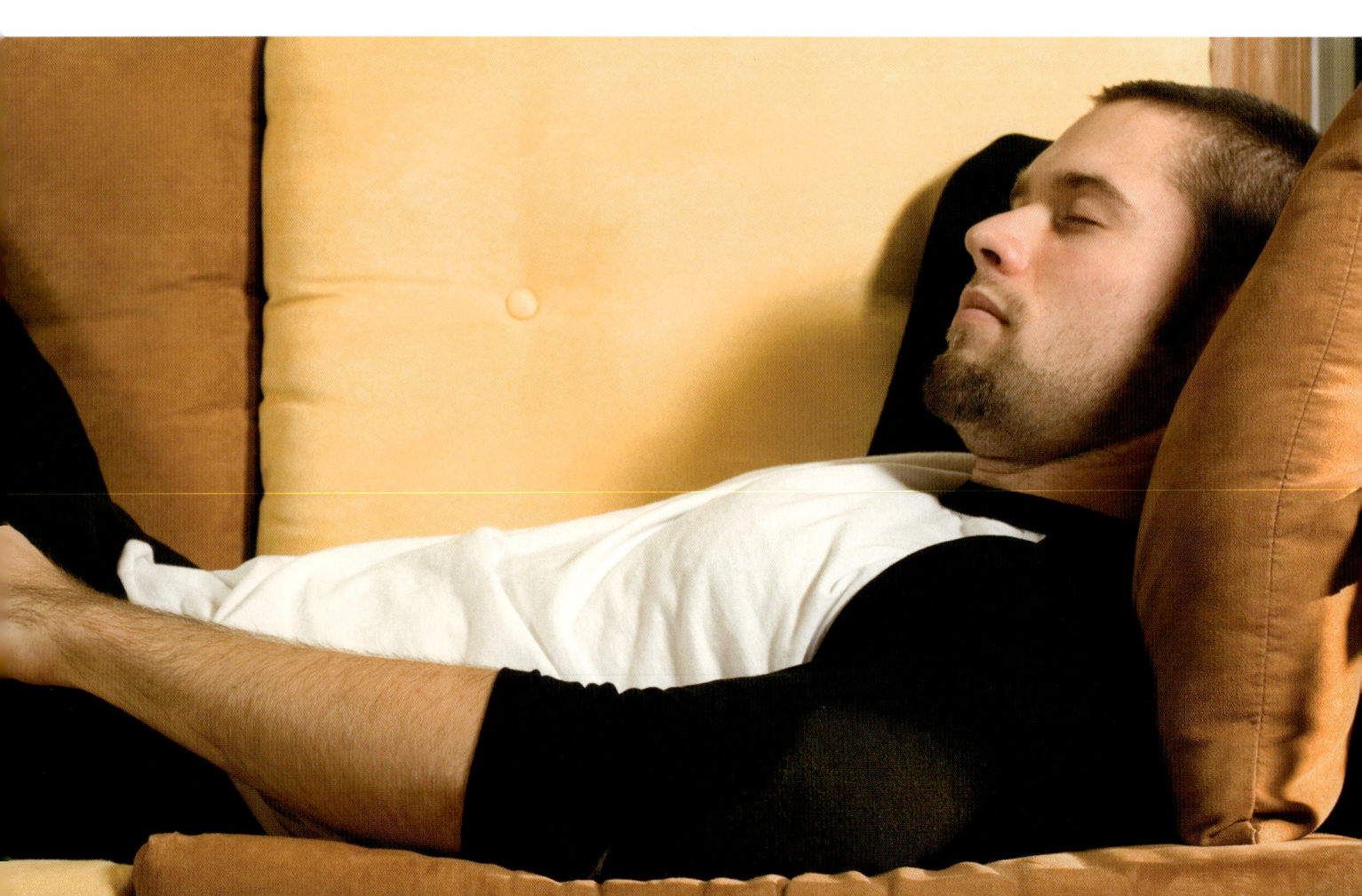

WEEKLY REST

And on the seventh day God ended His work which He had done, and He rested on the seventh day from all His work which He had done. Then God blessed the seventh day and sanctified it, because in it He rested from all His work which God had created and made.

GENESIS 2:2–3

As you have already seen, the seven-day rhythm of life began with God at creation. It's important to realize that God didn't rest on the seventh day because He was tired. He took time to enjoy the life He had just created. You, too, should follow God's example and honor the weekly rhythms He instilled within you and the world around you. This is crucial to living a CREATION Life.

Maybe you think taking a weekly rest is a distraction. Wouldn't you be able to get more done if you simply worked more hours? During World War II, the country of Great Britain had the same idea. In order to be more productive they instituted a 74-hour work week. They soon found that their people could not maintain the pace. After experimenting and adjusting, they found that a 48-hour work week, with regular breaks plus one day of rest each week, resulted in maximum efficiency.[94] During the French Revolution, France changed its calendar and instituted a 10-day week. Workers still only got one of those days off. Chaos ensued, and eventually the whole calendar was abolished as the seven-day week returned.[95]

The world naturally operates on a seven-day rhythm. You can find this cycle in plants, animals and humans. For example, Gallup researchers found that for each additional day that a person exercised, they received the benefit of boosted energy levels. This boost continued to increase for up to six days, after which participants reached a point of diminishing returns.[96]

Medical research has demonstrated seven-day rhythms in connection with a variety of other physiological functions. These include heart rate, natural hormones in human breast milk and urine, swelling after surgery, rejection of transplanted organs, human and animal cancers and their response to treatment, and inflammatory responses and the drugs used to treat them. For instance, a patient will tend to have an increase in swelling on the seventh and the 14th day after surgery. Similarly, a patient who has had a kidney transplant is more likely to reject the organ seven days or 14 days after surgery.[97-103]

German scientists call the thing that sets a biorhythm a "zeitgeber" or "time-giver." The zeitgeber that initiates and maintains the seven-day rhythm is not yet understood, but some chronobiologists think that a regular day of rest might be the secret. It is possible that human beings have a physiological need to take a specific day off each week.

One thing is for sure: taking off one whole day in seven brings renewal to your physical and spiritual life. Unlike days, months and years, this biorhythm has no astronomical marker. There is no plausible explanation for its presence, except that our Creator built it into our physiology. There are lots of ways you can spend the Sabbath, such as connecting with others, in worship, in various types of recreation or personal reflection. And of course, it can be a special time to focus on nurturing your spiritual values. Isn't it cool that science is discovering the health benefits related to keeping God's fourth commandment?

 **God intended for the Sabbath to be a special day for you. What are you doing in order to connect with Him on this special day of rest?**

GO DEEPER

The Bible tells us to *"Remember the Sabbath day, to keep it holy"* (Exodus 20:8). What makes this day different from every other day, and how are you keeping it holy? Consider the following list of activities. Do you think you should do these on the Sabbath?

- Watch my favorite movie or TV show

- Study for an important test

- Hang out at the mall with my friends

- Get a part-time job to help out at home

- Clean my room

- Go to church

- Play a video game

- Help a neighbor with their yard work

- Take a meal to a needy family

- Work on my hobbies

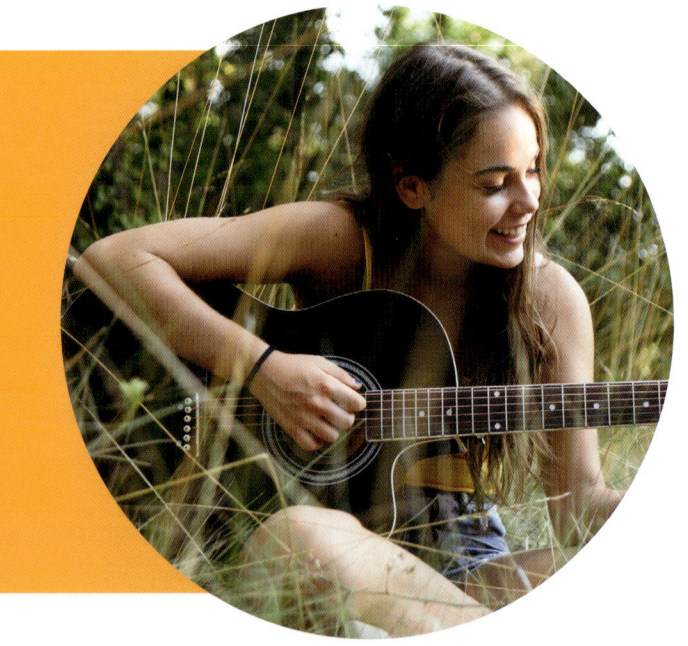

RECREATION

When you were younger, nobody had to tell you how to play. You naturally engaged in games, sports and pretend play that was fun and enjoyable. Of course, now that you're in high school, you really don't have time for all that kiddie stuff, do you? Well, you should. Taking time each day to enjoy some recreation is not only fun, it's a great way for you to get energized and feel refreshed. *Merriam-Webster's Dictionary* defines recreation as "a refreshment of strength and spirits after work."[104]

When you take time to have fun through participating in activities you enjoy, it's like you're hitting the reset button on your life. Don't just think of it as recreation; think of it as "re-creation."

Looking for some ideas? Start by getting outside. Activities such as swimming, hiking, sports or mountain biking are all great forms of recreation. Outdoor activities have the added benefit of providing you with sunshine, fresh air and exercise.

Hobbies are another way to fit recreation into your schedule. These could even give you the opportunity to show off your creative side: painting, drawing, cooking, music and photography are activities that will give you a welcome break from your daily routine. Other recreational hobbies might include reading, gardening or taking care of a pet. The list is endless. The point is finding something you enjoy.

Even better is to choose those activities or hobbies that allow you to socialize and connect with others. Friendships benefit your body, mind and spirit in many ways. You will explore this more deeply in the Interpersonal Relationships section.

Choose the kinds of recreation that actually reenergize and refresh you. But most importantly, whatever you do, have fun doing it.

What are some activities or hobbies you could do to "re-create" your life?

ANNUAL REST

It's no question that your body was made to work both physically and mentally, but you were also made to rest. As you get older, you will have more demands and responsibilities placed upon you. After college, you may feel like you're entering the "rat race," trying to get ahead in life. One great way to fight these feelings is by taking an annual period of rest, including a regularly scheduled vacation. In 2009, the travel company Expedia conducted an International Vacation Deprivation Survey, which found that roughly one-third of employed U.S. adults (34 percent) reported feeling better about their job and more productive after a vacation. Respondents also reported feeling closer to their family after a vacation.[105]

Right now, you might not be too concerned with the importance of taking a regular vacation, but as you age, you will find that skipping out on vacations can have serious repercussions on your health. During a 20-year follow-up of women participants, the Framingham Heart Study found an association between infrequent vacationing and increased incidence of death from coronary causes.[106] Another study found that men who developed psychosomatic illnesses were less likely to take vacations than were men who never developed such illnesses.[107] In another study of more than 12,000 men, it was discovered that annual vacations were associated with a reduced risk of all causes of mortality, and the specific cause of death most strongly associated with inadequate vacationing was coronary heart disease.[108]

Vacations can come in all shapes and sizes. Even a short vacation such as two to four days can help you get your groove back. If you are feeling fatigued or are experiencing neck pain, headaches or backaches, this is probably the signal that it's time for a break.

Most people have no problem working. What they need to do is learn how to rest. Getting enough sleep, enjoying weekly down time, remembering the Sabbath and taking relaxing vacations are crucial components to overall good health.

So, the next time you feel the need for rest, remember you don't have to feel guilty. You can enjoy the wonderful, restorative properties that God has ordained through the power of rest.

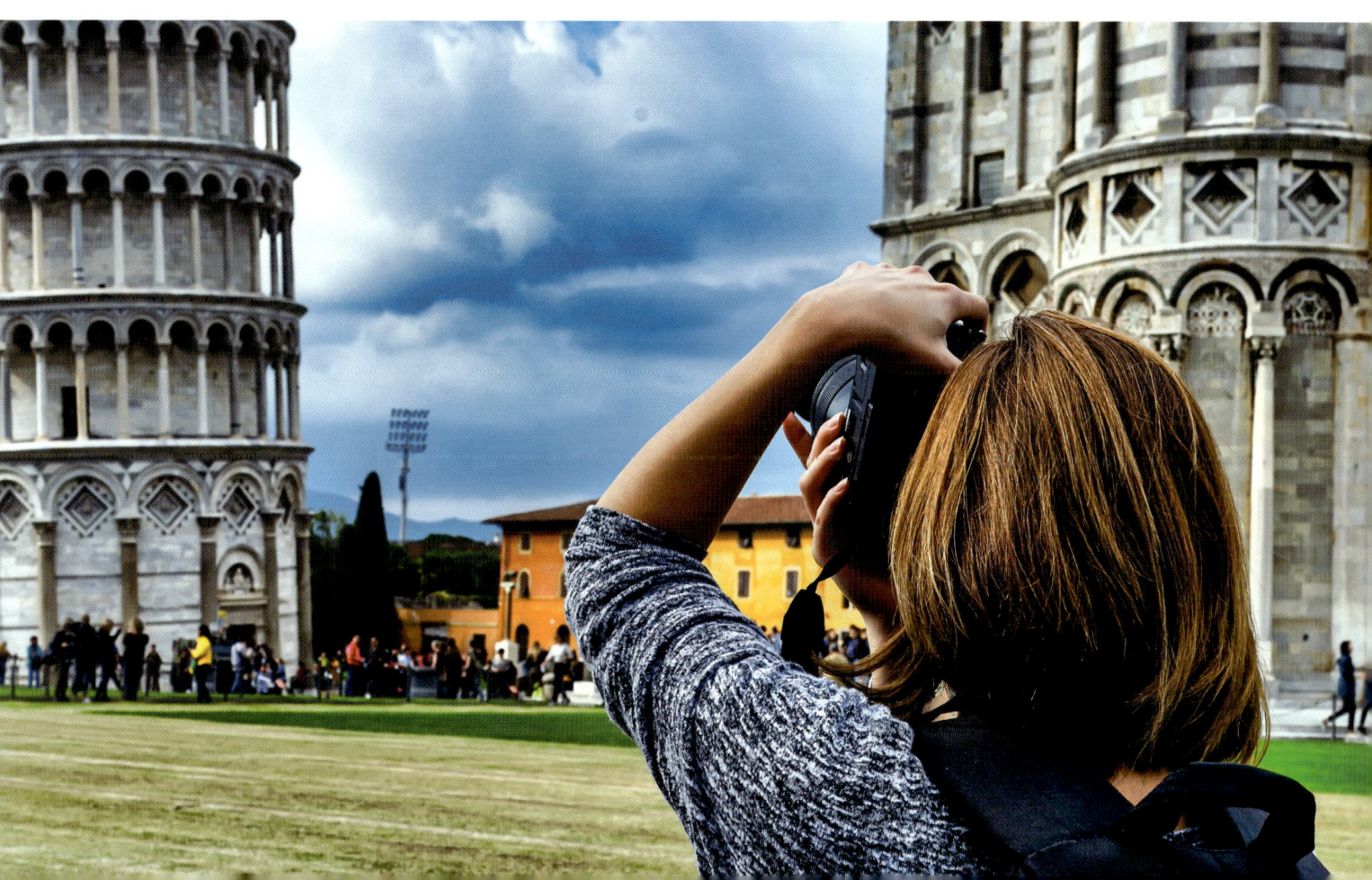

TRUE REST

"Come to Me, all who are weary and heavy-laden, and I will give you rest. Take My yoke upon you and learn from Me, for I am gentle and humble in heart, and you will find rest for your souls. For My yoke is easy and My burden is light." MATTHEW 11:28–30

Today's teens are struggling with a number of important issues. Strained relationships, financial problems and academic pressures all create heavy burdens of emotional and mental stress. Right now, you may feel weary and overwhelmed just thinking about all of the things you have to deal with as a student. You may not be sure of how you're going to handle everything. That's what makes Jesus' promise so important. Jesus desires for you to find the source of true rest whatever your situation may be. Of course, your circumstances may have you so frazzled that you are unable to hear His voice and respond to His offer. If that is the case, then remember — God is the source of true rest in every way. He invites you to come to Him and find the rest you need. Jesus doesn't want to add to your fears and concerns; He wants to relieve you of them. He promises that if you simply come to Him, then you will find what your soul is looking for. You will find true rest in Him.

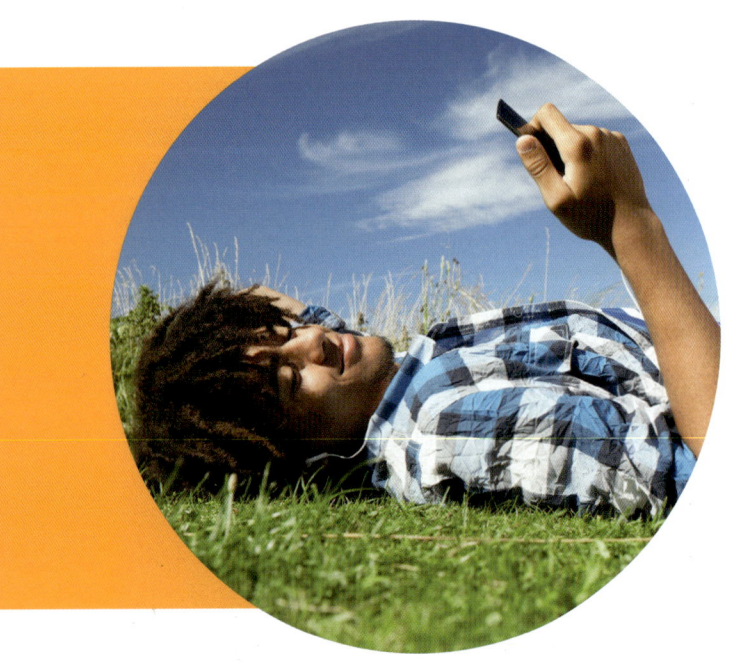

10 POWER TIPS FOR REST

Remember, what you do during the day will greatly affect how you sleep at night. Here are a few power tips to give you the best rest:

1. **Maintain a healthy circadian rhythm by getting daily sunlight.** Research shows that getting daytime sunlight helps you sleep better at night.[109] Put some regular outdoor activities into your schedule such as sports, walking or even washing your parents' car.

2. **Enjoy fresh air to improve circulation, which is vital to a good night's rest.** Fresh air greatly improves bodily oxygenation and circulation, especially when it comes with outdoor activity. In addition, fresh, outdoor air is likely to increase exposure to sunlight. Remember, negative charges in fresh air have been shown to improve one's sense of well-being, decrease anxiety through a relaxing effect, lower body temperature and lower one's resting heart rate.

3. **Stay active.** If your body is physically tired at the end of the day, you will sleep better. Research has confirmed that regular physical activity aids nighttime sleep.

4. **Eat early and eat light.** Your last meal of the day should be finished at least three hours before bedtime. For your best sleep, talk with your family about making it a light meal, too. In reality, this is very hard since many Americans lean toward eating a large meal that includes foods that are difficult to digest. Remember your digestive system needs rest, too. Restful sleep will be enhanced by a light dinner such as fruits, vegetables and whole grain. Limiting your intake of liquids before bedtime will also help you avoid additional trips to the bathroom.

5. **Regulate your sleep patterns to help you sleep better.** Try going to bed at the same time each night and getting up at the same time each morning. This way your body will get into a pattern that helps you sleep better. On the weekends, don't sleep in more than 30 minutes past your normal wake-up time or you will throw off your weekly sleep pattern. A brief nap in the early afternoon on the weekend is a better option than sleeping in excessively.

6. **Keep conflict, stress, anxiety and worry outside your bedroom.** Your mind is powerful; if actively engaged, it will overpower your body's ability to sleep. Put your mind to rest before you go to bed. Don't stay up worrying about what you cannot resolve today. On the other hand, resolve interpersonal relationship issues as much as you can *before* going to bed. A clear conscience is part of a healthy lifestyle and improves your quality of sleep and the rate at which you fall asleep.

7. **Relax before bedtime.** Begin to "wind down" before bedtime. Decide when you will go to bed and then, about 20 minutes prior, find an activity that is calming and relaxing.

8. **Avoid caffeine, tobacco and other stimulants.** Each of these is not only strongly addictive but will also keep you awake at night.[110] Playing video games, surfing the Internet or anything electronic can stimulate your internal stress hormones and rob you of a good night's sleep.

9. **Get your sleep primarily at night.** Remember, God created you to sleep at night, and the darkness of night helps your body to release melatonin, which will promote deep restful and restorative sleep. Naps can definitely be beneficial, but use them with discretion. If you find you are napping three or more times a week, examine your nighttime sleep habits in order to ensure you are not robbing yourself of this most critical and beneficial form of sleep.

10. **Take a hot shower or bath one to two hours before your bedtime.** Research published in the journal *Sleep* found that women with insomnia who took a hot bath within one to two hours of going to bed had a better night's sleep. The bath increased their core temperature, which then quickly dropped once they got out of the bath. This helped them to sleep better.[111]

CREATE A GOOD SLEEP ENVIRONMENT

Creating a good sleep environment is essential to getting good quality sleep. The following tips can help:

1. **Keep it dark.** Light can disturb your sleep. If too much light is a problem, invest in a sleep mask.

2. **Keep it quiet.** Noise can wake you up and make it a struggle for you to go back to sleep.

3. **Use your bed only for sleep.** Don't lie in bed to study or watch TV, or you will teach your body to associate your bed with sleeplessness.

4. **Circulate fresh air.** High air quality helps to maximize the restorative and regenerative properties of sleep.

5. **Get a comfortable bed and pillow.** Having a mattress and pillow that is right for you can make a world of difference in getting a good night's sleep.

6. **If you snore, get a sleep study.** If you snore loudly, find yourself waking up in the night gasping for air or have excessive daytime sleepiness, you should ask your doctor about having a sleep study done. It may even be an indicator of sleep apnea, so take it seriously.

REFERENCES

1. Zee, Phyllis C. and Fred W. Turek. "Sleep and Health: Everywhere and in Both Directions." *Archives of Internal Medicine* 166, no. 16 (2006): 1686-1688. https://doi.org/10.1001/archinte.166.16.1686.

2. Carskadon, Mary A., Kim Harvey, Paula Duke, Thomas F. Anders, Iris F. Litt, and William C. Dement. "Pubertal Changes in Daytime Sleepiness." *Sleep* 2, no. 4 (1980): 453-460. https://doi.org/10.1093/sleep/2.4.453.

3. Noland, Heather, James H. Price, Joseph Dake, and Susan K. Telljohann. "Adolescents' Sleep Behaviors and Perceptions of Sleep." *Journal of School Health* 79, no. 5 (2009): 224-230. https://doi.org/10.1111/j.1746-1561.2009.00402.x.

4. Spiegel, Karine, Esra Tasali, Plamen Penev, and Eve Van Cauter. "Brief Communication: Sleep Curtailment in Healthy Young Men is Associated with Decreased Leptin Levels, Elevated Ghrelin Levels, and Increased Hunger and Appetite." *Annals of Internal Medicine* 141, no. 11 (2004): 846-850. https://doi.org/10.7326/0003-4819-141-11-200412070-00008.

5. Ayas, Najib T., David P. White, JoAnn E. Manson, Meir J. Stampfer, Frank E. Speizer, Atul Malhotra, and Frank B. Hu. "A Prospective Study of Sleep Duration and Coronary Heart Disease in Women." *Archives of Internal Medicine* 163, no. 2 (2003): 205-209. https://doi.org/10.1001/archinte.163.2.205.

6. Perl, James. *Sleep Right in Five Nights: A Clear and Effective Guide for Conquering Insomnia.* New York: William Morrow and Company, 1993. 32.

7. Blahd, William. "The Healing Power of Sleep." WebMD. Last modified October 6, 2016. http://www.webmd.com/sleep-disorders/features/healing-power-sleep.

8. Marschall-Kehrel, Daniela. "Update on Nocturia: The Best of Rest is Sleep." *Urology* 64, no. 6 (2004): 21-24. https://doi.org/10.1016/j.urology.2004.10.072.

9. Stickgold, R., J. A. Hobson, R. Fosse, and M. Fosse. "Sleep, Learning, and Dreams: Off-line Memory Reprocessing." *Science* 294, no. 5544 (2001): 1052-1057. https://doi.org/10.1126/science.1063530.

10. Ayas, Najib T., David P. White, Wael K. Al-Delaimy, JoAnn E. Manson, Meir J. Stampfer, Frank E. Speizer, Sanjay Patel, and Frank B. Hu. "A Prospective Study of Self-Reported Sleep Duration and Incident Diabetes in Women." *Diabetes Care* 26, no. 2 (2003): 380-384. https://doi.org/10.2337/diacare.26.2.380.

11. Fallone, Gahan, Christine Acebo, Ronald Seifer, and Mary A. Carskadon. "Experimental Restriction of Sleep Opportunity in Children: Effects on Teacher Ratings." *Sleep* 28, no. 12 (2005): 1561-1567. https://doi.org/10.1093/sleep/28.12.1561.

12. Howell, Andrew J., Jesse C. Jahrig, and Russell A. Powell. "Sleep Quality, Sleep Propensity, and Academic Performance." *Perceptual and Motor Skills* 99, no. 2 (2004): 525-535. https://doi.org/10.2466/pms.99.2.525-535.

13. Brown, Franklin C., Walter C. Buboltz Jr., and Barlow Soper. "Relationship of Sleep Hygiene Awareness, Sleep Hygiene Practices, and Sleep Quality in University Students." *Behavioral Medicine* 28, no. 1 (2002): 33-38. https://doi.org/10.1080/08964280209596396.

14. Buboltz Jr., Walter C., Franklin Brown, and Barlow Soper. "Sleep Habits and Patterns of College Students: A Preliminary Study." *Journal of American College Health* 50, no. 3 (2001): 131-135. https://doi.org/10.1080/07448480109596017.

15. Pilcher, June J. and Amy S. Walters. "How Sleep Deprivation Affects Psychological Variables Related to College Students' Cognitive Performance." *Journal of American College Health* 46, no. 3 (1997): 121-126. https://doi.org/10.1080/07448489709595597.

16. Van Dongen, Hans, Greg Maislin, Janet M. Mullington, and David F. Dinges. "The Cumulative Cost of Additional Wakefulness: Dose-Response Effects on Neurobehavioral Functions and Sleep Physiology from Chronic Sleep Restriction and Total Sleep Deprivation." *Sleep* 26, no. 2 (2003): 117-126. https://doi.org/10.1093/sleep/26.2.117.

17. Nedley, Neil. *Proof Positive: How to Reliably Combat Disease and Achieve Optimal Health Through Nutrition and Lifestyle.* Edited by David DeRose. Ardmore: Neil Nedley, 1999, 502.

18. Williamson, Ann M. and Anne-Marie Feyer. "Moderate Sleep Deprivation Produces Impairments in Cognitive and Motor Performance Equivalent to Legally Prescribed Levels of Alcohol Intoxication." *Occupational and Environmental Medicine* 57, no. 10 (2000): 649-655. http://dx.doi.org/10.1136/oem.57.10.649.

19. American Academy of Sleep Medicine. Accessed July 19, 2018. http://www.aasmnet.org/Resources/FactSheets/DrowsyDriving.pdf.

20. Knipling, Ronald R. and Jing-Shiarn Wang. "Revised Estimates of the U.S. Drowsy Driver Crash Problem Size Based on General Estimates System Case Reviews." *Annual Proceedings of the Association for the Advancement of Automotive Medicine* 39 (1995): 451-466.

21. Edgerton, Robyn, ed., *CREATION Health Seminar Personal Study Guide.* Altamonte Springs: Florida Hospital Mission Development, 2016.

22. Ibid.

23. Monk, Timothy H., Daniel J. Buysse, Jaime M. Potts, Jean M. DeGrazia, and David J. Kupfer. "Morningness-Eveningness and Lifestyle Regularity." *Chronobiology International* 21, no. 3 (2004): 435-443. https://doi.org/10.1081/CBI-120038614.

24. Ranganathan, Deepa. "Can a Night Owl Become a Morning Person – A Slate Experiment." Slate. Last modified June 13, 2008. http://www.slate.com/articles/health_and_science/medical_examiner/2008/06/can_a_night_owl_become_a_morning_person.html.

25. National Sleep Foundation. "2005 Sleep in America Poll – Segment Profiles." *Sleep Foundation*, March 2005. https://sleepfoundation.org/sites/default/files/Sleep_Segments.pdf.

26. Krauss Whitbourne, Susan. "Morning Person or Evening Person? Time to Find Out." Psychology Today. Last modified September 1, 2012. https://www.psychologytoday.com/us/blog/fulfillment-any-age/201209/morning-person-or-evening-person-its-time-find-out.

27. Pilcher, June J. and Amy S. Walters. "How Sleep Deprivation Affects Psychological Variables Related to College Students' Cognitive Performance." *Journal of American College Health* 46, no. 3 (1997): 121-126. https://doi.org/10.1080/07448489709595597.

28. Harrison, Yvonne and James A. Horne. "Sleep Loss and Temporal Memory." *The Quarterly Journal of Experimental Psychology* 53, no. 1 (2000): 271-279. https://doi.org/10.1080/713755870.

29. Gais, Steffen, Brian Lucas, and Jan Born. "Sleep After Learning Aids Memory Recall." *Learning & Memory* 13, no. 3 (2006): 259-262. https://www.doi.org/10.1101/lm.132106.

30. Stickgold, Robert. "Sleep-Dependent Memory Consolidation." *Nature* 437, no. 7063 (2005): 1272-1278. https://doi.org/10.1038/nature04286.

31. Tamminga, Carol A., R. Shadmehr, and H. H. Holcomb. "Images in Neuroscience. Cognition: Procedural Memory." *The American Journal of Psychiatry* 157, no. 2 (2000): 162. https://doi.org/10.1176/appi.ajp.157.2.162.

32. Ibid.

33. Stickgold, Robert, J. Allen Hobson, Roar Fosse, and Magdalena Fosse. "Sleep, Learning, and Dreams: Off-Line Memory Reprocessing." *Science* 294, no. 5544 (2001): 1052-1057. https://doi.org/10.1126/science.1063530.

34. Wagner, Ullrich, Steffen Gais, Hilde Haider, Rolf Verleger, and Jan Born. "Sleep Inspires Insight." *Nature* 427, no. 6972 (2004): 352-355. https://doi.org/10.1038/nature02223.

35. Buboltz Jr., Walter C., Franklin Brown, and Barlow Soper. "Sleep Habits and Patterns of College Students: A Preliminary Study." *Journal of American College Health* 50, no. 3 (2001): 131-135. https://doi.org/10.1080/07448480109596017.

36. Carskadon, Mary A. "Adolescent Sleepiness: Increased Risk in a High-Risk Population." *Alcohol, Drugs & Driving* 5, no. 4 (1990): 317-328.

37. "Working Group Report on Problem Sleepiness." National Center on Sleep Disorders Research and Office of Prevention, Education, and Control. Accessed July 6, 2012. http://www.nhlbi.nih.gov/health/prof/sleep/pslp_wg.pdf.

38. Teter, Christian J., Sean Esteban McCabe, James A. Cranford, Carol J. Boyd, and Saliy K. Guthrie. "Prevalence and Motives for Illicit Use of Prescription Stimulants in an Undergraduate Student Sample." *Journal of American College Health* 53, no. 6 (2005): 253-262. https://doi.org/10.3200/JACH.53.6.253-262.

39. Teter, Christian J., Sean Esteban McCabe, Kristy LaGrange, James A. Cranford, and Carol J. Boyd. "Illicit Use of Specific Prescription Stimulants Among College Students: Prevalence, Motives, and Routes of Administration." Pharmacotherapy: *The Journal of Human Pharmacology and Drug Therapy* 26, no. 10 (2006): 1501-1510. https://doi.org/10.1592/phco.26.10.1501.

40. Breus, Michael J., "Your Performance and The Freshman 8." The Huffington Post. Last modified December 6, 2017. http://www.huffingtonpost.com/dr-michael-j-breus/your-performance-and-the-_b_709679.html.

41. Wingard, Deborah L. and Lisa F. Berkman. "Mortality Risk Associated with Sleeping Patterns Among Adults." *Sleep* 6, no. 2 (1983): 102-107. https://doi.org/10.1093/sleep/6.2.102.

42. "Melatonin." *Alternative Medicine Review* 10, no. 4 (2005): 326-336. http://www.altmedrev.com/archive/publications/10/4/326.pdf.

43. Spiegel, Karine, Esra Tasali, Plamen Penev, and Eve Van Cauter. "Brief Communication: Sleep Curtailment in Healthy Young Men is Associated with Decreased Leptin Levels, Elevated Ghrelin Levels, and Increased Hunger and Appetite." *Annals of Internal Medicine* 141, no. 11 (2004): 846-850. https://doi.org/10.7326/0003-4819-141-11-200412070-00008.

44. Copinschi, Georges. "Metabolic and Endocrine Effects of Sleep Deprivation." *Essential Psychopharmacology* 6, no. 6 (2005): 341-347.

45. Taheri, Shahrad, Ling Lin, Diane Austin, Terry Young, and Emmanuel Mignot. "Short Sleep Duration is Associated with Reduced Leptin, Elevated Ghrelin, and Increased Body Mass Index." *PLOS Medicine* 1, no. 3 (2004): e62. https://doi.org/10.1371/journal.pmed.0010062.

46. Kohatsu, Neal D., Rebecca Tsai, Terry Young, Rachel VanGilder, Leon F. Burmeister, Ann M. Stromquist, and James A. Merchant. "Sleep Duration and Body Mass Index in a Rural Population." *Archives of Internal Medicine* 166, no. 16 (2006): 1701-1705. https://doi.org/10.1001/archinte.166.16.1701.

47. Hubina, Erika, Miklós Góth, and Márta Korbonits. "Ghrelin – A Hormone With Multiple Functions." *Orvosi Hetilap* 146, no. 25 (2005): 1345-1351.

48. U.S. Department of Health and Human Services. *Your Guide to Healthy Sleep.* Bethesda: National Institutes of Health, 2005. Accessed October 4, 2018. http://www.nhlbi.nih.gov/health/public/sleep/healthy_sleep.pdf.

49. Obal Jr., Ferenc and James M. Krueger. "GHRH and Sleep." *Sleep Medicine Reviews* 8, no. 5 (2004): 367-377. https://doi.org/10.1016/j.smrv.2004.03.005.

50. U.S. Department of Health and Human Services. *Your Guide to Healthy Sleep.* Bethesda: National Institutes of Health, 2005. Accessed October 4, 2018. http://www.nhlbi.nih.gov/health/public/sleep/healthy_sleep.pdf.

51. Roehrs, Timothy and Thomas Roth. "Caffeine: Sleep and Daytime Sleepiness." *Sleep Medicine Reviews* 12, no. 2 (2008): 153-162. https://doi.org/10.1016/j.smrv.2007.07.004.

52. Ibid.

53. Bourg Carter, Sherrie "Has Sleep and Stress Become a Vicious Cycle in Your Life?" Psychology Today. Last modified May 27, 2011. https://www.psychologytoday.com/us/blog/high-octane-women/201105/has-sleep-and-stress-become-vicious-cycle-in-your-life.

54. Leproult, Rachel, Georges Copinschi, Orfeu Buxton, and Eve Van Cauter. "Sleep Loss Results in an Elevation of Cortisol Levels the Next Evening." *Sleep* 20, no. 10 (1997): 865-870. https://doi.org/10.1093/sleep/20.10.865.

55. Spiegel, Karine, Rachel Leproult, and Eve Van Cauter. "Impact of Sleep Debt on Metabolic and Endocrine Function." *The Lancet* 354, no. 9188 (1999): 1435-1439. https://doi.org/10.1016/S0140-6736(99)01376-8.

56. Kashani, Mariam, Arn Eliasson, and Marina Vernalis. "Perceived Stress Correlates with Disturbed Sleep: A Link Connecting Stress and Cardiovascular Disease." *Stress: The International Journal on the Biology of Stress* 15, no. 1 (2012): 45-51. https://doi.org/10.3109/10253890.2011.578266.

57. Sharafkhaneh, Amir, Nilgun Giray, Peter Richardson, Terry Young, and Max Hirshkowitz. "Association of Psychiatric Disorders and Sleep Apnea in a Large Cohort." *Sleep* 28, no. 11 (2005): 1405-1411. https://doi.org/10.1093/sleep/28.11.1405.

58. Young, Terry, Paul E. Peppard, and Daniel J. Gottlieb. "Epidemiology of Obstructive Sleep Apnea: A Population Health Perspective." *American Journal of Respiratory And Critical Care Medicine* 165, no. 9 (2002): 1217-1239. https://doi.org/10.1164/rccm.2109080.

59. U.S. Department of Health and Human Services. *Your Guide to Healthy Sleep.* Bethesda: National Institutes of Health, 2005. Accessed October 4, 2018. http://www.nhlbi.nih.gov/health/public/sleep/healthy_sleep.pdf.

60. Pilcher, June J., Douglas R. Ginter, and Brigitte Sadowsky. "Sleep Quality Versus Sleep Quantity: Relationships Between Sleep and Measures of Health, Well-Being and Sleepiness in College Students." *Journal of Psychosomatic Research* 42, no. 6 (1997): 583-596. https://doi.org/10.1016/S0022-3999(97)00004-4.

61. Gangwisch, James E., Lindsay A. Babiss, Dolores Malaspina, Blake J. Turner, Gary K. Zammit, and Kelly Posner. "Earlier Parental Set Bedtimes as a Protective Factor Against Depression and Suicidal Ideation." *Sleep* 33, no. 1 (2010): 97-106. https://doi.org/10.1093/sleep/33.1.97.

62. Ibid.

63. Emmons, Robert A. and Michael E. McCullough. "Counting Blessings Versus Burdens: An Experimental Investigation of Gratitude and Subjective Well-Being in Daily Life." *Journal of Personality and Social Psychology* 84, no. 2 (2003): 377-389. https://doi.org/10.1037/0022-3514.84.2.377.

64. Scheier, Michael F. and Charles S. Carver. "Optimism, Coping, and Health: Assessment and Implications of Generalized Outcome Expectancies." *Health Psychology* 4, no. 3 (1985): 219-247.

65. Baldwin, Bernell. "Why is Fresh Air Fresh?" *Journal of Health and Healing* 11, no. 4: 26–27.

66. Soyka, Fred and Alan Denis Edmonds. *The Ion Effect: How Air Electricity Rules Your Life and Health.* New York: Bantam Books, 1978. 21.

67. Baldwin, Bernell. "Why is Fresh Air Fresh?" *Journal of Health and Healing* 11, no. 4: 26–27.

68. Duffee, R. A. and R. H. Koontz. "Behavioral Effects of Ionized Air on Rats." *Psychophysiology* 1, no. 4 (1965): 347-359. https://doi.org/10.1111/j.1469-8986.1965.tb03267.x

69. Jordan, Juliana and Boris Sokoloff. "Air Ionization, Age, and Maze Learning of Rats." *Journal of Gerontology* 14, no. 3 (1959): 344-348. https://doi.org/10.1093/geronj/14.3.344.

70. Reilly, T. and I. C. Stevenson. "An Investigation of the Effects of Negative Air Ions on Responses to Submaximae Exercise at Different Times of Day." *Journal of Human Ergology.* 22 no. 1 (1993): 1-9. https://doi.org/10.11183/jhe1972.22.1.

71. Mitchell, Bailey W. and Daniel J. King. "Effect of Negative Air Ionization on Airborne Transmission of Newcastle Disease Virus." *Avian Diseases* 38, no.4 (1994): 725-732. https://doi.org/10.2307/1592107.

72. Giannini, A. J., B. T. Jones, and R. H. Loiselle. "Reversibility of Serotonin Irritation Syndrome with Atmospheric Anions." *The Journal of Clinical Psychiatry* 47, no. 3 (1986): 141-143.

73. Gabbay, Jacob, Orna Bergerson, Nissim Levi, Shmuel Brenner, and Ilana Eli. "Effect of Ionization on Microbial Air Pollution in the Dental Clinic." *Environmental Research* 52, no. 1 (1990): 99-106. https://doi.org/10.1016/S0013-9351(05)80154-9.

74. Cohen, Lorenzo, Carla Warneke, Rachel T. Fouladi, M. Alma Rodriguez, and Alejandro Chaoul–Reich. "Psychological Adjustment and Sleep Quality in a Randomized Trial of The Effects of a Tibetan Yoga Intervention in Patients with Lymphoma." *Cancer: Interdisciplinary International Journal of the American Cancer Society* 100, no. 10 (2004): 2253-2260. https://doi.org/10.1002/cncr.20236.

75. Bauman, Richard. "Taking a Daily Vacation." Vibrant Life. Accessed July 19, 2018. http://www.vibrantlife.com/?p=188.

76. Ariga, Atsunori and Alejandro Lleras. "Brief and Rare Mental "Breaks" Keep You Focused: Deactivation and Reactivation of Task Goals Preempt Vigilance Decrements." *Cognition* 118, no. 3 (2011): 439-443.

77. "Brief Diversions Vastly Improve Focus, Researchers Find." ScienceDaily. Accessed June 18, 2018. www.sciencedaily.com/releases/2011/02/110208131529.htm.

78. Puetz, Timothy W., Patrick J. O'Connor, and Rod K. Dishman. "Effects of Chronic Exercise on Feelings of Energy and Fatigue: A Quantitative Synthesis." *Psychological Bulletin* 132, no. 6 (2006): 866-876.

79. Barton, Jo and Jules Pretty. "What is the Best Dose of Nature and Green Exercise For Improving Mental Health? A Multi-Study Analysis." *Environmental Science & Technology* 44, no. 10 (2010): 3947-3955.

80. Takahashi, Masaya, Akinori Nakata, Takashi Haratani, Yasutaka Ogawa, and Heihachiro Arito. "Post-Lunch Nap as a Worksite Intervention to Promote Alertness on the Job." *Ergonomics* 47, no. 9 (2004): 1003-1013.

81. Tucker, Matthew A., Yasutaka Hirota, Erin J. Wamsley, Hiuyan Lau, Annie Chaklader, and William Fishbein. "A Daytime Nap Containing Solely Non REM Sleep Enhances Declarative But Not Procedural Memory." *Neurobiology of Learning and Memory* 86, no. 2 (2006): 241-247.

82. Backhaus, Jutta and Klaus Junghanns. "Daytime Naps Improve Procedural Motor Memory." *Sleep Medicine* 7, no. 6 (2006): 508-512.

83. Takahashi, Masaya, and Heihachiro Arito. "Maintenance of Alertness and Performance by a Brief Nap After Lunch Under Prior Sleep Deficit." *Sleep* 23, no. 6 (2000): 813-819.

84. Takahashi, Masaya, Hideki Fukuda, and Heihachiro Arito. "Brief Naps During Post-Lunch Rest: Effects on Alertness, Performance, and Autonomic Balance." *European Journal of Applied Physiology and Occupational Physiology* 78, no. 2 (1998): 93-98.

85. Hayashi, Mitsuo, Makiko Watanabe, and Tadao Hori. "The Effects of a 20 Min Nap in the Mid-Afternoon on Mood, Performance and EEG Activity." *Clinical Neurophysiology* 110, no. 2 (1999): 272-279. https://doi.org/10.1016/S1388-2457(98)00003-0.

86. Tamaki, Munehisa, A. I. Shirota, Hideki Tanaka, Mitsuo Hayashi, and Tadao Hori. "Effects of a Daytime Nap in the Aged." *Psychiatry and Clinical Neurosciences* 53, no. 2 (1999): 273-275. https://doi.org/10.1046/j.1440-1819.1999.00548.x.

87. Luo, Zili and Shojiro Inoué. "A Short Daytime Nap Modulates Levels of Emotions Objectively Evaluated by the Emotion Spectrum Analysis Method." *Psychiatry and Clinical Neurosciences* 54, no. 2 (2000): 207-212. https://doi.org/10.1046/j.1440-1819.2000.00660.x.

88. Taub, John M., Peter E. Tanguay, and Roger R. Rosa. "Effects of Afternoon Naps on Physiological Variables Performance and Self-Reported Activation." *Biological Psychology* 5, no. 3 (1977): 191-210. https://doi.org/10.1016/0301-0511(77)90002-3.

89. Hayashi, Mitsuo and Tadao Hori. "The Effects of a 20-Min Nap Before Post-Lunch Dip." *Psychiatry and Clinical Neurosciences* 52, no. 2 (1998): 203-204. https://doi.org/10.1111/j.1440-1819.1998.tb01031.x.

90. Tietzel, Amber J. and Leon C. Lack. "The Short-Term Benefits of Brief and Long Naps Following Nocturnal Sleep Restriction." *Sleep* 24, no. 3 (2001): 293-300. https://doi.org/10.1093/sleep/24.3.293.

91. Tietzel, Amber J. and Leon C. Lack. "The Recuperative Value of Brief and Ultra–Brief Naps on Alertness and Cognitive Performance." *Journal of Sleep Research* 11, no. 3 (2002): 213-218. https://doi.org/10.1046/j.1365-2869.2002.00299.x.

92. Zili Luo and Shojiro Inoué. "A Short Daytime Nap Modulates Levels of Emotions Objectively Evaluated by the Emotion Spectrum Analysis Method." *Psychiatry and Clinical Neurosciences* 54, no 2 (2000): 207-212. https://doi.org/10.1046/j.1440-1819.2000.00660.x.

93. Clavreul, Genevieve E. "Why Power Napping Might Be Right For the Nurses at Your Hospital." Working Nurse. Accessed July 20, 2018. http://www.workingnurse.com/articles/Why-Power-Napping-Might-be-Right-for-the-Nurses-at-Your-Hospital.

94. Ludington, Aileen and Hans Diehl. *Dynamic Living: How to Take Charge of Your Health.* Hagerstown: Review and Herald Publishing Association, 1995. 189.

95. Ibid.

96. Rath, Tom, James K. Harter, and Jim Harter. *Wellbeing: The Five Essential Elements*. New York: Simon and Schuster, 2010. 78, 211.

97. Baldwin, Bernell. "Seven-day Rhythms," *Journal of Health and Healing* 9, no. 4: 3, 14.

98. Rawson, M. J., G. Cornélissen, J. Holte, G. Katinas, E. Eckert, J. Siegelová, and F. Halberg. "Circadian and Circaseptan Components of Blood Pressure and Heart Rate During Depression." *Scripta Medica (BRNO)* 73, no. 2 (2000): 117-124.

99. Agrimonti, F., R. Frairia, D. Fornaro, M. Torta, G. Borretta, G. Trapani, et al. "Circadian and Circaseptan Rhythmicities in Corticosteroid-Binding Globulin (CBG) Binding Activity of Human Milk." *Chronobiologia* 9, no. 3 (1982): 281-290. https://doi.org/10.1159/000410981.

100. Levi, Francis and Franz Halberg. "Circaseptan (About-7-Day) Bioperiodicity—Spontaneous and Reactive—and the Search for Pacemakers." *Ricerca in Clinica e in Laboratorio* 12, no. 2 (1982): 323-370.

101. Pöllmann, L. and G. Hildebrandt. "Long-Term Control of Swelling After Maxillo-Facial Surgery: A Study Of Circaseptan Reactive Periodicity." *International Journal of Chronobiology* 8, no. 2 (1982): 105-114.

102. Besarab, A., L. Wesson, B. Jarrell, and J. F. Burke. "Effect of Delayed Graft Function and ALG on The Circaseptan (About 7-Day) Rhythm of Human Renal Allograft Rejection." *Transplantation* 35, no. 6 (1983): 562-566.

103. Baldwin, Bernell. "Seven-day Rhythms." *Journal of Health and Healing* 9, no. 4 (1984): 3, 14.

104. *Merriam-Webster*, s.v. "recreation," Accessed September 19, 2018, https://www.merriam-webster.com/dictionary/recreation.

105. Expedia. "Expedia.com – 2009 International Vacation Deprivation Survey Results." Accessed August 2, 2013. https://media.expedia.com/media/content/expus/graphics/promos/vacations/Expedia_International_Vacation_Deprivation_Survey_2009.pdf.

106. Eaker, Elaine D., Joan Pinsky, and William P. Castelli. "Myocardial Infarction and Coronary Death among Women: Psychosocial Predictors From a 20-Year Follow-Up of Women in the Framingham Study." *American Journal of Epidemiology* 135, no. 8 (1992): 854-864. https://doi.org/10.1093/oxfordjournals.aje.a116381.

107. Vaillant, George E. "Natural History of Male Psychological Health: IV. What Kinds of Men Do Not Get Psychosomatic Illness." *Psychosomatic Medicine* 40, no. 5 (1978): 420-431. http://dx.doi.org/10.1097/00006842-197808000-00006.

108. Gump, Brooks B. and Karen A. Matthews. "Are Vacations Good for Your Health? The 9-Year Mortality Experience After the Multiple Risk Factor Intervention Trial." *Psychosomatic Medicine* 62, no. 5 (2000): 608-612. http://dx.doi.org/10.1097/00006842-200009000-00003.

109. Schenck, Carlos H., Mark W. Mahowald, and Robert L. Sack. "Assessment and Management of Insomnia." *Journal of the American Medical Association* 289, no. 19 (2003): 2475-2479. https://doi.org/10.1001/jama.289.19.2475.

110. U.S. Department of Health and Human Services. Your Guide to Healthy Sleep. National Institutes of Health & National Heart, Lung, and Blood Institute, NIH Publication No. 06-5271, November 2005. http://www.nhlbi.nih.gov/health/public/sleep/healthy_sleep.pdf.

111. Dorsey, Cynthia M., Martin H. Teicher, Mairav Cohen-Zion, Louis Stefanovic, Andrew Satlin, Wendy Tartarini, David Harper, and Scott E. Lukas. "Core Body Temperature and Sleep of Older Female Insomniacs Before and After Passive Body Heating." *Sleep* 22, no. 7 (1999): 891-898. https://doi.org/10.1093/sleep/22.7.891.

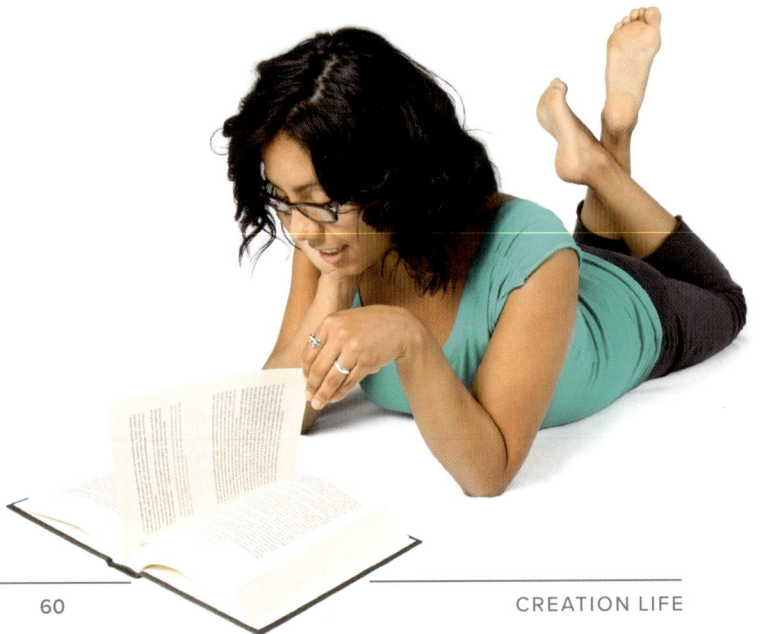

REST

ENVIRONMENT

Influence your surroundings

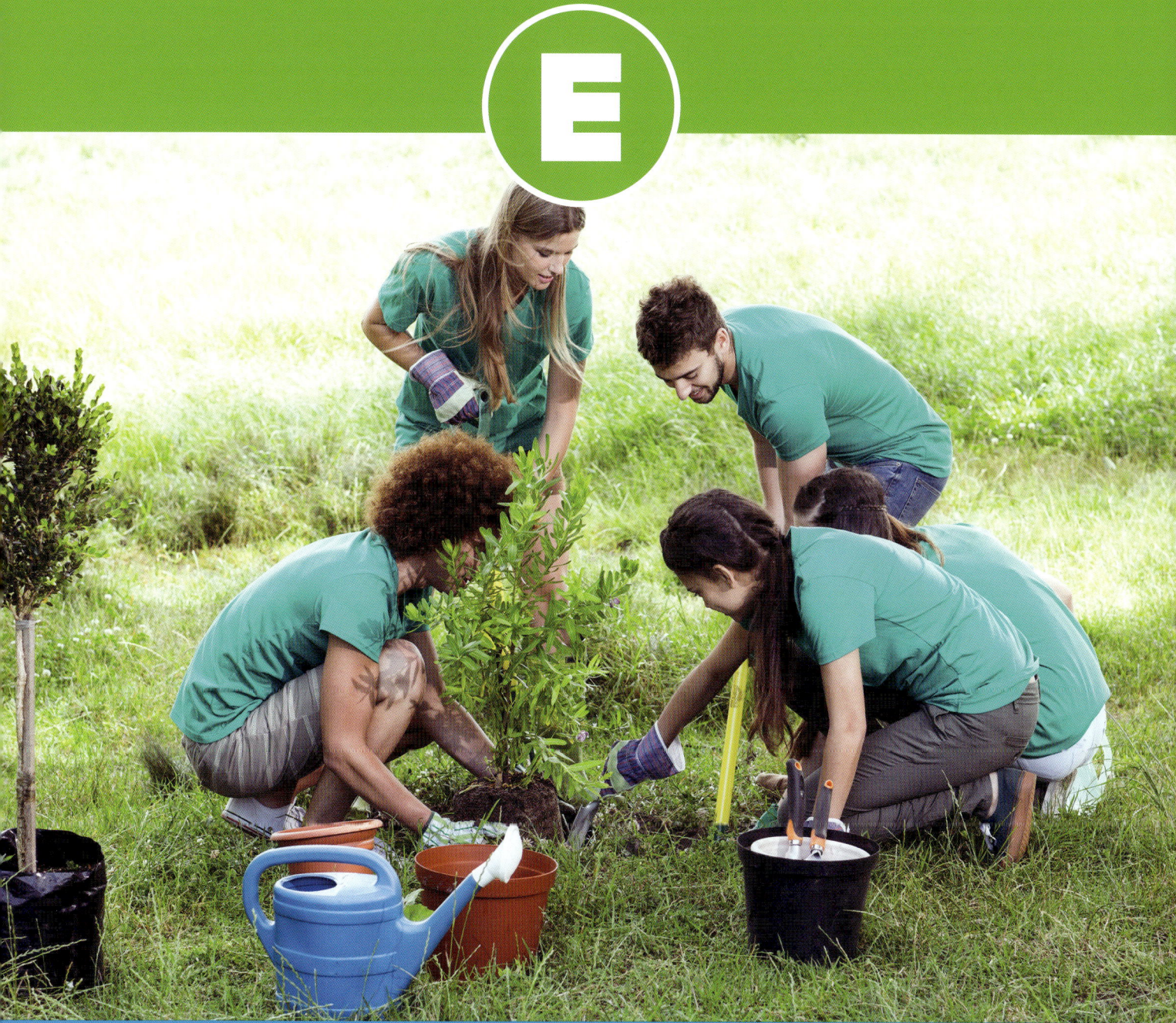

THE BIG PICTURE

Take a quick look around you. What do you see? Are you inside, outside or upside down? Are you at home, in school or parasailing in the Bahamas? Are you hot, cold, wet, dry, cool, calm or collected? Do you hear any sounds, notice any interesting scents in the air?

The purpose of this exercise is to get you thinking about your environment. Your environment is more than just the world you encounter when you walk outside your front door; it's everything that lies outside of you, either immediately or in the world at large. Where you are right now, the air you are breathing, the sights, smells, colors and sounds that are all around you... all of this is a part of your environment.

"The environment is everything that isn't me."

ALBERT EINSTEIN

Maybe you're wondering why all this matters. What makes environment so special, and what, if anything, does it have to do with your health? Quite a lot actually. Environment is the third principle of CREATION Life because everything that lies outside of you affects what's inside of you. The world around you is coming inside of you all the time through your skin, mouth and even your mind. All of your senses influence your mood and ultimately your health and well-being. In this section, you will see the important roles your larger environment (air and water quality) and your immediate environment (light, sound, aroma and touch) play in giving you optimal health and happiness. You will also be encouraged to make changes to your surroundings to create the best possible environment for yourself and those around you.

Your ENVIRONMENT is everything that surrounds and influences you in a physical, mental or spiritual way. You are in a constant process of taking in your environment through your five senses. Through this process, the stimuli in your environment affect who you are on the inside.

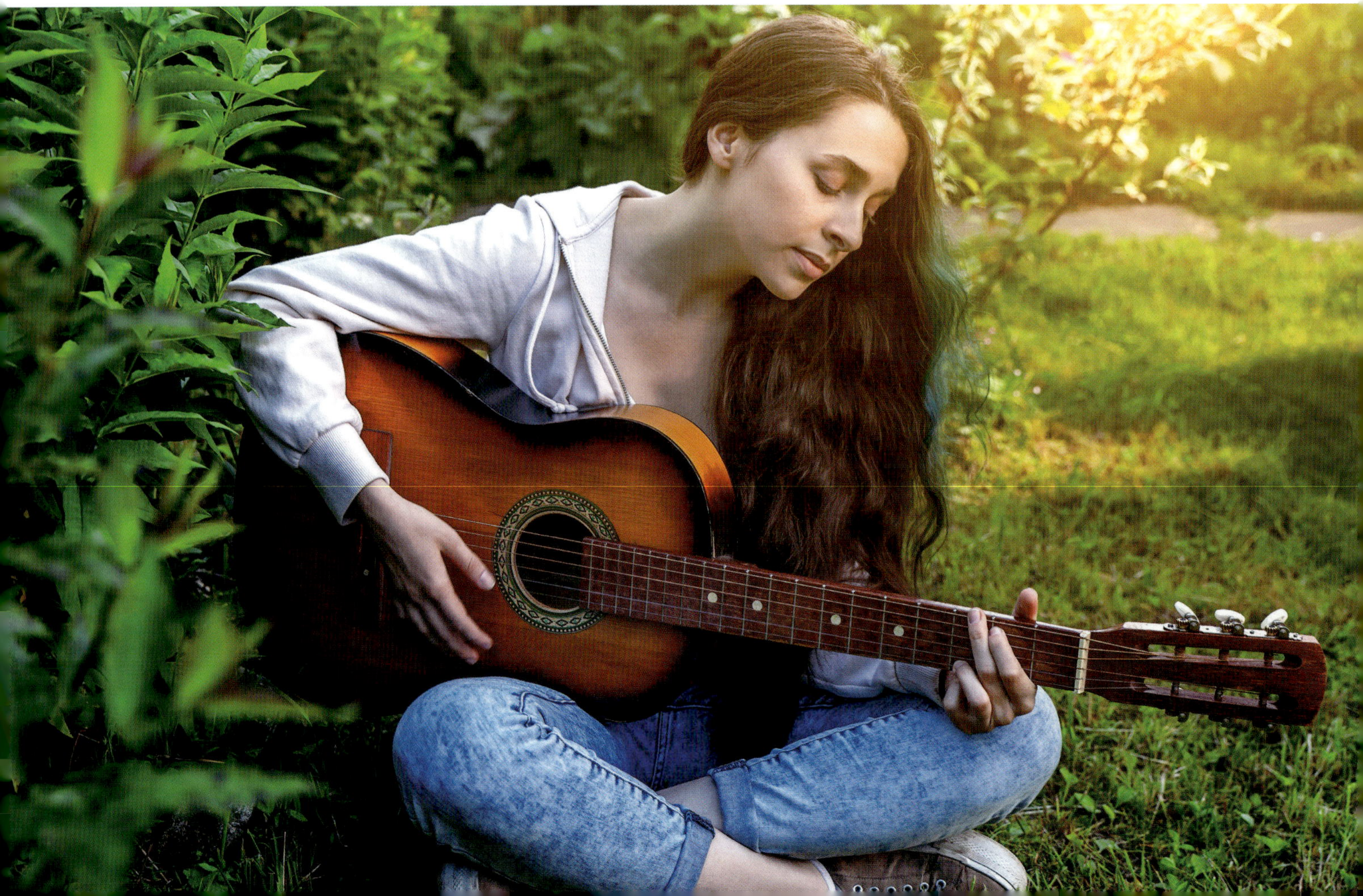

THE GIFT OF ENVIRONMENT

The Lord God planted a garden toward the east, in Eden; and there He placed the man whom He had formed. Out of the ground the Lord God caused to grow every tree that is pleasing to the sight and good for food; the tree of life also in the midst of the garden, and the tree of the knowledge of good and evil.

GENESIS 2:8–9

When Adam was created, God formed him in the open field. He used the dust of the ground to fashion a man and breathed the breath of life deep into his lungs, but God didn't leave Adam out in the open to fend for himself. He knew His creation needed a home, a place where he would be provided for and protected. God wanted to place Adam in the ideal environment.

First, He chose the perfect spot. The Bible says a river flowed through the garden, providing the man with the water he would need to survive (Genesis 2:10). Then God caused trees to grow up from the ground. These trees gave Adam food and shade, but they were also beautiful for him to look upon. Everything was perfect in Adam's new garden home.

God still reveals Himself through His creation. Adam could see that God was truly a loving Father. God met Adam's physical needs, but He also delighted in providing a beautiful, nurturing environment for Adam to make his home.

God's beautiful, life-promoting environment was His gift to you at creation. The earth was designed to sustain you, give you air to breathe, sunshine to provide warmth, food to eat and water to drink. God wants you to treasure the environment as the precious gift that it is. By spending time in creation your heart will naturally be drawn closer to the Creator. Take time to enjoy your surroundings and reflect on the One who created you and your environment.

The Bible says the "invisible attributes" of God, His eternal power and divine nature, are clearly seen in and understood through His creation (Romans 1:20). What evidence of God do you see exhibited in nature?

OUTSIDE

American poet Joyce Kilmer once wrote, "I think that I shall never see a poem lovely as a tree." These words perfectly capture the joy humans receive from being surrounded by the beauty of nature. Getting outdoors into the wonderful world God created is a great way for you to feel refreshed and restored. However, for the majority of people this is increasingly difficult. As urban and suburban areas have become more predominant, most people fail to see the critical role that natural elements play in their quality of life.

University of Michigan researcher Rachel Kaplan says that experiencing nature, whether through passive observance or active participation, is an important component of your psychological well-being.[1] Another University of Michigan researcher, Stephen Kaplan, states that the pressures of modern life contribute to the experience of mental fatigue, which can lead to less tolerance, less effectiveness and poorer health. By providing deeply needed restorative experiences, natural settings can play a central role in reducing these devastating effects.[2]

Take trees for example. Trees are a major capital asset in cities and towns — as much an integral part of the scene as streets, sidewalks and buildings — and they represent a major component called the "green infrastructure."[3] By getting outside you will be able to enjoy the trees and other natural resources. This section will help you appreciate the wonders and beauties of creation as well as explain the wonderful benefits you receive from spending time in a natural environment.

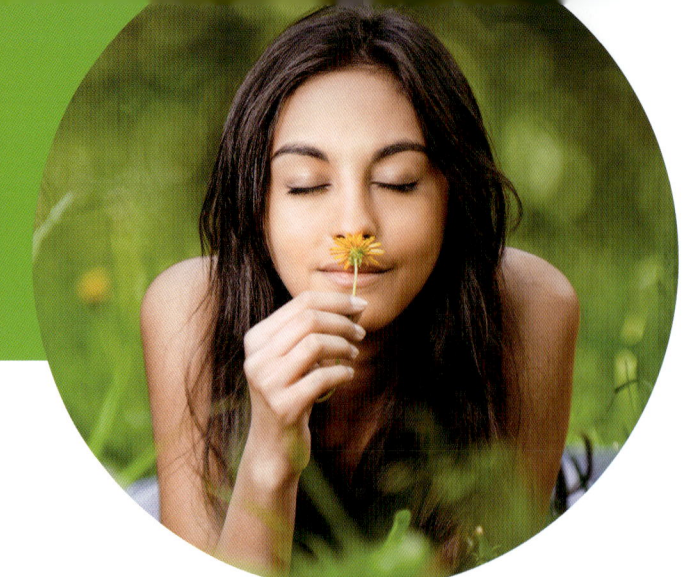

ENVIRONMENT

RURAL SETTINGS

High school can be a stressful time for students. You have to juggle your free time between schoolwork, hanging out with your friends and being there for your family. Could living in a natural setting alleviate some of that stress? Researchers Nancy Wells and Gary Evans believe so. They studied the effects of nature on stress in and around the rural homes of 337 children in third through fifth grades. Wells and Evans found that, "In a rural setting, levels of nearby nature moderate the impact of stressful life events on the psychological well-being of children. Specifically, the impact of life stress was lower among children with high levels of nearby nature than among those with little nearby nature."[4]

Another study published in the journal *Nature* found living in a more rural setting helps two of the brain's regions involved with emotion and stress. In three different experiments, the researchers found that rural-living and city-living people have very different responses to stress. The participants did math tasks under time pressure while the researchers examined their brains using functional magnetic resonance imaging (fMRI). The researchers found that those test subjects who lived in cities had increased activity in an area of the brain called the amygdala, a region involved in stress response, compared to those subjects who lived in towns and rural areas.[5]

Why does being in nature alleviate daily stress? Because it was designed this way by a loving Creator. Consider one of the primary colors of nature: the blue sky. There is scientific evidence that blue is not only soothing and relaxing, but is also associated with lower anxiety levels.[6] Blue is also associated with soothing feelings of security and comfort, which imply pleasure and relaxation. The presence of blue has also been shown to slow the pulse rate and lower body temperature.[7]

Research clearly supports a rural setting as a natural stress-reducing environment for those living there, but what if you don't live in a rural area? Can you still get stress-relieving benefits from your environment? The good news is there are still plenty of health benefits available through the environment around you, regardless of where you live. If you are fortunate enough to live in a rural setting, you will likely receive these stress-lowering benefits. However, if your home is in an urban or suburban area, don't feel discouraged. Consider finding ways to spend more time outdoors. Many local and state parks exist within a short driving distance, regardless of where you live. Spending a weekend in a natural setting can do wonders for your health and wellness. According to a report published by *The Trust for Public Land*, "City parks and open space improve our physical and psychological health, strengthen our communities and make our cities and neighborhoods more attractive places to live and work."[8]

FRESH AIR

As a young child, your parents may have told you, "Go outside and get some fresh air." When it comes to your health and well-being, this is very good advice. As you learned in the chapter on Rest, fresh air is negatively ionized, and breathing it provides you with many wonderful health benefits. Unfortunately, these benefits are destroyed when the air you breathe is recirculated inside a building, or worse — when it's full of pollution.

You may be surprised to learn that air pollution can be more of a concern indoors than out. In the last several years, a growing body of scientific evidence has indicated that the air within homes and buildings can be more polluted than the outdoor air in even the largest and most industrialized cities.[9] In fact, the air inside most homes is an average of two to five times more polluted than the air outside its walls. Indoor pollution has been identified as one of the top five environmental risks for public health.[10] Given this information, it's easy to see why indoor air pollution is something you should pay attention to.

Sometimes indoor air pollution is created from toxic chemical products such as household cleaners and pesticides. It is also present in home furnishings such as carpets, foams and composite wood products made from fume-emitting synthetic materials. You may also find it in poorly vented combustion appliances like gas ranges and furnaces. Combine these sources with energy efficient home construction that limits the amount of fresh air exchanged between the inside and outside, and air pollution can quickly build to unhealthy levels. Other pollutants such as tobacco smoke and fumes from paint, varnish or aerosol sprays not only deplete the healing effects of fresh air, they also come with their own laundry list of harmful side effects.

Researchers have documented that one common pollutant, ozone, causes serious health concerns. If you stayed awake in chemistry class you already know that ozone is a molecule made up of three oxygen atoms. You probably also know about the Earth's ozone layer, which absorbs much of the sun's harmful UV radiation. While ozone is great up in the atmosphere, it's bad

news for you down on the ground. Ozone is a by-product of internal combustion engines and power plant emissions; exposure to ozone causes eye irritation, shortness of breath, coughs, decreased lung function and decreased physical performance.[11-12] This is just one reason why it's important for you to get the cleanest, freshest air possible. And where is that air found in abundance? You'll find it in natural, outdoor environments — especially in areas such as the mountains, forests and seas. Breathing fresh air cleans out the stale air from your lungs that would otherwise promote disease.

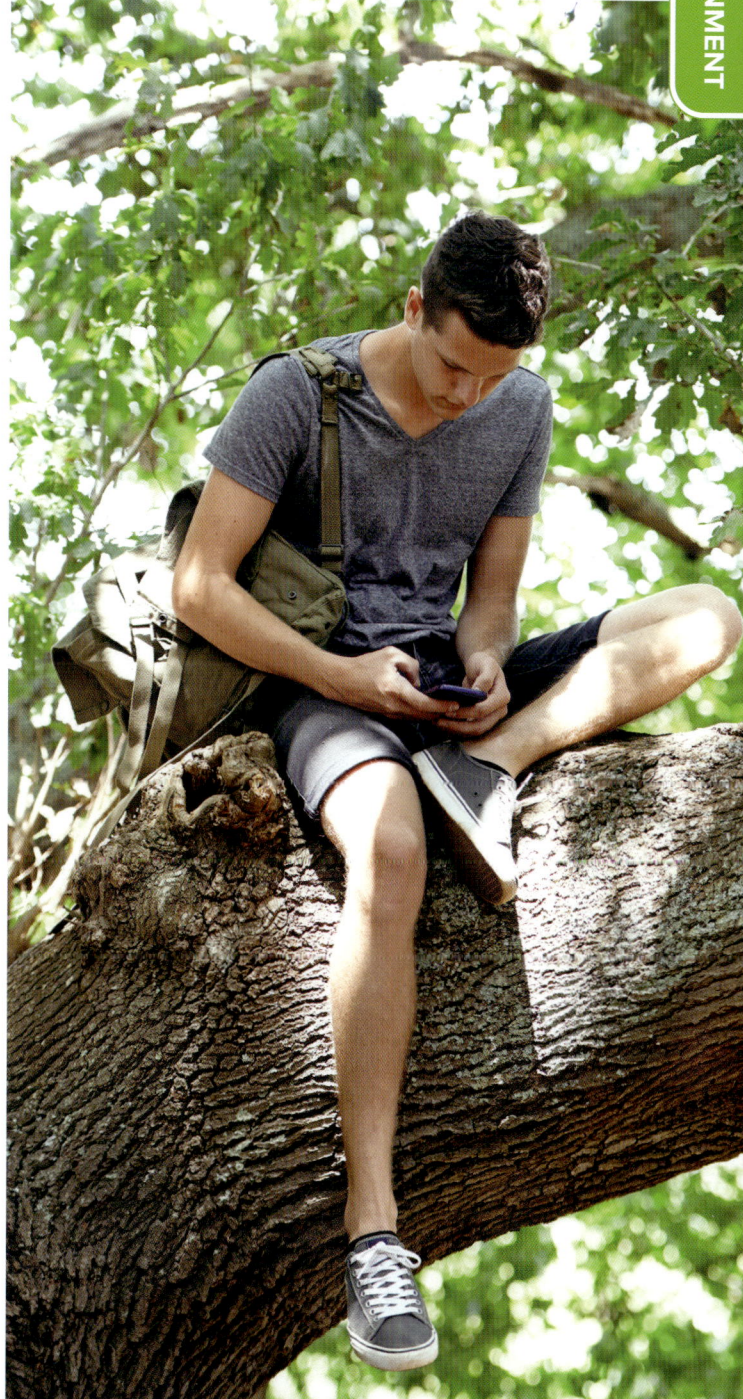

THE POWER OF SUNLIGHT

If you visit the small town of Barrow, Alaska in the wintertime, you would experience what is commonly called the "polar night." This is a period of time when the night lasts for over 24 hours. In Barrow, polar night begins in mid-November and lasts until January, producing over 60 days of twilight. Imagine being without sunlight for such a long period of time. Some people may view it as only a small annoyance, but for others, living without seeing the sun causes serious depression. This condition is called seasonal affective disorder (SAD), and it may include sad, anxious or "empty" feelings, feelings of hopelessness and/or pessimism, feelings of guilt, worthlessness or helplessness, irritability, restlessness, loss of interest or pleasure in activities you used to enjoy. Other symptoms may include fatigue and decreased energy, difficulty concentrating, remembering details and making decisions, difficulty sleeping or oversleeping, changes in weight and even thoughts of death or suicide.[13]

This connection between sunlight and mood has been the focus of much research, especially regarding SAD and its usual method of treatment. According to the MedlinePlus website, "SAD may be effectively treated with light therapy." Light therapy is when an artificial light source, such as a light box, is used to mimic exposure to natural outdoor light. However, the web site also says that nearly half of the people with SAD do not respond to light therapy alone. Antidepressant medicines and talk therapy are often used or combined with light therapy to reduce the symptoms of SAD.[14]

The reason for this may have something to do with the unique effect sunlight has on your physiology. Sunlight increases the production of serotonin, which some call the "happy hormone." This important brain chemical boosts your mood and is often seen as key to treating depression. In one study published in *The Lancet*, it was found that the turnover of serotonin in the brain was lowest in the winter. Researchers found that the brain's rate of production of serotonin was directly related to the prevailing duration of bright sunlight, and rose rapidly with increased luminosity.[15] Serotonin also promotes positive thinking,[16] while a reduction in serotonin levels has been connected to attention deficit hyperactivity disorder (ADHD),[17] irritability,[18] depression,[19] aggression,[20] anxiety,[21] lack of concentration,[22] chronic pain,[23] fatigue,[24] nausea,[25] obsessive-compulsive disorder,[26] fibromyalgia,[27] arthritis,[28] chronic fatigue syndrome[29] and heat intolerance.[30] Serotonin has also been connected with eating behavior and body weight.[31]

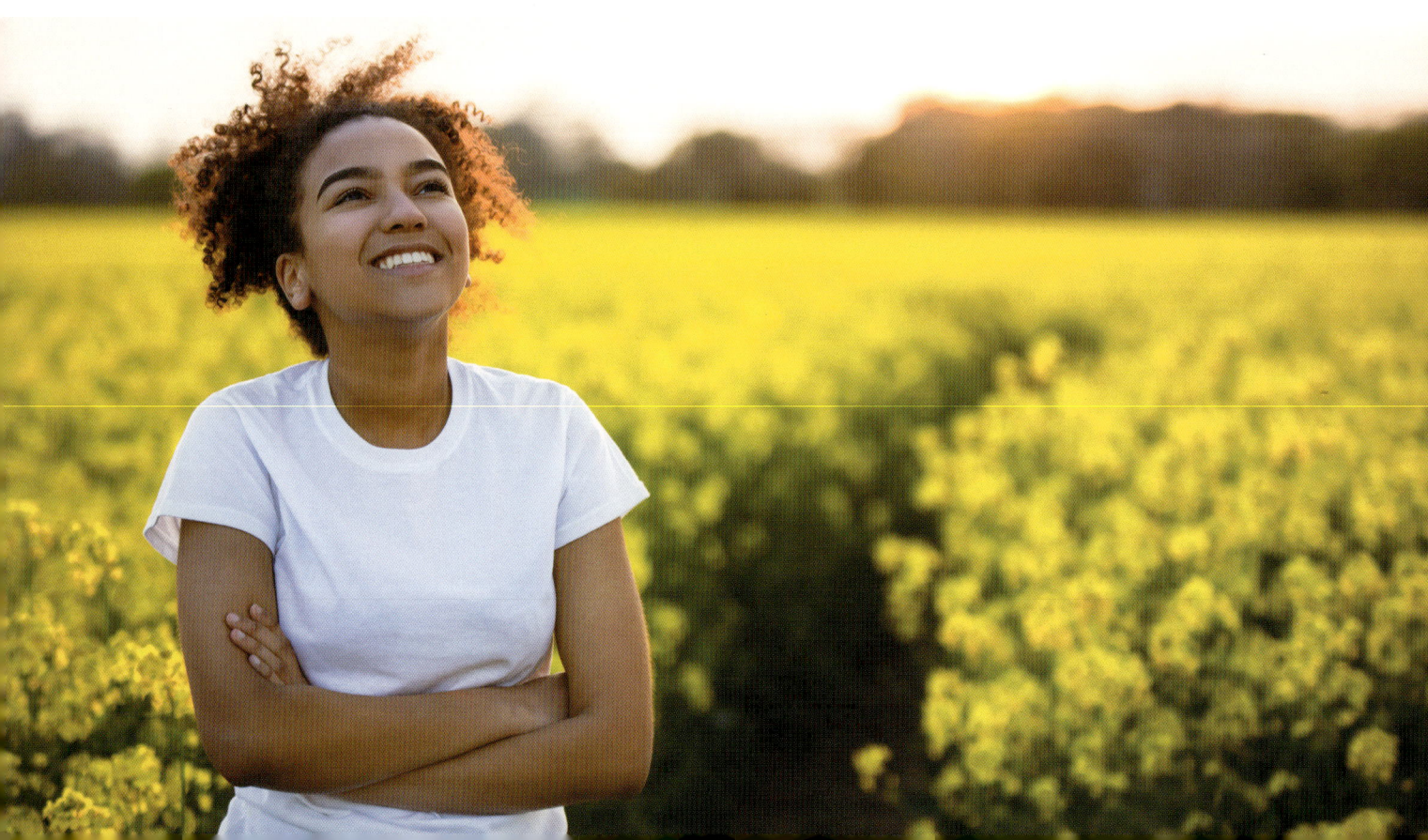

All this research may indicate a simple truth: you weren't designed to live in the dark. Sunshine is a powerful promoter of health and well-being, not just for you but the entire planet. As the primary energy source of the earth, sunshine is necessary for the growth of green plants, which provide you with healthy foods to eat and oxygen-rich air to breathe.

The presence of sunlight has also been shown to help surgical patients with stress and pain management. In one study, pain medication use was examined in 89 patients undergoing elective cervical and lumbar spinal surgery. The patients were housed on either the "bright" or "dim" side of the same hospital unit. Patients staying on the bright side of the hospital unit were exposed to an average of 46 percent higher-intensity sunlight than those staying on the dim side. The bright-side patients perceived less stress, marginally less pain, took 22 percent less analgesic medication per hour and had 21 percent less pain medication costs. "At discharge, patients on the bright side reported significantly less stress and a marginal decrease in pain than the patients on the dim side."[32]

Sunlight has also been found to increase feelings of relaxation. Results of previous studies suggest that emotional states, such as those characterized by relaxation, promote and facilitate activities requiring intense concentration.[33]

The presence of sunlight may also help motivate you to do your best at school. One study reported a dramatic increase in student performance when schoolrooms were exposed to abundant daylight.[34] Another study found the presence of windows in a classroom affected student perception in that the room was more motivating.[35] Other research showed that holding classes in a natural, outdoor setting improved science[36] and other standardized test scores, reduced discipline and classroom management problems, increased engagement and enthusiasm for learning and resulted in greater pride and ownership in accomplishments.[37]

Sunlight is also a great way for you to get enough vitamin D. Vitamin D isn't just one substance but is actually a group of substances that are vital to helping your intestines absorb important minerals such as calcium and phosphate. While vitamin D is present in some foods and can be taken in vitamin supplements, it is most easily synthesized when your skin is exposed to sunlight. Sunlight converts a chemical present in your skin into vitamin D3. This is then carried to your liver and kidneys where it becomes active vitamin D. Because your body produces vitamin D in this manner, it has earned the nickname the "sunshine vitamin." It is important for many reasons, including building strong bones and muscles and impacting your immune system.[38] Several recently published studies offer some of the strongest evidence yet of the power of the "sunshine vitamin" against Multiple Sclerosis (MS),[39] rheumatoid arthritis,[40] type 1 diabetes,[41] and certain other diseases.[42] Research studies confirm the inverse relationship between sunlight and blood pressure.[43-44] There is also evidence that vitamin D protects against some cancers.[45-46]

Unfortunately, sunlight has a bad reputation. As you may know, excessive amounts of sunlight have shown to increase the risk of skin cancer and cataracts in your eyes. It is understood that the most common types of skin cancer are linked to sunburn. Although these cancers are treatable and do not usually result in death, it is still best to avoid getting a sunburn. Getting moderate amounts of sunlight can be extremely beneficial and may even help prevent certain types of cancer. One study suggested that adequate moderate sunlight exposure appeared to protect against melanoma.[47] It may be that the increased production of vitamin D helps to protect the body from one of the deadliest skin cancers. Another study that looked at overall cancer rates in several states concluded that although frequent sun exposure statistically causes 2,000 U.S. cancer fatalities per year, it also acts to prevent another 138,000 U.S. annual cancer deaths and could possibly prevent 30,000 more deaths if Americans practiced regular, moderate sunning.[48] For the best health, don't avoid the sun. Be sure to get adequate sunshine without getting sunburned.

NATURE BREAK

So, you've been studying the rise and fall of the Roman Empire for the past three hours and your brain feels like it's full of oatmeal? Clearly you need a break, but here's the question; where should you take it? Researcher Gary Felsten wanted to know the best location for students to take a study break, so he asked them what they preferred. Students were told to imagine themselves cognitively fatigued. This is when your brain slows down after thinking for a long time. The students then rated the different places on their campus as to how mentally restorative each setting was. The settings varied by their views of nature: some had no views of nature, some had window views of nature with built structures present and some had views of simulated nature depicted through large murals. Students rated the settings with views of dramatic nature murals — especially those with water — more restorative than settings with window views of real but mundane nature with built structures present. Students rated the settings that lacked views of real or simulated nature the least restorative. These findings suggest that large nature murals in indoor settings used for study breaks may provide cognitively fatigued students with opportunities for restoration when other views of nature are unavailable or limited.[49]

In two more studies, a research team found that walking in nature or viewing pictures of nature can improve directed-attention abilities. Direct attention is a cognitive mechanism that is restored by interactions with nature. In the first study, students did a task that assessed their direct attention. Some went on a walk in a downtown area with few natural surroundings; others did the task and then walked in an area that was tree-lined and secluded from cars and people. Both groups came back and did the task again. Then they repeated the procedure with the groups trading walking places. The researchers found that performance on the task significantly improved when all of the students walked in nature, but not when they walked downtown.[50]

In the second study, the students did a test and a task before and after they viewed either pictures of nature or urban areas. They viewed pictures for about 10 minutes. In this study the students made improvements on both measures only after viewing pictures of nature compared to urban areas.[51]

These results showed that directed attention has an important role in short-term memory[52] and school success.[53] Another study found that college students "who had natural views from their dormitory windows were better able to direct attention than those with less natural views on some of the measures used to test the capacity to direct attention."[54] This study was based on a theoretical view, which suggests that under increased demands for attention, individuals' capacity to direct attention may become fatigued. Once fatigued, attentional restoration must occur in order to return to an effectively functioning state. An attention-restoring experience can be as simple as looking at nature.[55]

For those students that struggle to pay attention in class, nature may be a wonderful remedy. In one study, parents were surveyed regarding their ADHD-diagnosed child's attentional functioning after activities in several settings. Results showed that children function better than usual after activities in "green" settings. Research also indicates that the "greener" a child's play area, the less severe his or her attention deficit symptoms.[56]

So, the next time you need a break from studying, seek an environment that includes the presence of nature, either outdoors or through paintings or photographs. This will be a greater benefit to your fatigued mind and ultimately help you perform your best in school. Even something as simple as studying and doing your schoolwork in a room where plants are present can have a positive effect. Researchers found that after taking a break in a room filled with interior plants, workers did better in a proofreading test and showed increased concentration and attention to detail.[57]

TAKE FIVE MINUTES

Simply being able to see nature impacts your satisfaction with life. In a 2009 meta-analysis study involving 1,252 participants, researchers looked at the best dose of nature and green exercise for improving mental health. Amazingly, it was found that the greatest improvements in mood and self-esteem come from as little as five minutes of green exercise.[58] What are some ways you can add five minutes in nature to your regular routine?

INDOORS

Even though being outdoors refreshes and makes them happy, Americans spend 90 percent of their time indoors behind cinder block walls, under artificial lights and breathing recirculated air.[59] This makes it all the more important for you to make your indoor environment as vibrant and uplifting as possible, but where do you start? Work and home environments probably impact your health the most because you spend most of your time in them. So, paying attention and striving to create a healthy environment in both places gives rich rewards.

> *"He who knows what sweets and virtues are in the ground, the waters, the plants, the heavens and how to come at these enchantments, is the rich and royal man."*
>
> RALPH WALDO EMERSON

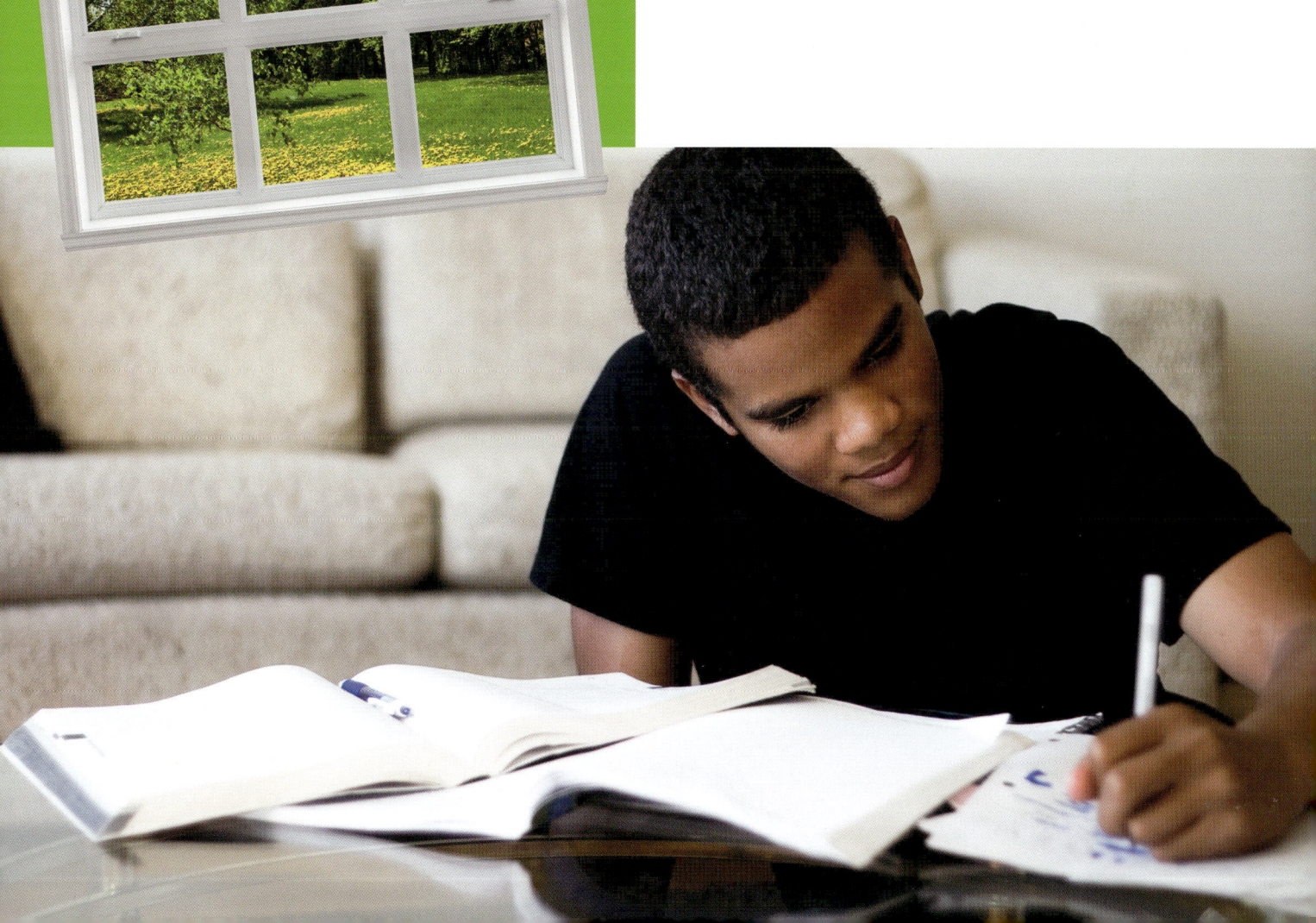

HOMEWORK

Thomas Fuller famously said, "Charity begins at home." Well, so does your indoor environment. Apart from school, your home is the place where you spend the majority of your time. You eat, sleep and play there. Ideally, your home should be like an oasis in the desert — a place of refreshment and restoration that exists in sharp contrast to the harshness of the world at large. Maybe you already see your home this way; however, if this is not the case, then you might need to do a little "homework." Don't worry. This isn't like writing a 20-page paper for English class on the colloquialism found in *Huckleberry Finn*. Instead, you should begin to identify those factors that are keeping your indoor environment from being the best it can be. Ask yourself the following questions:

- Does excessive clutter keep me from experiencing the maximum benefits of an organized living space?

- Does sharing a living space with a particular family member create conflict that makes it difficult to live in peace and harmony?

- Are there repairs or home improvements that need to be made in order to create a safer, better living space?

At this point in life you are under a parent or guardian's supervision. You may not have much of a vote in what kind of environment your entire home has, but one thing you can do is take responsibility for your own space, specifically your bedroom. Your room is a reflection of you. If it's messy and unorganized, this is the impression you are making to your parents, siblings and anyone else who may visit.

? What message does the current state of your bedroom say about you? How does your room make you feel inside and out? Are you happy with the current state of your environment or is it time for a change?

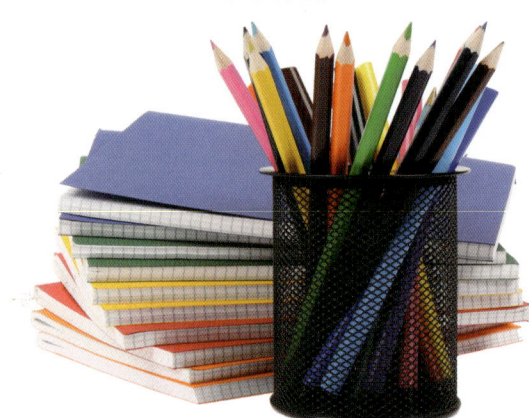

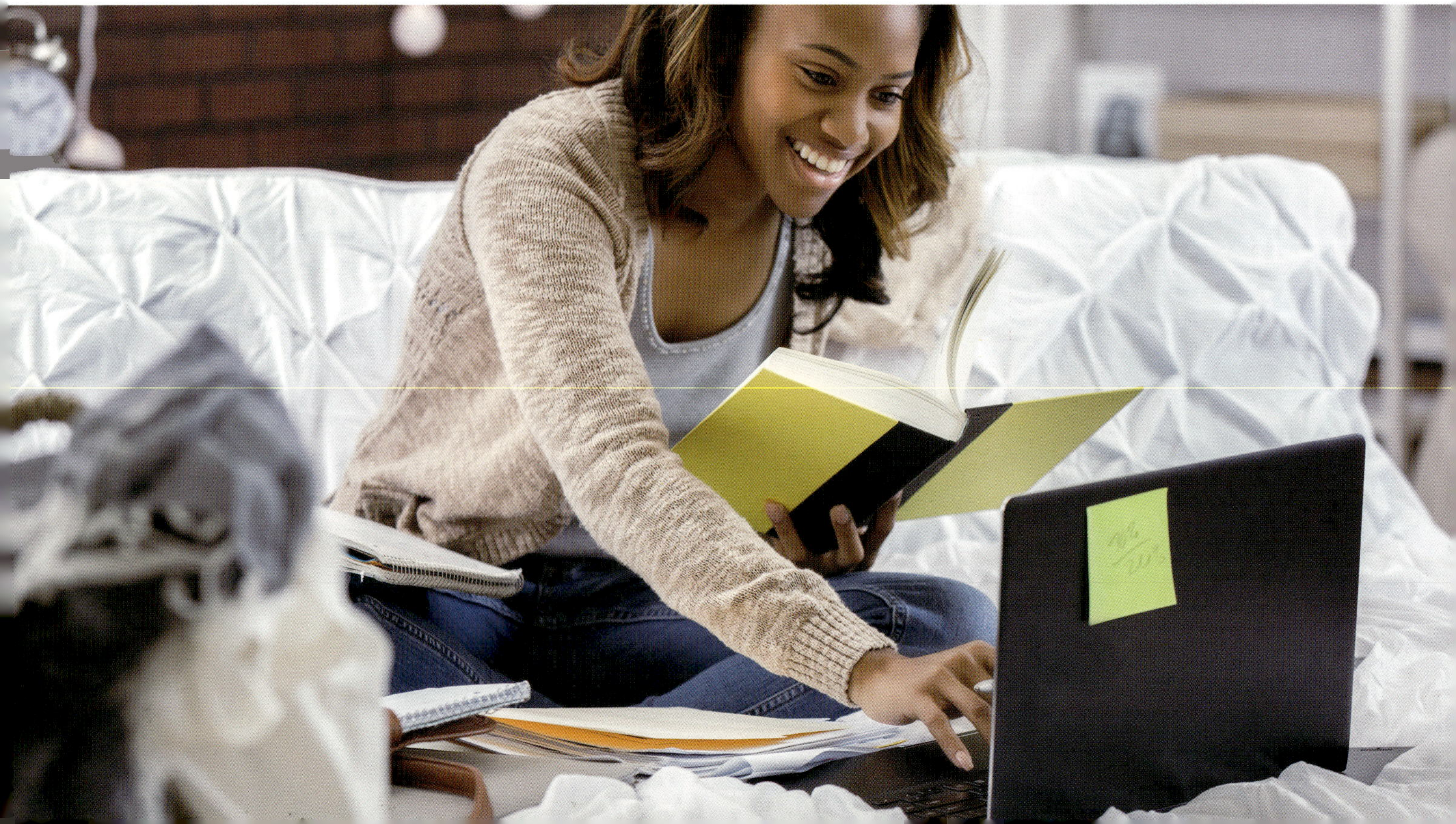

CLUTTER

Your room should make you feel good; it should recharge and revive you daily as a place of comfort and peace. Everything in your environment can either help or challenge your peace. Organization, cleanliness and order all promote much-needed health and peace. Clutter, messes and a lack of organization in your room can be a great source of stress or may even be caused by stress. Learning how to manage clutter now may even better prepare you for your future. For example, some surveys indicate that people with cluttered desks and offices are less likely to get promoted.[60] This is because clutter sends the wrong message. It also promotes disorder and stress in your mind, giving you less time and energy for other tasks. Think about it — even spending five minutes a day trying to find something in a cluttered room adds up to over 30 hours a year of wasted time.

Clutter in your life can also hurt your relationships or cause hard feelings among those who deal with the messes you make. You may have already experienced this with your parents or siblings, but in the future, you will most likely have roommates to contend with too. Learning to keep your room in order, as well as taking basic steps to clean up after yourself, will create a much better living environment for you and everyone who lives with you.

Clutter also impacts your social life. If your room looks like a disaster area, you might be less likely to have friends over to your house; in fact, your parents may forbid it. If your room stays messy for too long, you could push your parents to the breaking point. Imagine finding yourself grounded and missing out on enriching opportunities to be with your friends, all because of the deplorable state of your room. Start taking responsibility for your environment now so you can enjoy the benefits of a clean and organized living space. By keeping your bedroom neat and tidy, you will help to create a place where not only you, but also your family and friends are blessed — a place that nurtures and restores everyone who enters it.

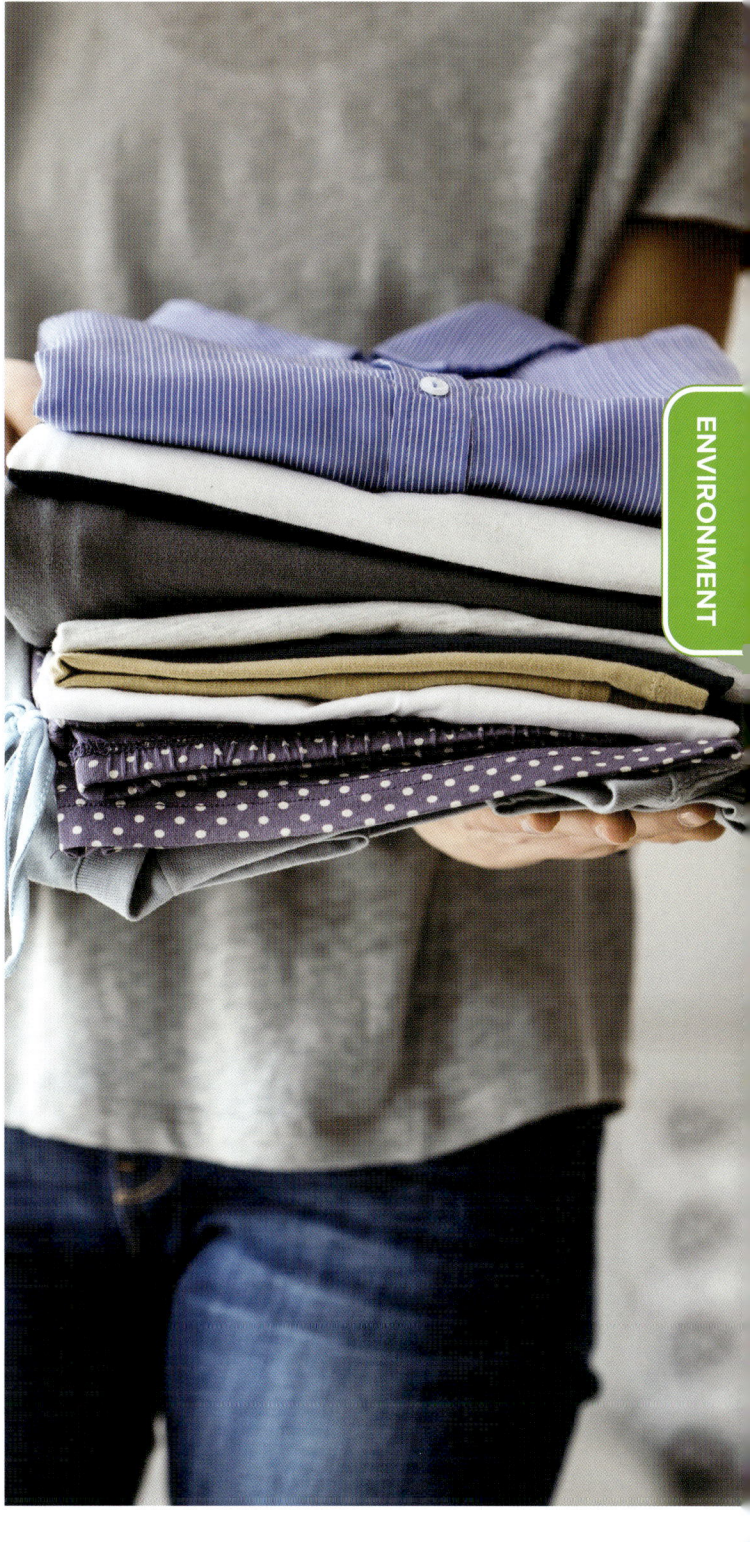

"Better keep yourself clean and bright; you are the window through which you must see the world."

GEORGE BERNARD SHAW

MEDIA JUNKIES

Every day, teenagers view countless hours of media. From the shows you watch, the games you play to the websites you visit, the media you consume impacts you in a powerful way, whether you realize it or not. Take TV for example. In most homes the TV is often on for many hours a day.[61] Consider the images it feeds your brain. Are they positive and health promoting? In many cases they are not. Even the news, though informative, can have negative effects on the mind. In one study, research showed that after watching just a few minutes of the news, participants said they felt more anxious and sad, which subsequently led to greater fear and personal worries.[62]

Of course, the news is just one source from a virtual buffet of media to choose from. Today's technology allows you 24-hour media access, and all this access means teens are using media at a record high. A national survey by the Kaiser Family Foundation found the amount of time young people spend with entertainment media has increased dramatically. Today, eight to 18-year-olds spend an average of seven hours and 38 minutes using entertainment media in a typical day. That's more than 53 hours a week. They also spend much of that time "media multitasking," or using more than one medium at a time. This means they actually manage to pack a total of 10 hours and 45 minutes worth of media content into those seven hours.[63]

Many of the movies, video games and websites in your environment contain images and concepts that you do not wish to model or become. Violence is often a major component, especially in video games and movies. Behavioral and cognitive studies have linked exposure to violent media with aggressive behavior. Violent video games show increased activity in areas of the brain linked to aggression and decreased responses in regions that contribute to self-control.[64] So, playing these kinds of games may contribute to making you less able to control your temper. It's worth considering: if you have an anger problem and you play violent video games, you may be making it worse.[65]

In one review study, consistent evidence was found that violent imagery in television, film, video and computer games has substantial short-term effects on thoughts and emotions, increasing the likelihood of fearful or aggressive behavior in younger children. This was found to be especially true in boys.[66]

Does this mean you should never play another video game or watch a movie for the rest of your life? For many teens in today's society this is unlikely; however, it is important for you to consider what your consumption of media may be doing to your mind. If you are in a constant state of checking social media sites, streaming videos or playing games, they are affecting you. There

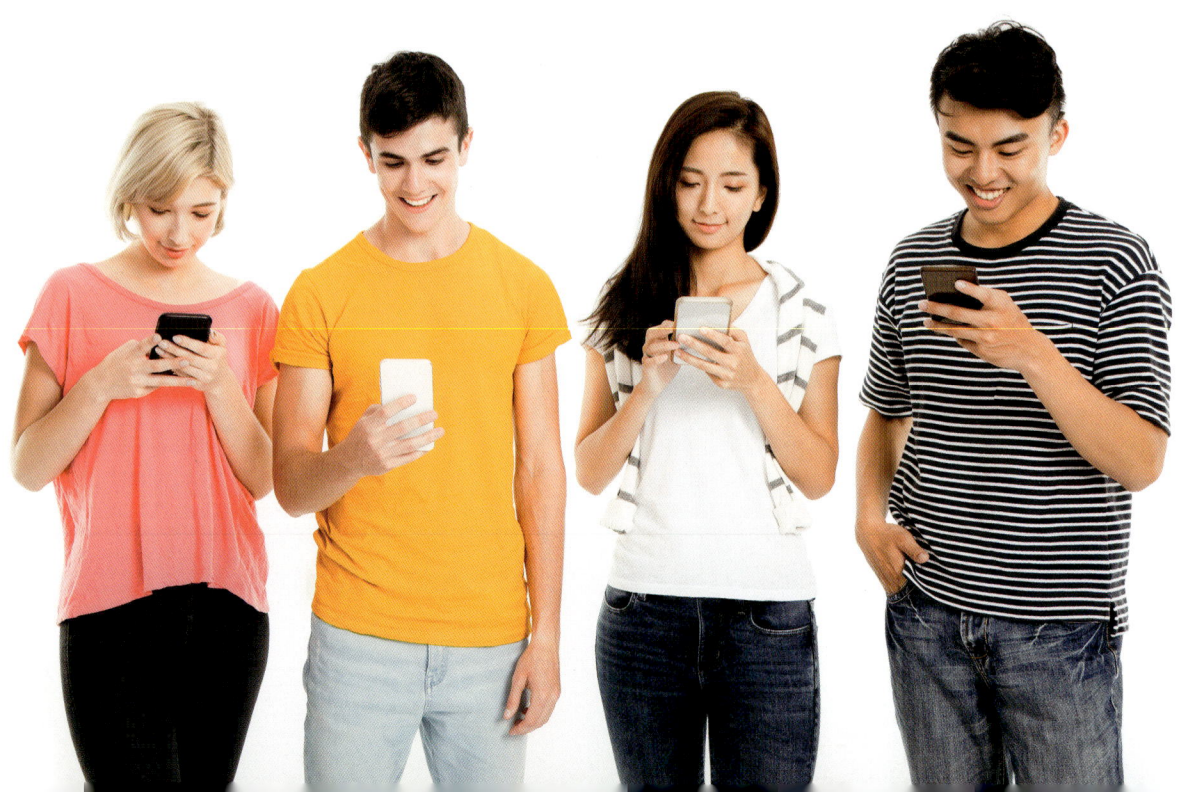

is even a risk of addiction. Dr. Michael Bengtson, professor and chief of child and adolescent psychiatry at the University of South Florida's Morsani College of Medicine, commented on the reality of social media addiction. "Addiction doesn't have to involve a substance or a drug. It can be a behavioral addiction, like gambling. That's where social media seems to fit in."[67] Bengston goes on to explain that interaction with social media activates the brain's reward center. People who are addicted to social media feel "gratification" when their posts or photos get lots of "likes." While this type of addiction may not be as destructive as alcohol or drug abuse, it can hinder your ability to establish meaningful personal relationships.[68]

Spending time in the virtual environment of media also means you are less aware of your natural environment. Nowadays, you don't have to look too far for an example. You've probably seen two people sitting across from each other in a restaurant, each of them typing away on their phones, seemingly unaware of the person in front of them. Don't let media control your life or lead you to lose track of the natural environment around you.

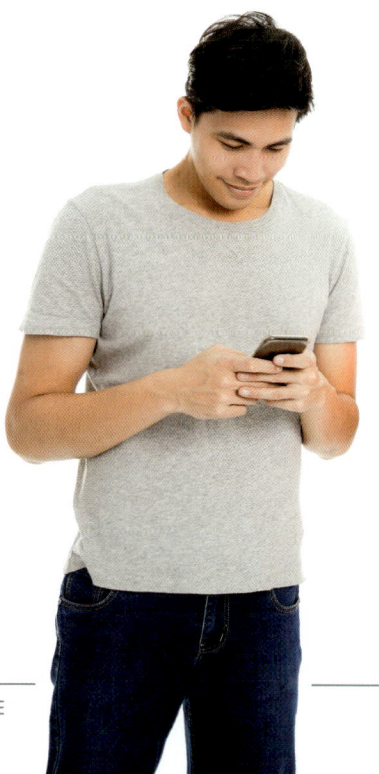

UNPLUG

If you think your environment may be oversaturated with media, here are a few tips to disconnect and get back to reality:

1. **Close your screens.** If you are using a computer for schoolwork, then keep the windows closed and try to focus on one thing at a time. You may also want to turn off your phone so you aren't tempted to check your notifications or messages. Don't worry. It will all still be there when you're done.

2. **Disable push notifications.** Devices have made it able for you to stay connected 24/7, but that also means a life of constant distractions. By turning off or limiting the notifications on your phone you can access media on your terms rather than letting it rule your life.

3. **Set a limit.** Can't go a minute without checking out the latest viral video? Then give yourself a daily time limit on all media. Tell yourself you'll spend no more than one-and-a-half to two hours a day with the media of your choice. And once your time is up, find something else to do.

4. **Shut it down.** Remember, you don't have to use media every day. In some situations, it might be better not to use it at all. If you're visiting with a friend, at a family meal or on a vacation, try shutting down all media completely. Engaging with the people and places around you will help to make those times more special.

SIGHTS

Your eyes see a wealth of information every day. This input will either help to promote your well-being or become a detriment to it. For example, it's often difficult for residents of some apartment complexes to find satisfaction with their living spaces. Cramped rooms and noisy neighbors can make apartment living a real challenge. But in one study, it was found that when residents living in an apartment complex could look out onto more natural settings as opposed to built settings, they had more satisfaction. This satisfaction was even greater when residents could see even a few trees than when their view was of large open spaces.[69] Just the sight of nature may positively impact your life and give you greater satisfaction.

Researchers have also documented that hospital patients with a view of trees outside their windows had shorter hospital stays... and took fewer analgesic medications than patients who had undergone the same operation but had a view of a brick wall outside their window.[70] Having windows that look out onto the beauty of nature has also been shown to reduce the need for healthcare services.[71]

In the inner city, residents of buildings with more landscaping get to know their neighbors better, socialize with them more, have stronger feelings of community and feel safer and better adjusted than residents who live in buildings with little or no vegetation.[72] Landscaping also reduced reports of property crime and violent crime in public housing developments.[73] Another study found that the levels of aggression and violence were significantly lower in areas near nature.[74] Residents are able to cope better with the demands of living in poverty; they feel more hopeful about the future, better able to manage their most important problems[75] and find greater satisfaction with the neighborhood when nature plays a significant role in their environment.[76] The enjoyable scenery[77-78] and the presence of hills are also associated with increased physical activity. Older people who are blessed to live near green open spaces tend to live longer.[79]

If you don't have access to a view of the natural world, then why not bring the natural world inside? Flowers and plants are a wonderfully easy way to enhance your environment and make any space more beautiful, but flowers go one step further by positively impacting your happiness as well. Two studies conducted at Rutgers University showed the incredible effect flowers have on your mood. In the first study, researchers found that upon receiving flowers, all study participants expressed "true" or "excited" smiles, demonstrating extraordinary delight and gratitude. This reaction was immediate, universal and occurred in all of the age groups who were studied.[80] The first study also found that flowers had a long-term positive effect on the participants' moods. Specifically, they reported feeling less depressed, anxious and agitated after receiving flowers. They also demonstrated

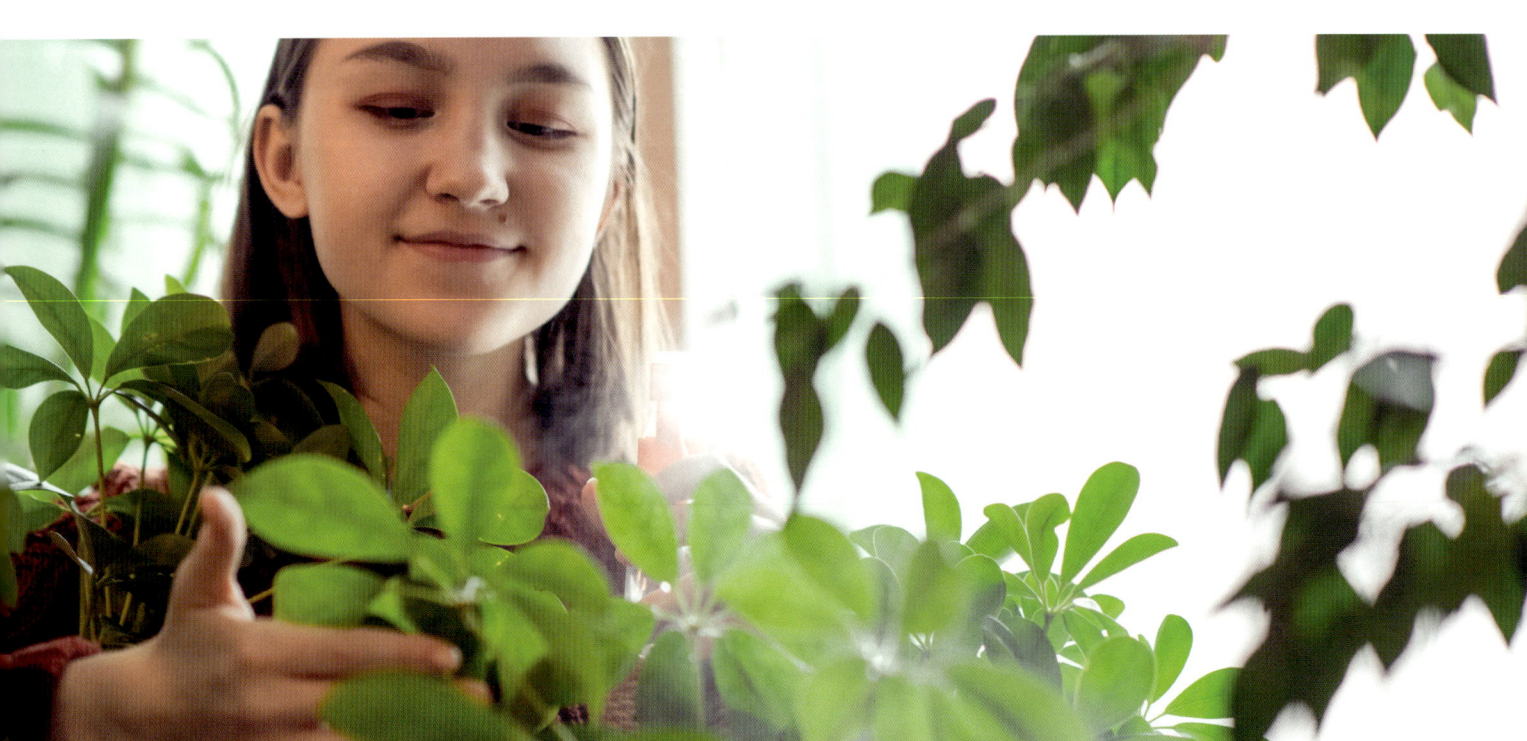

a higher sense of enjoyment and life satisfaction.[81] In the second Rutgers study, researchers discovered that flowers helped connect people; specifically, the presence of flowers led to increased contact with family and friends.[82]

You may not think flowers have much of a role in your daily life, but because society is increasingly more connected to technology, people's desires for the tranquility and stress relief brought about by nature has become even more popular. Research from Harvard looked at how flowers can be used effectively in day-to-day living. A behavioral research study conducted by Nancy Etcoff, PhD, of Harvard Medical School and Massachusetts General Hospital, found that people feel more compassionate toward others, have less worry and anxiety and feel less depressed when flowers are present in the home. "Other research has proven that flowers make people happy when they receive them," said Etcoff. "What we didn't know is that spending a few days with flowers in the home can affect a wide variety of feelings."[83]

Another Harvard study on the home ecology of flowers found that flowers help chase away anxieties and worries. Overall, participants in the study simply felt less negative after being around flowers at home for just a few days. The flowers were especially a pick-up in the morning when many people have a hard time getting going.[84]

These benefits were found to be true for plant owners as well. The average anxiety levels of individuals working in a building with plants was found to be lower than that of individuals working without plants.[85] Plants and flowers may also encourage you to think creatively. A Texas A&M University research team investigated one workplace and found that employees had an increase in innovative thinking, ideas and original solutions when their office environment included flowers and plants.[86] Your state of mind may often reflect the state of your environment.

If you feel overly stressed, try gazing upon the beauties of nature. Studies find that simply viewing a garden or other natural setting can quickly reduce blood pressure and pulse rate, and increase the brain activity that uplifts your mood.[87]

NATURAL AIR FRESHENERS

Research done by NASA shows that living, green and flowering plants remove several toxic chemicals from the air in building interiors. NASA found that the following eleven plants are the top picks for removing formaldehyde (found in virtually all indoor environments), benzene (a commonly used solvent that is present in many common items), and carbon monoxide from the air:

- Bamboo Palm
- Chinese Evergreen
- English Ivy
- Gerbera Daisy
- Janet Craig
- Marginata
- Mass Cane/Corn Plant
- Mother-in-Law's Tongue
- Pot Mum
- Peace Lily
- Warneckii

By enjoying these plants in your home, you will not only improve the quality of the air, but also make it a more pleasant environment in which to live.[88]

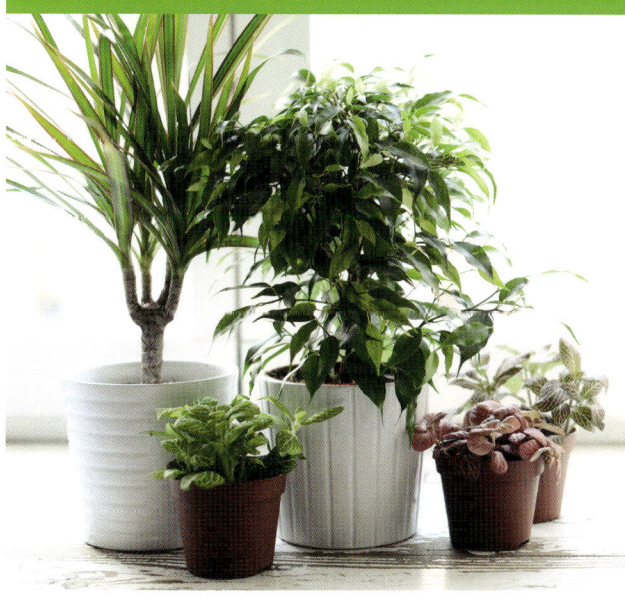

SOUNDS

Not only the sights you see, but the sounds you hear impact your health. Many times your environment is cluttered with the noise of ringing phones, chaotic conversations and blaring music. Chronic noise exposure, whether at high or low levels, has a harmful effect. Research shows noise elevates stress and decreases the level of your perceived quality of life.[89] Noise can also contribute to deficits in long-term memory, speech perception and standardized reading test scores.[90] Even low levels of noise can reduce your productivity.[91] The harmful effects of loud noise also include hearing loss (temporary and permanent) as well as increased blood pressure, decreased concentration and a negative effect on your mood.[92]

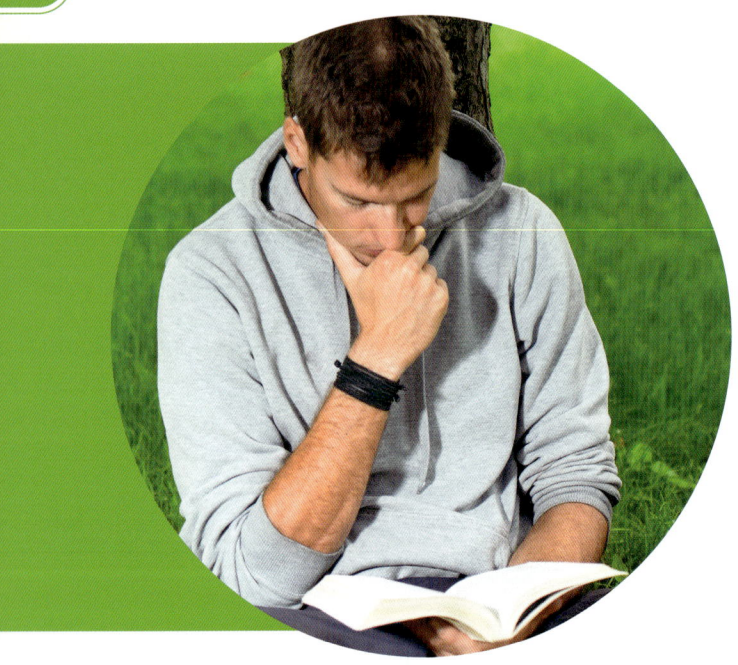

> "We need to find God, and He cannot be found in noise and restlessness. God is the friend of silence. See how nature — trees, flowers, grass — grows in silence; see the stars, the moon and the sun, how they move in silence... We need silence to be able to touch souls."
>
> MOTHER TERESA

Noisy environments can have serious repercussions. Take a normal classroom at school, for example. Julian Treasure — author, speaker and chairman of The Sound Agency — has pointed out that noisy classrooms are not only a great detriment to learning, but are also causing permanent hearing loss. The World Health Organization recommends a noise level of 35 decibels for classrooms. This is similar to the noise level in a library. However, one study found that the average noise volume in classrooms is 65 decibels. That's a level associated with permanent hearing loss. Treasure says that the speech intelligibility of a student sitting in the fourth row of a traditional classroom is just 50 percent. This means they only hear half of what their teacher says.[93]

Since noise pollution is so detrimental to your health, it makes sense to seek out environments that are as quiet and serene as possible. This is why many hospitals have recognized that a quiet environment is a healing environment. According to one report, patients complain twice as often about noise in hospitals as they do about any other part of their stay.[94] This has led hospitals like St. Charles Health in Bend, Oregon to make several adjustments in order to create quieter floors. "Quiet is also good for healing. As the noise level goes up, patients become anxious, which can lead to elevated heart rates and blood pressure. The physiological aspects of healing are impacted negatively by noise."[95]

One great example of how positive sounds impact your health is the numerous benefits related to singing. Research has shown that singing in a choir leads to increased positive emotional effects and increased function of the immune system. So, just joining a choir at school or church will not only help you feel better emotionally, but will also help your body to fight off disease and illness. Also, individuals who participate in singing lessons have increases in the hormone oxytocin. Oxytocin is responsible for the feelings of well-being associated with interacting with close friends. (You'll learn more about oxytocin in the Trust in God chapter). People who take singing lessons also feel more energetic and relaxed.[96] Researchers have also found that those who simply listen to choral music experience a decrease in the stress hormone cortisol.[97] If you're looking to feel less stressed, consider adding some choral works to your listening playlist.

Of course, you'll need a way to listen to that music. You'll probably reach for the nearest pair of headphones, and why not? Headphones are a popular accessory, and they let you hear your favorite songs whenever you want. But if you find yourself rocking out to really loud music on a regular basis, you may want to think twice before popping in those ear buds. Listening to music at high volumes for long periods of time can cause noise-induced hearing loss. This is a permanent, irreversible condition resulting from a one-time exposure to either a sound at or above 120 decibels or by listening to loud sounds at or above 85 decibels over an extended period of time.[98] Headphones and ear buds easily achieve this volume level, so it's best to limit your exposure and keep the volume low.

HEARING LOSS

Because the damage from noise exposure is usually gradual, you might not notice signs of hearing loss until more pronounced symptoms of permanent loss become evident. Noticeable signs of hearing loss can include the following:

- Muffled or distorted hearing

- Difficulty hearing sounds such as birds singing, crickets chirping, alarms, telephones or doorbells

- Difficulty understanding speech during telephone conversations or while participating in group conversations

- Pain or ringing in the ears after exposure to excessively loud sounds

If you experience any of these signs, see a doctor right away. The only accurate way to determine the extent and degree of hearing loss is through evaluation by an expert trained to test hearing (audiologist) or other qualified professional.[99]

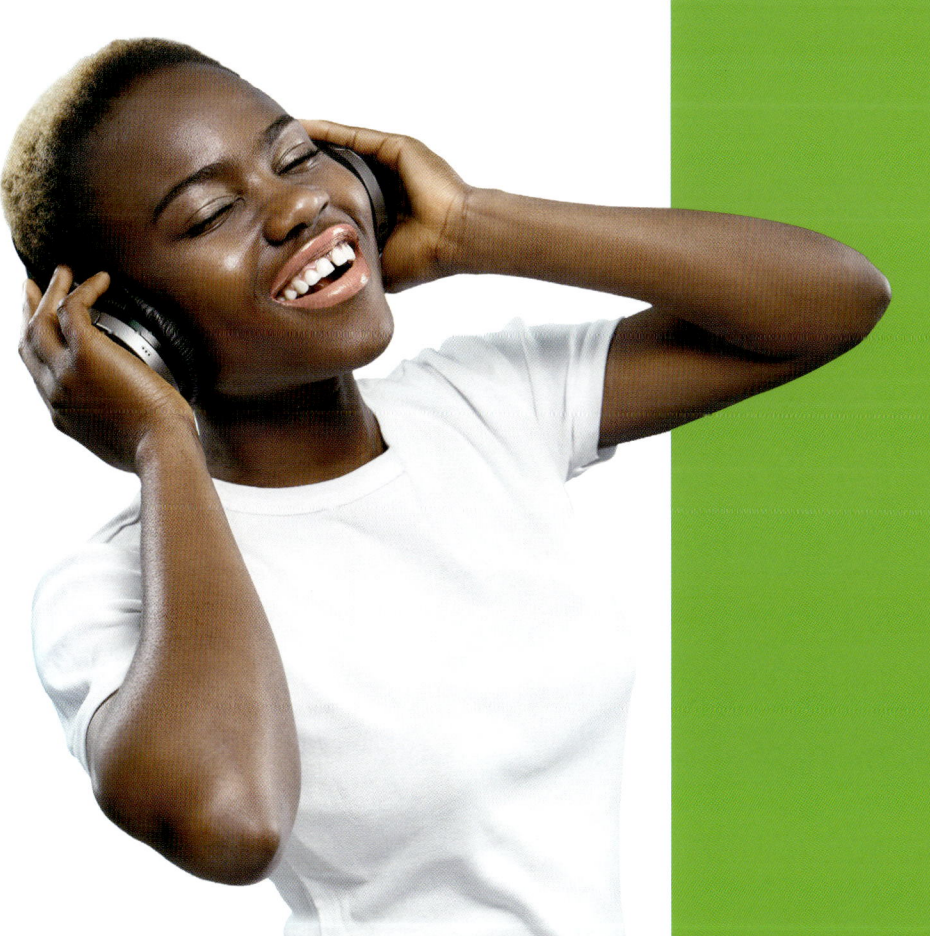

NATURAL REMEDIES

God has provided many powerful and healing agents in our natural environment. Everything, from the beauty you see in the world around you to the natural solutions that exist in plants, sunlight, water and minerals can help to heal you physically, mentally and spiritually.

Strong evidence also points to the healing benefits of herbs and other remedies readily available in nature — such as garlic, golden seal, tea tree oil and what some might call one of the best-kept secret in the world of healing — charcoal.

Now don't go breaking out that old bag of briquettes your dad keeps in the garage just yet. The kind of charcoal you need to look for is called "activated charcoal," and though it's similar to common charcoal, it's made especially for use as a medicine. Activated charcoal has the amazing ability to attract other substances to its surface and hold them there through the process of adsorption. This means it can adsorb many times its own weight in gases, heavy metals, poisons and other chemicals. Activated charcoal is often used in water filtration systems, but it has many medical uses as well. Many people use it to treat poisonings, reduce intestinal gas and lower cholesterol levels.[107] It is harmless and safe for internal use if used for short periods of time. Charcoal actually has the ability to draw harmful inflammatory toxins out of a wound, through the skin and into the bandage.[108]

Another healing remedy found in nature comes from a plant that has been used medicinally since the beginning of the First Century AD. Aloe vera is well-known for its use in treating burns,[109] but the aloe vera plant has other uses as well. Aloe vera can help in cancer treatment,[110] can increase the absorption of vitamins C and E[111] and is potentially helpful for wounds, edema and pain relief in diabetics.[112] It even improves the skin.[113]

SCENTS

Your sense of smell does a lot more than just alert you to the presence of freshly baked cinnamon rolls in your vicinity. You can use it to enhance your quality of life. The world is full of wonderful scents, many of which may have a powerful impact on you. Have you ever noticed how certain stores have their own particular smells? That's because retailers use special odors to trigger emotions and encourage customers to spend more money.[100] For instance, customers often smell the fragrance of pumpkin pie or evergreen trees as they shop for seasonal gifts or décor. Movie theater popcorn contains chemicals that allow its aroma to fill the theater, making you crave it even more.[101] Using scents in casinos has even been shown to increase gambling.[102] Even that famous "new car smell" is an artificial scent added to enhance a car buyer's satisfaction.[103]

Scents can also be used to keep people calm in stressful situations. London's Heathrow Airport has reportedly used the scent of pine needles to reduce stress and tension for its many passengers.[104] Another study examined patients who were going to a closed MRI scan. This type of scan occurs in a small space, and often participants feel claustrophobic. However, the researchers were able to reduce the overall anxiety of the patients by 63 percent by using a vanilla-like odor.[105] In contrast, bad odors have been found to make people more aggressive.[106]

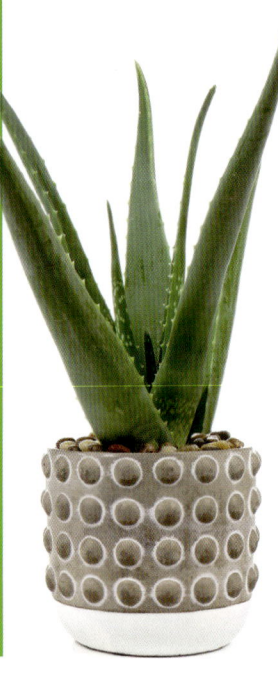

These examples show that your sense of smell has a powerful impact on your mindset and your mood. Smell can also affect your memory. This is because smell signals are projected into the emotion center of your brain. The field of aromatherapy uses this connection to enhance your sense of well-being. By understanding the power scents have in your life you can strive to enjoy the aromas of food, spices, nature or even taking time to literally "stop and smell the roses."

? Is your current environment helping you to grow spiritually? Do your surroundings draw you closer to God or make it harder to connect?

Your environment does not limit God's power or His presence. Jacob experienced God in the wilderness while sleeping on a rock for a pillow (Genesis 28:11–17). Jonah discovered in the belly of a great fish that God could still hear his prayers (Jonah 2:1). At the same time, God wants you to make an effort to seek Him. James 4:8 says, "Draw near to God and He will draw near to you." This means creating an environment where He is placed first and foremost in the center. God wants to be your main focus, not just of your environment but also of your entire life.

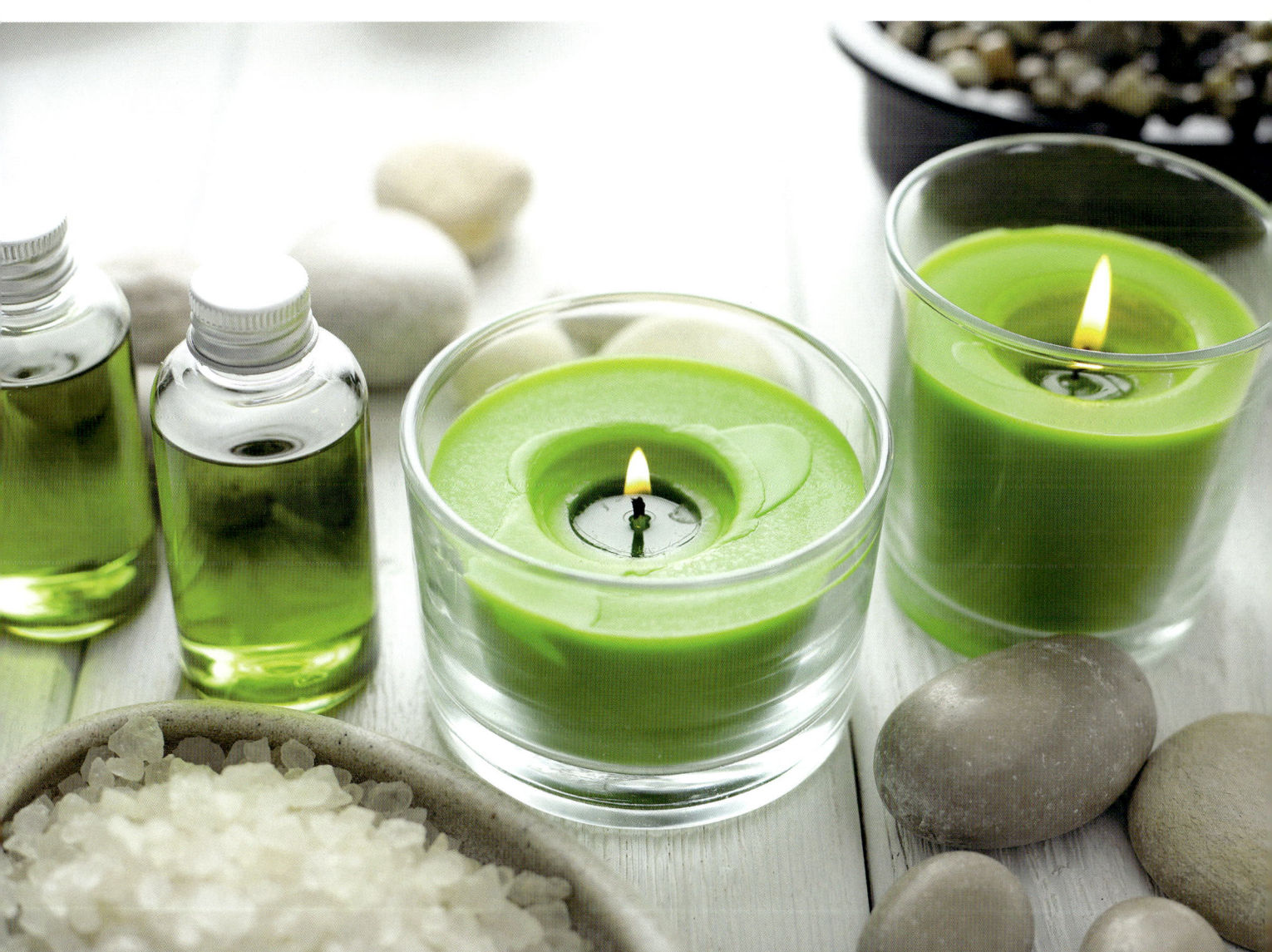

ENVIRONMENT ISSUES

When God created Adam and Eve, He gave them the following instructions:

Be fruitful and increase in number; fill the earth and subdue it. Rule over the fish in the sea and the birds in the sky and over every living creature that moves on the ground.

GENESIS 1:28

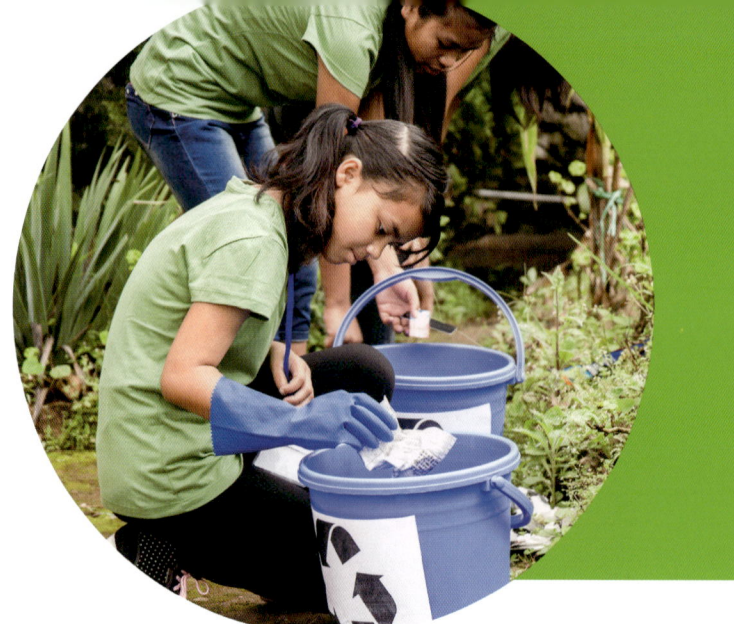

God gave humans the responsibility to rule over the earth and all of the creatures in it; however, some people have taken advantage of this gift. Today, the world is hurting from the overuse of natural resources and rampant pollution. God designed the natural environment to take care of you — to give you peace, tranquility, food, shelter and health — but He also designed you to take care of the environment. This is the God-given mandate humans have for taking care of the environment and for not abusing the wonderful gift God has given. The perfect way to think of your responsibilities is as a steward. A steward is a caretaker or guardian, one who has been placed into their position of power by someone else. Essentially, their job is to care for someone else's property.

The earth is the Lord's, and all it contains, The world, and those who dwell in it.

PSALM 24:1

Since the world and everything in it belongs to God, it makes sense to take stewardship very seriously. Being a careful steward of the environment isn't just the right thing to do for future generations; it's what God has created you to do. It's the job of a lifetime. As a steward of creation, you can make a tremendous difference in the world around you. Even the little things you do like recycling and repurposing add up and, over time, can make a huge difference in the world. Every action you take doesn't just impact your environment, it also impacts your health, your outlook and those around you.

GOING GREEN

So, how can you become a better steward of the world God has given you? An important first step is to think about everything you do in light of how it impacts your environment. For example, the next time you make a small purchase, say a bottle of water, try asking yourself, "Does this purchase help the environment or hurt it?" When it comes to the plastic in a water bottle, it may make more sense to buy a reusable bottle you can refill rather than a disposable one you may use only once. The truth is, in recent years humans have become much more wasteful. The most effective way to stop this trend is by preventing waste in the first place. Waste prevention is the practice of designing, manufacturing, purchasing or using materials (such as products and packaging) in ways that reduce the amount or toxicity of trash created."[114]

Waste is not just created when you throw something away. Throughout the entire life cycle of a product — from extraction of raw materials to transportation, to processing and manufacturing facilities, to manufacture and use — waste is generated. Reusing items or making them with less material can decrease waste in a big way. Ultimately, this means fewer materials will need to be recycled or sent to a landfill.

The benefits of preventing waste go beyond reducing reliance on other forms of waste disposal. It can also mean economic savings for communities, businesses, schools and you... the consumer.

RECYCLING

As you probably already know, recycling is a series of activities that includes collecting items that would otherwise be considered waste, sorting and processing them into raw materials and manufacturing the raw materials into new products. Collecting and processing secondary materials, manufacturing recycled-content products and then purchasing recycled products creates a loop that ensures the overall success and value of recycling.[115]

For recycling to work, everyone has to participate in each phase of the loop. From government and industry to organizations, small businesses and people at home, everyone needs to make recycling a part of their daily routine. You can recycle at home by finding out if there is a recycling program in your community. If so, participate in the program by separating and putting out your recyclables for curbside pickup or taking them to your local drop-off or buy-back center. You can also shop smarter by using products in containers that can be recycled in your community and items that can be repaired or reused. Also, support recycling efforts by buying and using products made from recycled materials.

REUSE

Reusing an item instead of throwing it away is always helpful to you and the environment. According to the Environmental Protection Agency (EPA), you can reuse items by repairing them, donating them to charity and community groups or selling them.[116] All of these are great ways to reduce waste. Try using a product more than once, either for the same purpose or for a different purpose, and if a product is strictly a "one-use" only item, consider buying something else. The EPA also says that reusing is preferable to recycling because items do not need to be reprocessed before they can be used again. "Ways to reuse would include refilling bottles, donating old books, magazines or surplus equipment, reusing boxes, turning empty jars into containers for leftover food, purchasing refillable pens and pencils, participating in a paint collection and reuse program."[117]

CREATING A SPIRITUAL ENVIRONMENT

"For in Him we live and move and have our being." ACTS 17:28

If your environment is everything that surrounds you and that you are constantly taking in through your five senses, then it stands to reason it will all have a huge impact on every area of your life, especially your spirituality. Everything that surrounds you is sending a message, and nothing in your environment is neutral.

You may find it easy to think about spiritual things when you are in a more spiritual environment such as church. But what about the rest of the week? Do you sense a connection to your Creator at school, at work and at home? If not, then you may need to take steps to create a more spiritual environment for yourself. For example, do you have a quiet place in your home where you can be alone and pray? It's very hard to focus your thoughts on prayer when you hear a loud television, music or conversation in the next room. Your mind will wander and you will have to work to keep from being distracted. If this sounds all too familiar, then you may want to follow the example of Jesus.

"Now in the morning, having risen a long while before daylight, He went out and departed to a solitary place; and there He prayed." MARK 1:35

Here you see Jesus getting up very early in the morning, going off by Himself, and praying to His Father. Jesus made it a point to find a "solitary place," free from distractions and interruptions, where He and God could have communion and fellowship. This is what creating a spiritual environment looks like.

What does your ideal spiritual environment look like? How can you place God at the center of everything?

REFERENCES

1. Kaplan, Rachel. "The Psychological Benefits of Nearby Nature." In *The Role of Horticulture in Human Well-being and Social Development*, edited by Diane Relf, 125-133. Arlington: Timber Press, 1992.

2. Kaplan, Stephen. "The Restorative Environment: Nature and Human Experience." In *The Role of Horticulture in Human Well-being and Social Development*, edited by Diane Relf, 134-142. Arlington: Timber Press, 1992.

3. Hartel, Dudley R. "Trees as Capital Assets." *City Trees* (2004): https://urbanforestrysouth. org/resources/library/ttresources/ TTResource.2004-12-08.4926.

4. Wells, Nancy M. and Gary W. Evans. "Nearby Nature: A Buffer of Life Stress Among Rural Children." *Environment and Behavior* 35, No. 3 (2003): 311-330. https://doi.org/10.1177/0013916503 035003001.

5. Lederbogen, Florian, Peter Kirsch, Leila Haddad, Fabian Streit, Heike Tost, Philipp Schuch, Stefan Wust, Jens C. Pruessner, Marcella Rietschel, Michael Deuschle, and Andreas Meyer-Linderberg. "City Living and Urban Upbringing Affect Neural Social Stress Processing in Humans." *Nature* 474, No. 7352 (2011): 498-501. https://doi.org/10.1038/ nature10190.

6. Jacobs, Keith W. and James F. Suess. "Effects of Four Psychological Primary Colors on Anxiety State." *Perceptual and Motor Skills* 41, no. 1 (1975): 207-210. https://doi.org/10.2466/pms.1975.41.1.207.

7. Wexner, Lois B. "The Degree to Which Colors (Hues) are Associated with Mood-tones." *Journal of Applied Psychology* 38, no. 6 (1954): 432-435. http://dx.doi.org/10.1037/h0062181.

8. Sherer, Paul. *The Benefits Of Parks: Why America Needs More City Parks And Open Space*. San Francisco: The Trust for Public Land, 2006. http:// eastshorepark.org/benefits_of_parks%20tpl.pdf.

9. *Healthy Housing Reference Manual*. Atlanta: U.S. Department of Health and Human Services, 2006. https://www.cdc.gov/nceh/publications/books/ housing/housing_ref_manual_2012.pdf.

10. Wallace, Lance A. "Total Exposure Assessment Methodology (TEAM) Study: Summary And Analysis. Volume 1." *Environmental Protection Agency. Washington, DC (USA): Office of Acid Deposition, Environmental Monitoring, and Quality Assurance* No. PB-88-100060/XAB; EPA-600/6-87/002A (1987): https://www.osti.gov/ biblio/5936245.

11. Linder, J., D. Herren, C. Monn, and H. U. Wanner. "Effect of Ozone on Physical Performance Capacity." *Sozial-und Praventivmedizin* 32, No. 4-5 (1987): 251-252.

12. American Family Physician. "Outdoor Air Pollution." Last modified March 15, 2001. https:// www.aafp.org/afp/2001/0315/p1221.html.

13. Medline Plus. "Seasonal Affective Disorder." Accessed September 19, 2013. http://www.nlm.nih. gov/medlineplus/seasonalaffectivedisorder.html.

14. Ibid.

15. Lambert, G. W., C. Reid, D. M. Kaye, G. L. Jennings, and M. D. Esler. "Effect of Sunlight and Season on Serotonin Turnover in the Brain." *The Lancet* 360, No. 9348 (2002): 1840-1842. https://doi. org/10.1016/S0140-6736(02)11737-5.

16. Ibid.

17. Kent, L., U. Doerry, E. Hardy, R. Parmar, K. Gingell, Z. Hawi, A. Kirley, N. Lowe, M. Fitzgerald, M. Gill, and N. Craddock. "Evidence That Variation at the Serotonin Transporter Gene Influences Susceptibility to Attention Deficit Hyperactivity Disorder (ADHD): Analysis and Pooled Analysis." *Molecular Psychiatry* 7, No. 8 (2002): 908-912. https://doi.org/10.1038/sj.mp.4001100.

18. Russo, Sascha, Ido P. Kema, Elizabeth B. Haagsma, Jim C. Boon, Pax HB Willemse, Johan A. den Boer, Elisabeth G.E. de Vries, and Jakob Korf. "Irritability Rather Than Depression During Interferon Treatment is Linked to Increased Tryptophan Catabolism." *Psychosomatic Medicine* 67, No. 5 (2005): 773-777. https://doi.org/10.1097/01. psy.0000171193.28044.d8..

19. Baldwin, D. and S. Rudge. "The Role of Serotonin in Depression and Anxiety." *International Clinical Psychopharmacology* 9, no. 4 (1995). 41-45. http:// dx.doi.org/10.1097/00004850-199501004-00006.

20. Coccaro, Emil F., Richard J. Kavoussi, Thomas B. Cooper, and Richard L. Hauger. "Central Serotonin Activity and Aggression: Inverse Relationship with Prolactin Response to D-Fenfluramine, but not CSF 5-HIAA Concentration, in Human Subjects." *The American Journal of Psychiatry* 154, No. 10 (1997): 1430-1435. https://doi.org/10.1176/ ajp.154.10.1430.

21. Baldwin, D. and S. Rudge. "The Role of Serotonin in Depression and Anxiety." *International Clinical Psychopharmacology* 9, no. 4 (1995): 41-45. http:// dx.doi.org/10.1097/00004850-199501004-00006.

22. Warner, Jennifer. "Seasonal Depression Tied to Serotonin." WebMD. Last modified September 19, 2007. https://www.webmd. com/mental-health/news/20070919/ seasonal-depression-tied-to-serotonin.

23. Sommer, Claudia. "Serotonin in Pain and Analgesia." *Molecular Neurobiology* 30, no. 2 (2004): 117-125. https://doi.org/10.1385/MN:30:2:117.

24. Davis, J. Mark, Nathan L. Alderson, and Ralph S. Welsh. "Serotonin and Central Nervous System Fatigue: Nutritional Considerations." *The American Journal of Clinical Nutrition* 72, no. 2 (2000): 573S-578S. https://doi.org/10.1093/ajcn/72.2.573S.

25. Grundy, David. "5-HT System in the Gut: Roles in the Regulation of Visceral Sensitivity and Motor Functions." *European Review for Medical and Pharmacological Sciences* 12, no. Suppl 1 (2008): 63-67. https://www.europeanreview.org/wp/wp-content/uploads/517.pdf.

26. Pigott, Teresa A. and Sheila M. Seay. "A Review of the Efficacy of Selective Serotonin Reuptake Inhibitors in Obsessive-Compulsive Disorder." *The Journal of Clinical Psychiatry* 60, no. 2 (1999): 101-106. http://dx.doi.org/10.4088/JCP.v60n0206.

27. Juhl, John H. "Fibromyalgia and the Serotonin Pathway." *Alternative Medicine Review* 3, no. 5 (1998): 367-375. http://www.altmedrev.com/archive/publications/3/5/367.pdf.

28. Kling, Anders, Solbritt Rantapää-Dahlqvist, Hans Stenlund, and Tom Mjörndal. "Decreased Density of Serotonin 5-HT2A Receptors in Rheumatoid Arthritis." *Annals of the Rheumatic Diseases* 65, no. 6 (2006): 816-819. http://dx.doi.org/10.1136/ard.2005.042473.

29. Sharpe, M., K. Hawton, A. Clements, and P. J. Cowen. "Increased Brain Serotonin Function in Men with Chronic Fatigue Syndrome." *BMJ* 315, no. 7101 (1997): 164-165. https://doi.org/10.1136/bmj.315.7101.164.

30. Bridge, Mathew W., Andrew S. Weller, Mark Rayson, and David A. Jones. "Responses to Exercise in the Heat Related to Measures of Hypothalamic Serotonergic and Dopaminergic Function." *European Journal of Applied Physiology* 89, no. 5 (2003): 451-459. https://doi.org/10.1007/s00421-003-0800-z.

31. Leibowitz, Sarah F. and Jesline T. Alexander. "Hypothalamic Serotonin in Control of Eating Behavior, Meal Size, and Body Weight." *Biological Psychiatry* 44, no. 9 (1998): 851-864. https://doi.org/10.1016/S0006-3223(98)00186-3.

32. Walch, Jeffrey M., Bruce S. Rabin, Richard Day, Jessica N. Williams, Krissy Choi, and James D. Kang. "The Effect of Sunlight on Postoperative Analgesic Medication Use: A Prospective Study of Patients Undergoing Spinal Surgery." *Psychosomatic Medicine* 67, no. 1 (2005): 156-163. https://doi.org/10.1097/01.psy.0000149258.42508.70.

33. Boubekri, Mohamed, Robert B. Hull, and Lester L. Boyer. "Impact of Window Size and Sunlight Penetration on Office Workers' Mood and Satisfaction: A Novel Way of Assessing Sunlight." *Environment and Behavior* 23, no. 4 (1991): 474-493. https://doi.org/10.1177/0013916591234004.

34. Heschong, Lisa. *Daylighting in Schools: Investigation into Relationship Between Daylighting and Human Performance: A Report to Pacific Gas and Electric Company.* Fair Oaks: Heschong Mahone Group, 1999. Accessed July 31, 2018. https://files.eric.ed.gov/fulltext/ED444337.pdf.

35. Stone, Nancy J. "Windows and Environmental Cues on Performance and Mood." *Environment and Behavior* 30, no. 3 (1998): 306-321. https://doi.org/10.1177/001391659803000303.

36. American Institutes of Research. "Effects of Outdoor Education Programs for Children in California." Accessed September 20, 2013. http://www.air.org/files/Outdoorschoolreport.pdf.

37. Lieberman, Gerald A. and Linda L. Hoody. *Closing the Achievement Gap: Using the Environment as an Integrating Context for Learning. Results of a Nationwide Study.* State Education and Environment Roundtable, 1998. https://files.eric.ed.gov/fulltext/ED428943.pdf.

38. Sigmundsdottir, Hekla, Junliang Pan, Gudrun F. Debes, Carsten Alt, Aida Habtezion, Dulce Soler, and Eugene C. Butcher. "DCs Metabolize Sunlight-Induced Vitamin D3 to 'Program' T Cell Attraction to the Epidermal Chemokine CCL27." *Nature Immunology* 8, no. 3 (2007): 285-293. https://doi.org/10.1038/ni1433.

39. Munger, Kassandra L., Lynn I. Levin, Bruce W. Hollis, Noel S. Howard, and Alberto Ascherio. "Serum 25-Hydroxyvitamin D levels and Risk of Multiple Sclerosis." *Journal of the American Medical Association* 296, no. 23 (2006): 2832-2838. https://doi.org/10.1001/jama.296.23.2832.

40. Merlino, Linda A., Jeffrey Curtis, Ted R. Mikuls, James R. Cerhan, Lindsey A. Criswell, and Kenneth G. Saag. "Vitamin D Intake is Inversely Associated with Rheumatoid Arthritis: Results from the Iowa Women's Health Study." *Arthritis & Rheumatology* 50, no. 1 (2004): 72-77. https://doi.org/10.1002/art.11434.

41. Hyppönen, Elina, Esa Läärä, Antti Reunanen, Marjo-Riitta Järvelin, and Suvi M. Virtanen. "Intake of Vitamin D and Risk of Type 1 Diabetes: A Birth-Cohort Study." *The Lancet* 358, no. 9292 (2001): 1500-1503. https://doi.org/10.1016/S0140-6736(01)06580-1.

42. Holick, Michael F. "Vitamin D Deficiency." *The New England Journal of Medicine* 357, no. 3 (2007): 266-281. https://doi.org/10.1056/NEJMra070553.

43. Fiori, G., F. Facchini, D. Pettener, A. Rimondi, N. Battistini, and G. Bedogni. "Relationships Between Blood Pressure, Anthropometric Characteristics and Blood Lipids in High- and Low-Altitude Populations from Central Asia." *Annals of Human Biology* 27, no. 1 (2000): 19-28. https://doi.org/10.1080/030144600282343.

44. Rostand, Stephen G. "Ultraviolet Light May Contribute to Geographic and Racial Blood Pressure Differences." *Hypertension* 30, no. 2 (1997): 150-156. https://doi.org/10.1161/01.HYP.30.2.150.

45. Giovannucci, Edward, Yan Liu, and Walter C. Willett. "Cancer Incidence and Mortality and Vitamin D in Black and White Male Health Professionals." *Cancer Epidemiology, Biomarkers and Prevention* 15, no. 12 (2006): 2467-2472. https://doi.org/10.1158/1055-9965.EPI-06-0357.

46. Garland, Cedric F., Frank C. Garland, Eddie Ko Shaw, George W. Comstock, Knud J. Helsing, and Edward D. Gorham. "Serum 25-Hydroxyvitamin D and Colon Cancer: Eight-Year Prospective Study." *The Lancet* 334, no. 8673 (1989): 1176-1178. https://doi.org/10.1016/S0140-6736(89)91789-3.

47. Berwick, Marianne, Bruce K. Armstrong, Leah Ben-Porat, Judith Fine, Anne Kricker, Carey Eberle, and Raymond Barnhill. "Sun Exposure and Mortality from Melanoma." *Journal of the National Cancer Institute* 97, no. 3 (2005): 195-199. https://doi.org/10.1093/jnci/dji019.

48. Ainsleigh, H. Gordon. "Beneficial Effects of Sun Exposure on Cancer Mortality." *Preventive Medicine* 22, no. 1 (1993): 132-140. https://doi.org/10.1006/pmed.1993.1010.

49. Felsten, Gary. "Where to Take a Study Break on the College Campus: An Attention Restoration Theory Perspective." *Journal of Environmental Psychology* 29, no. 1 (2009): 160-167. https://doi.org/10.1016/j.jenvp.2008.11.006.

50. Berman, Marc G., John Jonides, and Stephen Kaplan. "The Cognitive Benefits of Interacting with Nature." *Psychological Science* 19, no. 12 (2008): 1207-1212. https://doi.org/10.1111/j.1467-9280.2008.02225.x.

51. Ibid.

52. Jonides, John, Richard L. Lewis, Derek Evan Nee, Cindy A. Lustig, Marc G. Berman, and Katherine Sledge Moore. "The Mind and Brain of Short-Term Memory." *Annual Review Psychology* 59 (2008): 193-224. https://doi.org/10.1146/annurev.psych.59.103006.093615.

53. Diamond, Adele, W. Steven Barnett, Jessica Thomas, and Sarah Munro. "Preschool Program Improves Cognitive Control." *Science* 318, no. 5855 (2007): 1387.

54. Tennessen, Carolyn M. and Bernadine Cimprich. "Views to Nature: Effects on Attention." *Journal of Environmental Psychology* 15, no. 1 (1995): 77-85. https://doi.org/10.1016/0272-4944(95)90016-0.

55. Ibid.

56. Taylor, Andrea Faber, Frances E. Kuo, and William C. Sullivan. "Coping with ADD: The Surprising Connection to Green Play Settings." *Environment and Behavior* 33, no. 1 (2001): 54-77. https://doi.org/10.1177/00139160121972864.

57. Oxford Brookes University. "Impact of Workplace Plants On: Perception and Use of Planted Space." Accessed February 1, 2009. http://greenplantsforgreenbuildings.org/pdf/perception.pdf.

58. Barton, Jo and Jules Pretty. "What is the Best Dose of Nature and Green Exercise for Improving Mental Health? A Multi-Study Analysis." *Environmental Science & Technology* 44, no. 10 (2010): 3947-3955. https://doi.org/10.1021/es903183r.

59. Environmental Protection Agency. "Indoor Air Pollution: An Introduction for Health Professionals" Accessed October 21, 2013. https://www.epa.gov/sites/production/files/2015-01/documents/indoor_air_pollution.pdf.

60. Ryan, Terri Jo. "Reducing Workplace Clutter Might Just Lead to That Promotion." Seattle Post-Intelligencer. Last modified August 14, 2005. http://www.seattlepi.com/business/article/Reducing-workplace-clutter-might-justlead-to-1180595.php.

61. Zuckerman, Diana M. and Barry S. Zuckerman. "Television's Impact on Children." *Pediatrics* 75, no. 2 (1985): 233-240.

62. Johnston, Wendy M. and Graham C. L. Davey. "The Psychological Impact of Negative TV News Bulletins: The Catastrophizing of Personal Worries." *British Journal of Psychology* 88, no. 1 (1997): 85-91. https://doi.org/10.1111/j.2044-8295.1997.tb02622.x.

63. Kaiser Family Foundation. "Generation M2: Media in the Lives of 8- to 18-Year-Olds." Last modified January 20, 2010. https://www.kff.org/other/event/generation-m2-media-in-the-lives-of/.

64. Weber, René, Ute Ritterfeld, and Klaus Mathiak. "Does Playing Violent Video Games Induce Aggression? Empirical Evidence of a Functional Magnetic Resonance Imaging Study." *Media Psychology* 8, no. 1 (2006): 39-60. https://doi.org/10.1207/S1532785XMEP0801_4.

65. Giumetti, Gary W. and Patrick M. Markey. "Violent Video Games and Anger as Predictors of Aggression." *Journal of Research in Personality* 41, no. 6 (2007): 1234-1243. https://doi.org/10.1016/j.jrp.2007.02.005.

66. Browne, Kevin D. and Catherine Hamilton-Giachritsis. "The Influence Of Violent Media On Children And Adolescents: A Public-Health Approach." *The Lancet* 365 no. 9460 (2005): 702-710. doi:10.1016/s0140-6736(05)17952-5.

67. Maher, Irene. "Social Media Can Become an Addiction, But You Can Break Free." Tampa Bay Times. Last modified July 25, 2013. http://www.tampabay.com/news/health/social-media-can-become-an-addiction-but-you-can-break-free/2133164.

68. Ibid.

69. Kaplan, Rachel. *Behavior and the Natural Environment*. Boston: Springer, 1983. https://doi.org/10.1007/978-1-4613-3539-9_5.

70. Ulrich, Roger S. "View Through a Window May Influence Recovery from Surgery." *Science* 224, no. 4647 (1984): 420-421. https://doi.org/10.1126/science.6143402.

71. Moore, Ernest O. "A Prison Environment's Effect on Healthcare Service Demands." *Journal of Environmental Systems* 11, no. 1 (1981): 17-34. https://doi.org/10.2190/KM50-WH2K-K2D1-DM69.

72. Kuo, Frances E., et al., "Fertile Ground for Community: Inner-City Neighborhood Common Spaces." *American Journal of Community Psychology* 26, no. 6 (1998): 823–851. http://illinois-online.org/krassa/ps450/Readings/Kuo%20Fertile%20Ground%20Innercity%20Common%20Space.pdf.

73. Kuo, Frances E. and William C. Sullivan. "Environment and Crime in the Inner City: Does Vegetation Reduce Crime?." *Environment and Behavior* 33, no. 3 (2001): 343-367. https://doi.org/10.1177/0013916501333002.

74. Kuo, Frances E. and William C. Sullivan. "Aggression and Violence in the Inner City: Effects of Environment via Mental Fatigue." *Environment and Behavior* 33, no. 4 (2001): 543-571. https://doi.org/10.1177/00139160121973124.

75. Kuo, Frances E. "Coping with Poverty: Impacts of Environment and Attention in the Inner City." *Environment and Behavior* 33, no. 1 (2001): 5-34. https://doi.org/10.1177/00139160121972846.

76. Kaplan, Rachel. *Behavior and the Natural Environment*. Boston: Springer, 1983. https://doi.org/10.1007/978-1-4613-3539-9_5.

77. King, Abby C., Cynthia Castro, Sara Wilcox, Amy A. Eyler, James F. Sallis, and Ross C. Brownson. "Personal and Environmental Factors Associated with Physical Inactivity Among Different Racial–Ethnic Groups of U.S. Middle-Aged and Older-Aged Women." *Health Psychology* 19, no. 4 (2000): 354-364. https://doi.org/10.1037/0278-6133.19.4.354.

78. Humpel, Nancy, Neville Owen, and Eva Leslie. "Environmental Factors Associated with Adults' Participation in Physical Activity: A Review." *American Journal of Preventive Medicine* 22, no. 3 (2002): 188-199. https://doi.org/10.1016/S0749-3797(01)00426-3.

79. Takano, Takehito, Keiko Nakamura, and Masafumi Watanabe. "Urban Residential Environments and Senior Citizens' Longevity in Megacity Areas: The Importance of Walkable Green Spaces." *Journal of Epidemiology & Community Health* 56, no. 12 (2002): 913-918. http://dx.doi.org/10.1136/jech.56.12.913.

80. Haviland-Jones, Jeannette, Holly Hale Rosario, Patricia Wilson, and Terry R. McGuire. "An Environmental Approach to Positive Emotion: Flowers." *Evolutionary Psychology* 3, no. 1 (2005). https://doi.org/10.1177/147470490500300109.

81. Ibid.

82. Ibid.

83. Etcoff, Nancy. "Harvard Study Investigates the Home Ecology of Flowers." Harvard University. Accessed March 21, 2008. http://www.steppingstonesmentalhealth.com/energyequation/docs/Ecology_of_Flowers.pdf.

84. Ibid.

85. Oxford Brookes University. "Impact of Workplace Plants On: Perception and Use of Planted Space." Accessed September 23, 2013. http://greenplantsforgreenbuildings.org/pdf/perception.pdf.

86. Chalquist, Craig. "A Look at the Ecotherapy Research Evidence." *Ecopsychology* 1, no 2. (2009): https://doi.org/10.1089/eco.2009.0003.com/health-benefits-a-research/workplace-productivity-study.html.

87. Ulrich, Roger S., Robert F. Simons, Barbara D. Losito, Evelyn Fiorito, Mark A. Miles, and Michael Zelson. "Stress Recovery During Exposure to Natural and Urban Environments." *Journal of Environmental Psychology* 11, no. 3 (1991): 201-230. https://doi.org/10.1016/S0272-4944(05)80184-7.

88. Wolverton, B. C., Anne Johnson, and Keith Bounds. *Interior Landscape Plants for Indoor Air Pollution Abatement*. John C. Space Center: National Aeronautics and Space Administration, 1989. Accessed July 24, 2018. https://ntrs.nasa.gov/archive/nasa/casi.ntrs.nasa.gov/19930073077.pdf.

89. Evans, Gary W., Monika Bullinger, and Staffan Hygge. "Chronic Noise Exposure and Physiological Response: A Prospective Study of Children Living Under Environmental Stress." *Psychological Science* 9, no. 1 (1998): 75-77. https://doi.org/10.1111/1467-9280.00014.

90. Evans, Gary W. and Lorraine Maxwell. "Chronic Noise Exposure and Reading Deficits: The Mediating Effects of Language Acquisition." *Environment and Behavior* 29, no. 5 (1997): 638-656. https://doi.org/10.1177/0013916597295003.

91. Evans, Gary W. and Dana Johnson. "Stress and Open-Office Noise." *Journal of Applied Psychology* 85, no. 5 (2000): 779-783. https://doi.org/10.1037/0021-9010.85.5.779.

92. Van Kempen, Elise E. M. M., Hanneke Kruize, Hendriek C. Boshuizen, Caroline B. Ameling, Brigit A. M. Staatsen, and Augustinus E. M. de Hollander. "The Association Between Noise Exposure and Blood Pressure and Ischemic Heart Disease: A Meta-Analysis." *Environmental Health Perspectives* 110, no. 3 (2002): 307-317. https://www.ncbi.nlm.nih.gov/pmc/articles/PMC1240772/pdf/ehp0110-000307.pdf.

93. Kate Torgovnick May, April 24, 2013 (4:28 p.m.), 9 Ways That Sound Affects Our Health, Wellbeing and Productivity," *TED Blog*, https://blog.ted.com/9-ways-that-sound-affects-our-health-wellbeing-and-productivity/.

94. "A Quiet Environment is a Healing Environment," *Flourish* 17, no. 4 (2012): 5, https://www.stcharleshealthcare.org/~/media/Files/Flourish/flourishwinter2012.pdf.

95. Ibid.

96. Grape, Christina, Maria Sandgren, Lars-Olof Hansson, Mats Ericson, and Töres Theorell. "Does Singing Promote Well-Being?: An Empirical Study of Professional and Amateur Singers During a Singing Lesson." *Integrative Physiological & Behavioral Science* 38, no. 1 (2002): 65-74. https://doi.org/10.1007/BF02734261.

97. Kreutz, Gunter, Stephan Bongard, Sonja Rohrmann, Volker Hodapp, and Dorothee Grebe. "Effects of Choir Singing or Listening on Secretory Immunoglobulin A, Cortisol, and Emotional State." *Journal of Behavioral Medicine* 27, no. 6 (2004): 623-635. https://doi.org/10.1007/s10865-004-0006-9.

98. Centers for Disease Control and Prevention. "What Noises Cause Hearing Loss?" Last modified February 26, 2017. https://www.cdc.gov/nceh/hearing_loss/what_noises_cause_hearing_loss.html.

99. Ibid.

100. Ravin, Karen. "Sniff... And Spend." Los Angeles Times. Last modified August 20, 2007. http://articles.latimes.com/2007/aug/20/health/he-smell20.

101. Strauss, Ilana. "13 Things a Movie Theater Employee Won't Tell You." Reader's Digest. Accessed October 21, 2013. https://www.rd.com/advice/saving-money/13-things-a-movie-theater-employee-wont-tell-you/.

102. Hirsch, Alan R. "Effects of Ambient Odors on Slot Machine Usage in a Las Vegas Casino." *Psychology & Marketing* 12, no. 7 (1995): 585-594. https://doi.org/10.1002/mar.4220120703.

103. Lindstrom, Martin. "Broad Sensory Branding." *Journal of Product & Brand Management* 14, no. 2 (2005): 84-87. https://doi.org/10.1108/10610420510592554.

104. Brumfield, C. Russell, James Goloney, and Stephanie Gunning. *Whiff. The Revolution Of Scent Communication In The Information Age*. New York: Quimby Press, 2008.

105. Redd, William H., Sharon L. Manne, Bruce Peters, Paul B. Jacobsen, and Hilary Schmidt. "Fragrance Administration to Reduce Anxiety During MR Imaging." *Journal of Magnetic Resonance Imaging* 4, no. 4 (1994): 623-626. https://doi.org/10.1002/jmri.1880040419.

106. Rotton, James, James Frey, Timothy Barry, Michael Milligan, and Michael Fitzpatrick. "The Air Pollution Experience and Physical Aggression." *Journal of Applied Social Psychology* 9, no. 5 (1979): 397-412. https://doi.org/10.1111/j.1559-1816.1979.tb02714.x.

107. WebMD. "Activated Charcoal." Accessed October 21, 2013. http://www.webmd.com/vitamins-supplements/ingredientmono-269-ACTIVATED%20CHARCOAL.aspx?activeIngredientId=269&activeIngredientName=ACTIVATED%20CHARCOAL.

108. Beckett, R., T. J. Coombs, M. R. Frost, J. McLeish, and K. Thompson. "Charcoal Cloth and Malodorous Wounds." *The Lancet* 316, no. 8194 (1980): 594. https://doi.org/10.1016/S0140-6736(80)92031-0.

109. Mayo Clinic. "Aloe." Accessed April 13, 2009. https://www.mayoclinic.org/drugs-supplements-aloe/art-20362267.

110. Lissoni, Paolo, Luisa Giani, Stanislao Zerbini, Patrizia Trabattoni, and Franco Rovelli. "Biotherapy with the Pineal Immunomodulating Hormone Melatonin Versus Melatonin Plus Aloe Vera in Untreatable Advanced Solid Neoplasms." *Natural Immunity* 16, no. 1 (1998): 27-33. https://doi.org/10.1159/000069427.

111. Vinson, Joe A., Hassan Al Kharrat, and Lori Andreoli. "Effect of Aloe Vera Preparations on the Human Bioavailability of Vitamins C and E." *Phytomedicine* 12, no. 10 (2005): 760-765. https://doi.org/10.1016/j.phymed.2003.12.013.

112. Reynolds, T. and A. C. Dweck. "Aloe Vera Leaf Gel: A Review Update". *Journal Of Ethnopharmacology* 68, no 1-3 (1999): 3-37. https://doi.org/10.1016/s0378-8741(99)00085-9.

113. Danhof, Ivan E. and B. H. McAnalley. "Stabilized Aloe Vera, Its Effect on Human Skin Cells." *Drugs in the Cosmetic Industry* 133, no. 2 (1983): 52.

114. Upper Valley Lake Sunapee Regional Planning Committee. "Reduce, Reuse, Upcycle..." Waste Management. Accessed September 19, 2018. http://waste.uvlsrpc.org/reduce-reuse/.

115. United States Environmental Protection Agency. "Recycling Basics." Last modified August 1, 2018. https://www.epa.gov/recycle/recycling-basics.

116. Arlingtonva.us. "Reduce & Reuse." Trash & Recycling. Accessed September 20, 2018. https://recycling.arlingtonva.us/residential/trash-recycling/reduce-reuse/.

117. Ibid.

> *"Nature is the art of God."*
>
> DANTE ALIGHIERI

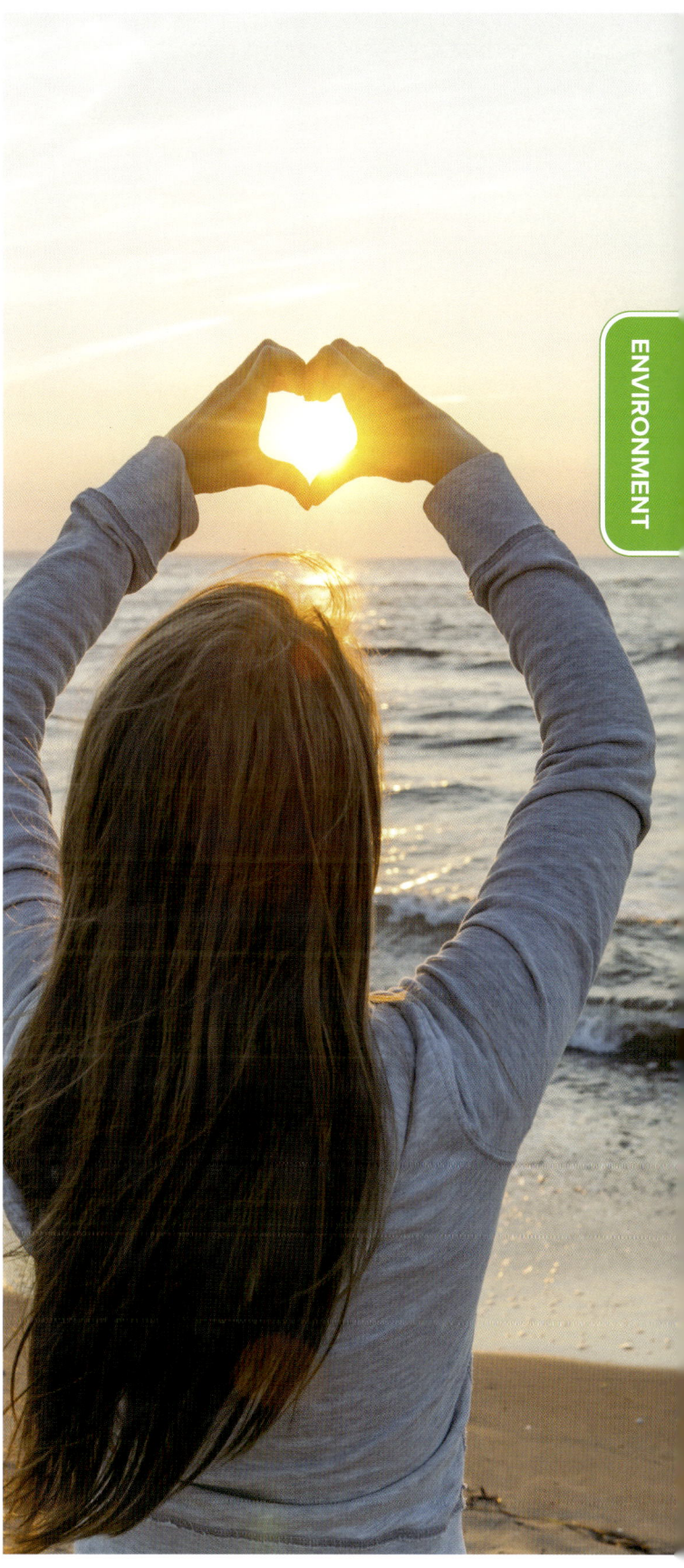

ENVIRONMENT

NOTES

ACTIVITY

Move your body, work your mind

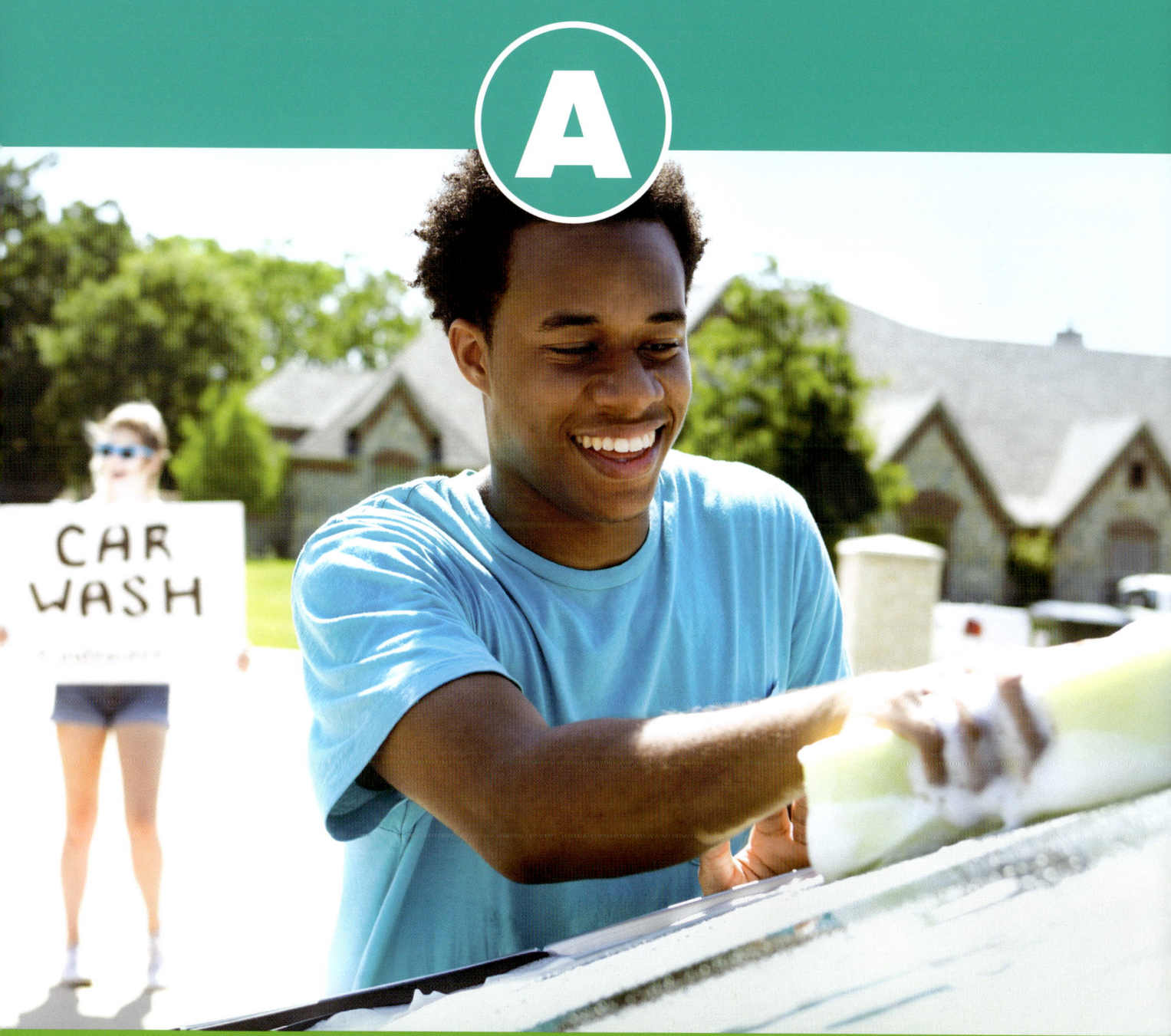

ACTIVITY [ak-tiv-i-tee] *noun* **1:** the movement of your body and the development of your mind. Exercising both can keep you alert and energized.

THE BIG PICTURE

If you're looking to get in shape, you have a lot of options available. Health clubs, exercise programs and even the latest fitness gadgets all promise big results. They tempt you with incredible before and after pictures — models with muscular bodies staring right into your eyes as if to say, "You can look just like me." The draw is so strong that when it comes to getting fit, people are willing to shell out some major bucks. How much? Enough to make fitness a multibillion-dollar industry, or as one article put it, "The fitness industry is in good shape."[1] In 2016, there were about 36,000 membership-based exercise facilities in the U.S. with 57.25 million members.[2] Sure that's a lot of sweatbands, but even though millions are members of health clubs, the population as a whole has never been unhealthier. From 1980 to 2008, the percentage of adolescents ages 12 to 19 who were obese more than tripled, increasing from five to 18 percent.[3] What's to blame for such a radical change that's left a third of American children and adolescents overweight or obese? It all comes down to keeping healthy lifestyle habits — not just eating healthy, but also getting plenty of physical activity.[4]

ACTIVITY includes both mental and physical movement and development. The mind and body are intimately connected. A fit mind promotes a fit body, and a fit body promotes a fit mind.

Activity is the fourth principle of CREATION Life. Exercise is a crucial part of having and maintaining an abundant life, but developing your body is only half the battle. You must also learn to develop and strengthen your mind. Mental activity should be as much a part of your routine as lifting weights or running laps. In fact, the mind and body are intimately connected to each other and as you will see, building up one helps to build up the other. In other words, you will get the best performance from your mind when you regularly exercise your body, and your body will be stronger when you regularly exercise your mind.

This section will encourage you to make physical and mental activities a greater part of your daily life by showing you the amazing benefits found in an active lifestyle. You will also explore the link between mental and physical activities and see how each one influences and enhances the other.

If you are not very physically or mentally active at this point in your life, don't worry. You'll soon see that getting more activity doesn't require a huge time commitment in order for you to benefit. For example, you can add plenty of physical activity to your life by just walking a little each day. According to the American Heart Association, just 30 minutes of walking a day will reduce your risk of heart disease. Studies show that for every hour of walking you do, your life expectancy may increase by two hours.[5]

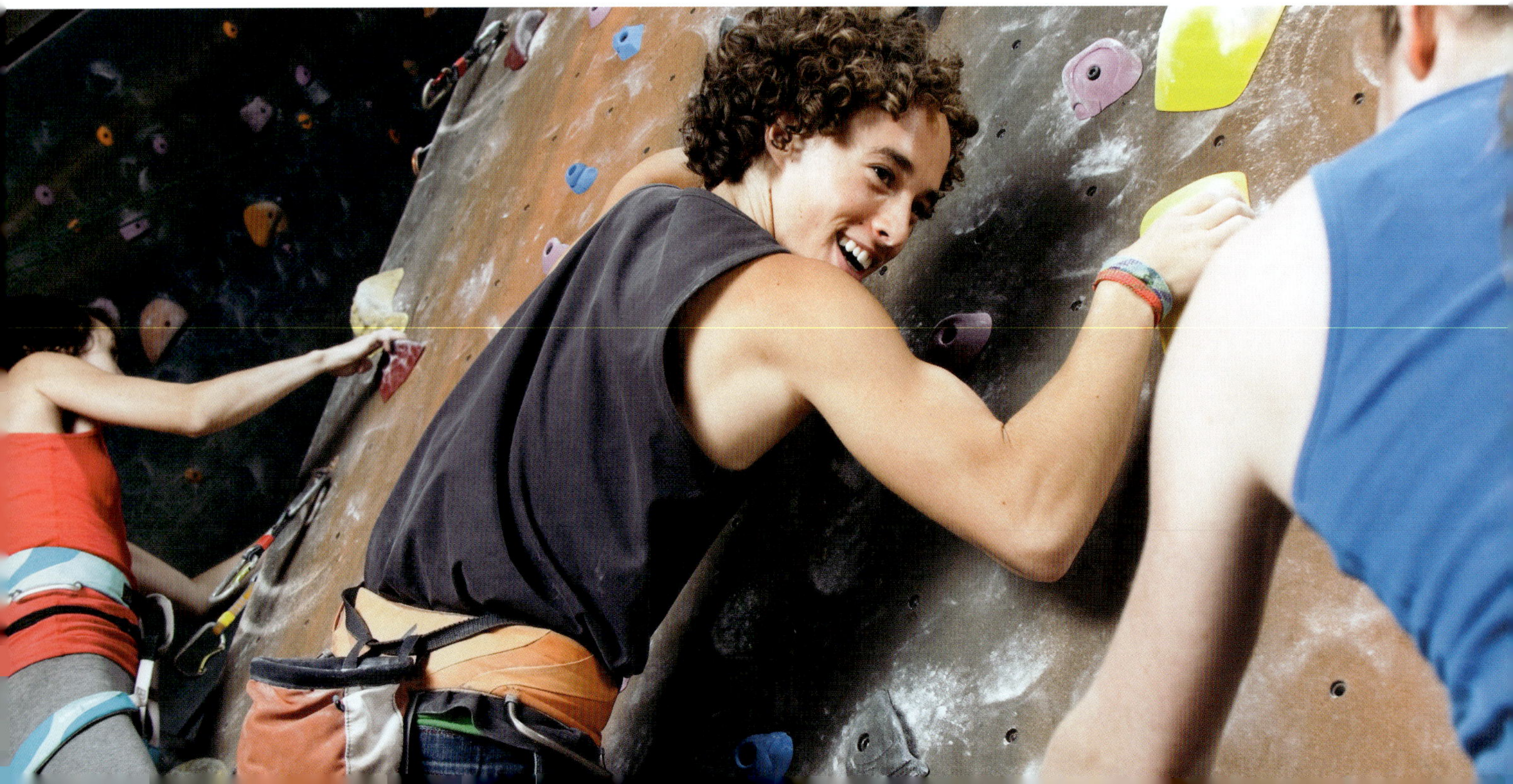

THE GIFT OF ACTIVITY

Then the Lord God took the man and put him into the garden of Eden to cultivate it and keep it. GENESIS 2:15

In the Bible's creation story, God placed Adam in the Garden of Eden with an active role. He was to "cultivate it and keep it." To "cultivate" something means to nurture and help it grow. To "keep" something means to watch over and protect it from harm. So, from the very beginning, Adam was quite active in Eden. He had a God-given task to perform daily as he helped the trees and plants to flourish. Even in paradise, there was work to be done.

Does this strike you as strange? After all, for many people the word "work" has negative connotations. Americans spend most of their days "at work," they can't wait to get "off work" and they even call exercising "working out." Ask someone to describe paradise and you'll most likely get images of lying on a tropical beach as far away from work as possible. But the Bible describes paradise as something quite different.

God created Adam with a purpose. Part of that purpose included work or staying active. Activity wasn't something that entered the world because of sin. It was always a part of God's plan. It didn't interfere with life; quite the contrary, it helped to make life worth living. When Adam dug his hands into the earth, pruned the trees of the garden or brought water to the plants, he was doing what God had created him to do. Adam was meant to take delight in his work, not view it as drudgery or as another mindless chore. Work was created to be a joy.

What is your personal view of work? Do you see it as a God-given gift or a "necessary evil" of life?

By enjoying his work, Adam was truly reflecting the image of God. God was the first workman, creating the world and all that was in it, and God delighted in the work of His hands. He saw how wonderful and incredible it was. And Adam, made in the image of God, was created to share those same feelings.

Your purpose in life includes being active. When done in connection with God's power, it's an energizing experience, a thrill ride that leaves you wanting more. God has a mission for you. Will you accept it? Will you live an active life and embrace work?

ACTIVITY

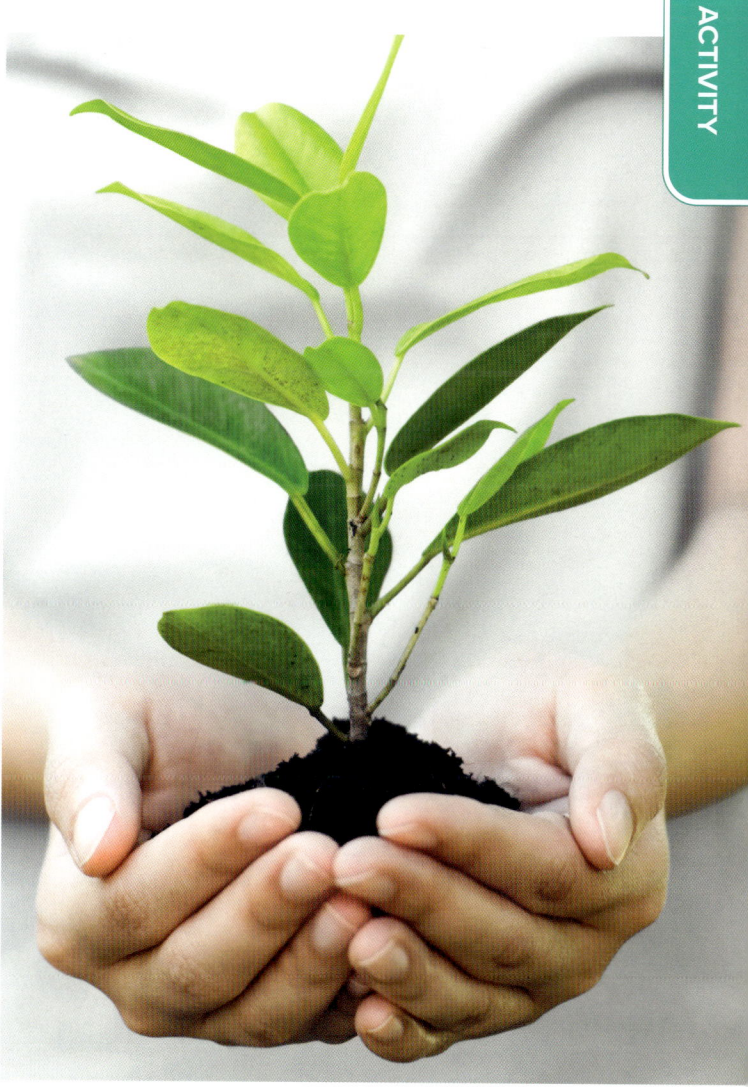

MENTAL ACTIVITY

The brain is sometimes referred to as "the strongest muscle in the body." Technically, the brain is not a muscle, but having a strong mind is key to success in all areas of your life. Planning positive mental activities into your routine will allow you to embrace and enjoy learning. Staying mentally active will also help keep you open-minded and more accepting of others, as opposed to being close-minded and judgmental. Mental activities help you show respect and curiosity for other ideas without feeling a need to conform. They provide you with confidence when confronted with unfamiliar situations, facts and figures.[6]

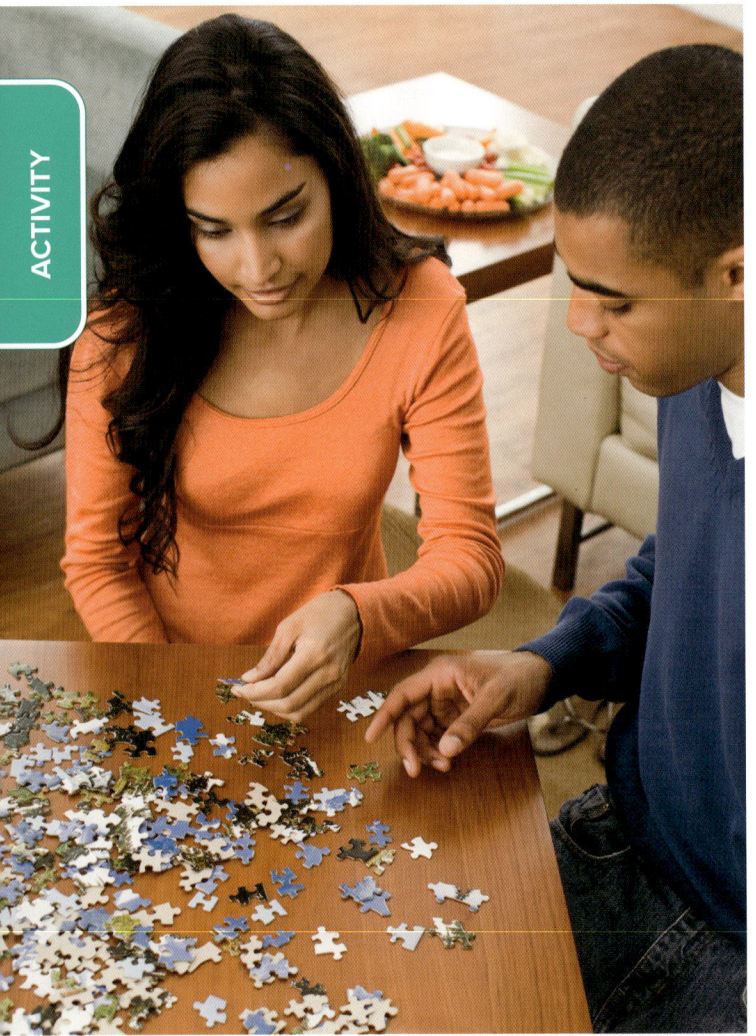

ACTIVITY

BIG HEADS

As a teenager, you are in a unique place in your life. The days of childhood are behind you, but you still haven't quite reached adulthood. Most likely, you've experienced a lot of physical changes during adolescence, but some of the most amazing changes are those you may not even be aware of. That's because they are happening deep inside your brain. Research shows that an adolescent's brain doesn't fully resemble an adult's brain until a person reaches his or her early twenties. This means you are still growing and developing mentally and emotionally, but when it comes to sheer intellectual power, the adolescent brain gives an adult's brain a run for the money. According to the National Institute of Mental Health, "The capacity of a person to learn will never be greater than during adolescence."[7] You're only young once, so take advantage of your brain's natural learning capacity now by engaging in the learning process and staying mentally active.

Of course, no one stays young forever. As some people get older, their minds and memories are often affected in tragic ways. They become more forgetful, less in tune with their surroundings and less able to perform certain mental tasks. Many have come to accept this as a natural result of the aging process, but this is not the case. Scientists have made an amazing discovery: the adult brain can grow in response to the regular demands placed on it. This was once thought impossible, but it seems that you can learn to exercise your brain much like you would exercise your body. Mental activity can actually change the physical structure of your brain much like the way exercise changes the physical structure of your body. "Until quite recently, most neuroscientists and psychologists believed that core aspects of cognitive processing were essentially fixed from a young age, with little or no room for improvement. Capacities like memory, attention and sensory processing were thought to be largely determined after a relatively brief period of early development…. We now understand that, with the right kind of stimulation and activity, the brain can dramatically change and remodel itself to become more efficient and effective in processing information, paying attention, remembering, thinking creatively and solving novel problems."[8]

One study that showed how mental activity affected the physical structure of the brain used structural magnetic resonance imaging (MRI) to measure the hippocampal volume of London taxi drivers. Hippocampal volume is an area of the brain that's involved in memory. The results of this study showed that people with intensive spatial training had significantly more hippocampal gray matter than usual. In other words, this area of the brain, which they used daily and extensively, was enlarged.[9] This has also been proven in other species, in particular with birds that have the ability to return to sites where they had previously found or stored food.[10] So, just as your heart, muscles and cardio-respiratory system respond to physical activity that increases their efficiency, power and size, the brain responds to and grows through mental activity.

Learning is critical in order for your brain to function optimally, not just now but for a lifetime. A large meta-analysis study done for the National Institutes of Health found that only two factors were associated with decreased risk of both Alzheimer's disease and cognitive decline. Those two factors were cognitive engagement — mental and physical activity.[11] Another study showed that older adults could indeed improve their brain abilities with the correct training. Certain mental exercises can help offset the expected decline in older adults' thinking skills, and they show promise for maintaining the cognitive abilities needed to do everyday tasks. Some of the benefits from training were even seen to be beneficial five years later.[12]

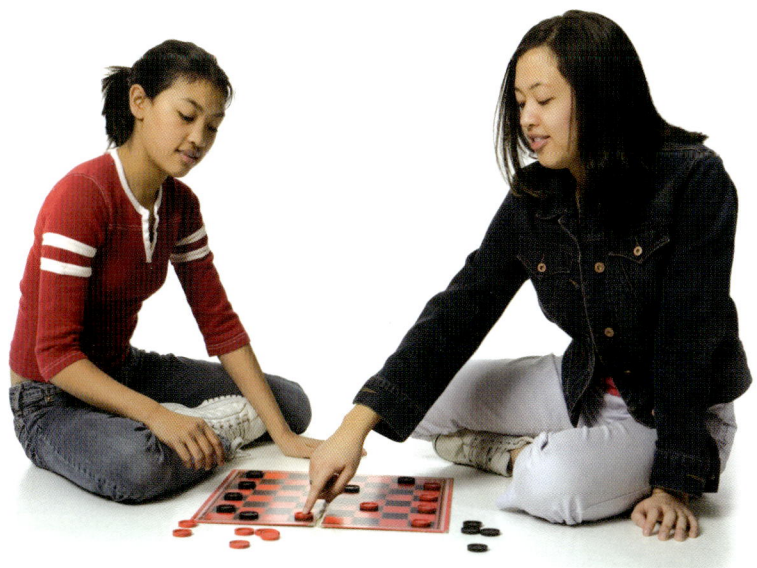

TRAINING YOUR GRAY MATTER

It is important to regularly exercise your brain, but it is also important to be careful regarding how you exercise it. When choosing mental activities for your brain, be careful to avoid those that require no real meaningful application or usefulness. Activities that increase brain fitness will include information and/or exercises that improve your performance in other meaningful endeavors. Some examples of these might include reading a book that interests or challenges you and has practical, enriching information. Books such as the classics and the Bible are excellent choices. Another activity that exercises your brain is memorization. You may wonder why in this day and age you should memorize anything, especially when you can easily find what you're looking for on the Internet, but memorizing poems or Bible verses causes you to focus on a text and reflect over and over on its meaning. You will also be able to recall the information whenever you need it. Other positive mental activities include doing jigsaw puzzles, learning a new language, increasing your vocabulary and practicing a task with your non-dominant hand.

In the Bronx Aging Study published in the *New England Journal of Medicine,* researchers followed almost 500 people for more than 20 years. In this study, those who participated in mentally stimulating activities, such as interactive games and other leisure activities multiple times a week, had a 65 to 75 percent better chance of remaining mentally sharp than people who did not do these activities.[13] Many fun games (such as chess) and puzzles (like crosswords and Sudoku) provide a fun mental challenge.

PHYSICAL ACTIVITY AND FITNESS

A physical activity is "any bodily movement produced by skeletal muscles that results in energy expenditure."[14] This could include any type of activity from strenuous exercise to reaching across the couch for the remote control. The real question is whether the activities you are doing are the kind that get your body working and your heart rate up. Jogging, swimming, playing basketball or doing aerobics are all great types of physical activities that benefit your body because they help you develop physical fitness. Physical fitness is defined as "a set of attributes that are either health or skill related. The degree to which people have these attributes can be measured with specific tests."[15]

HEALTH-RELATED FITNESS

Health-related physical fitness is the measure of your general well-being through exercise. There are five components of health-related physical fitness, which are used to measure your own total level of fitness. How fit you are depends on how well your body performs in each of these five categories:

1. **Cardiovascular Endurance** is also referred to as aerobic fitness and is a measure of a person's ability to continue an exercise that places demands on the circulatory and respiratory system over a prolonged period of time. This occurs in activities such as running, walking, cycling and swimming. To improve your cardiorespiratory endurance, you should do exercises that elevate your heart rate for a sustained period.

2. **Muscular Strength** is the maximal force that can be applied against a resistance. It is measured by the largest weight a person can lift or the largest body they can push or pull. Working your muscles against greater resistance is the key to gaining more muscular strength.

3. **Muscular Endurance** is the ability of the muscle to continue to perform without fatigue, for example the ability to do a series of push-ups over a certain period of time.

4. **Flexibility** is the measure of free movement in a person's joints. Good flexibility helps to prevent injuries and is especially important in activities such as gymnastics.

5. **Body Composition** is the percentages of muscle, fat, bone and other vital parts in the body. Usually, body composition is computed by measuring the percentage of body fat a person carries. Even if a person's total body weight doesn't change over time, it is important to know how much of that weight is fat and how much is lean mass.

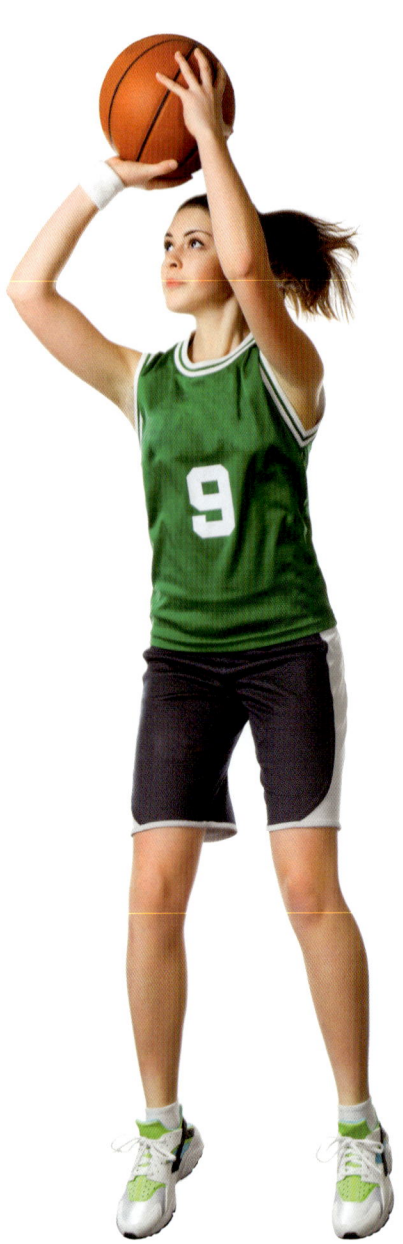

SKILL-RELATED FITNESS

Skill-related fitness is the ability to perform well in activities such as sports. There are six components to skill-related physical fitness:

1. **Agility** is the ability to rapidly and accurately change the direction of the whole body in space.

2. **Balance** is the ability to maintain equilibrium while stationary or moving.

3. **Coordination** is the ability to use the senses and body parts in order to perform motor tasks smoothly and accurately.

4. **Power** is the amount of force a muscle can exert.

5. **Reaction Time** is a measure of the body's ability to respond to stimuli.

6. **Speed** is the amount of time it takes the body to perform specific tasks.

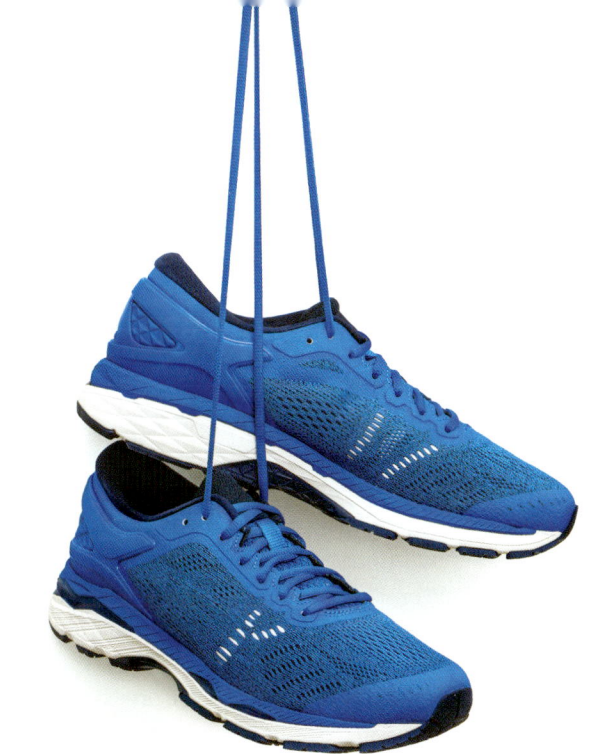

"The quality of life is determined by its activities."

ARISTOTLE

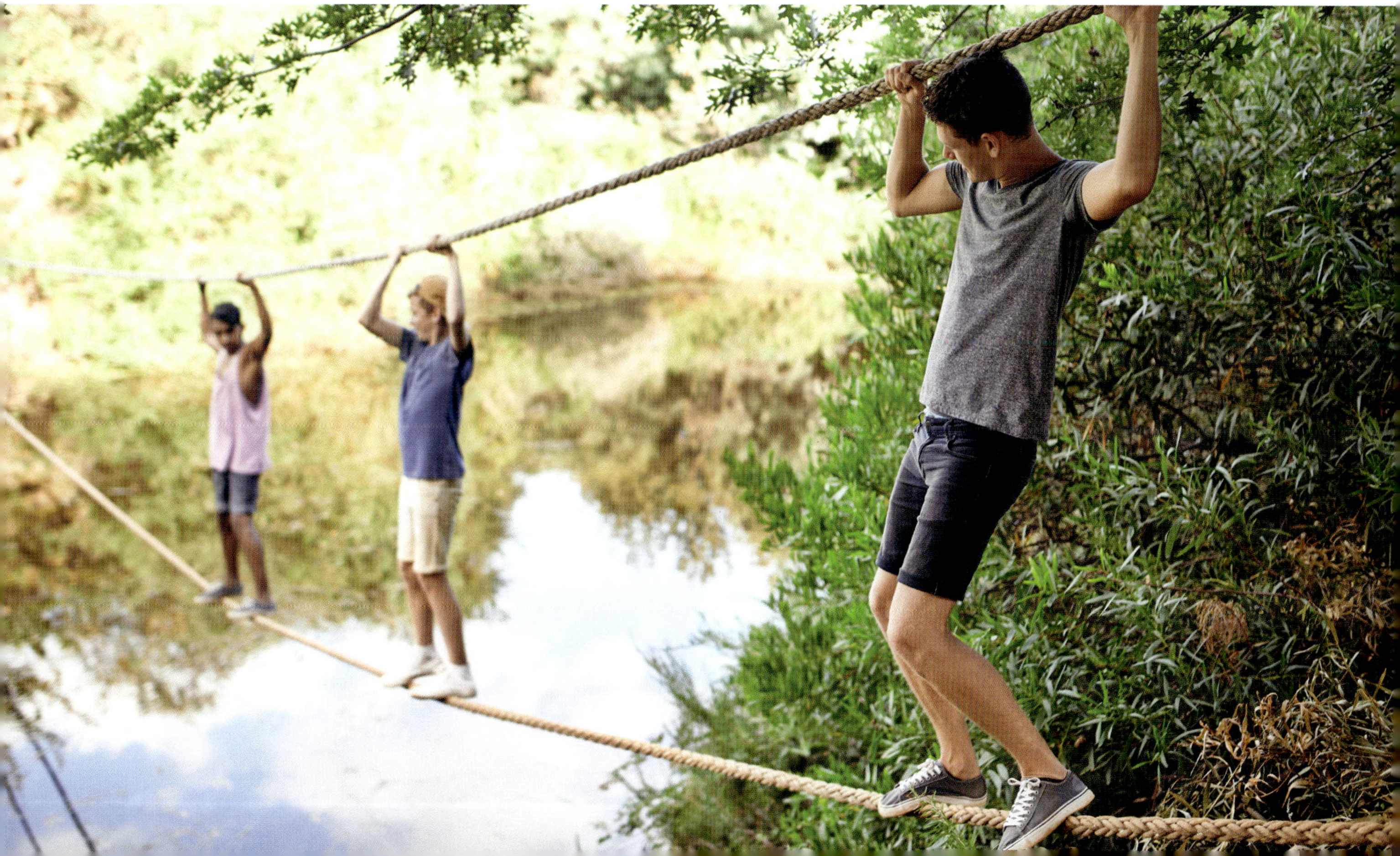

BENEFITS OF PHYSICAL ACTIVITY

Physical activity provides a number of positive benefits. For one thing, staying physically active will increase longevity. One large study conducted on 16,000 Harvard alumni showed that for every hour spent exercising, subjects could add four or more hours to their life.[16] This makes physical activity a great investment when it comes to how you choose to spend your time. Other studies show that low levels of activity and fitness are associated with increased mortality rates. It is estimated that of 250,000 deaths per year in the United States, approximately 12 percent of the total, are attributed to a lack of regular physical activity.[17] Research has shown that physical activity is a stronger predictor of your mortality rate than other factors such as having high blood pressure, high cholesterol or smoking. In one study, the researchers found that physically fit people with any combination of smoking, elevated blood pressure or elevated cholesterol levels had lower death rates overall than low-fit people with none of these problems. In other words, if a person smokes and has high blood pressure but is physically active, his or her chances of dying prematurely are lower than someone who does not smoke and does not have high blood pressure, but is physically inactive.[18]

How does physical activity help you live longer? Perhaps it has something to do with the many health and wellness benefits an active life provides. According to the Centers for Disease Control Prevention and the American College of Sports Medicine, physical activity lowers the risk of coronary heart disease, improves blood lipid profiles and gives you better resting blood pressure, glucose tolerance, insulin sensitivity, bone density, immune function and psychological function.[19] Another report in the *Journal of the American Medical Association* showed that exercise is protective against coronary heart disease and cancer.[20]

Physical activity may benefit more than just your longevity or your physical health. It may also help you fight stress and keep a positive outlook. Gallup researchers found that people who exercise at least two days a week are happier and are significantly less stressed than people who do not. And these benefits increase the more frequently you engage in physical activity.[21]

Why is physical activity such an excellent stress reliever? Dr. John J. Ratey, a noted author and clinical professor of psychiatry at Harvard Medical School, says that activity works on both the body and the brain by providing you with some much-needed distraction. Quite literally, exercise puts your mind on something else. Activity also helps to reduce muscle tension, build up the important mood hormones in your brain and improve your resilience.[22]

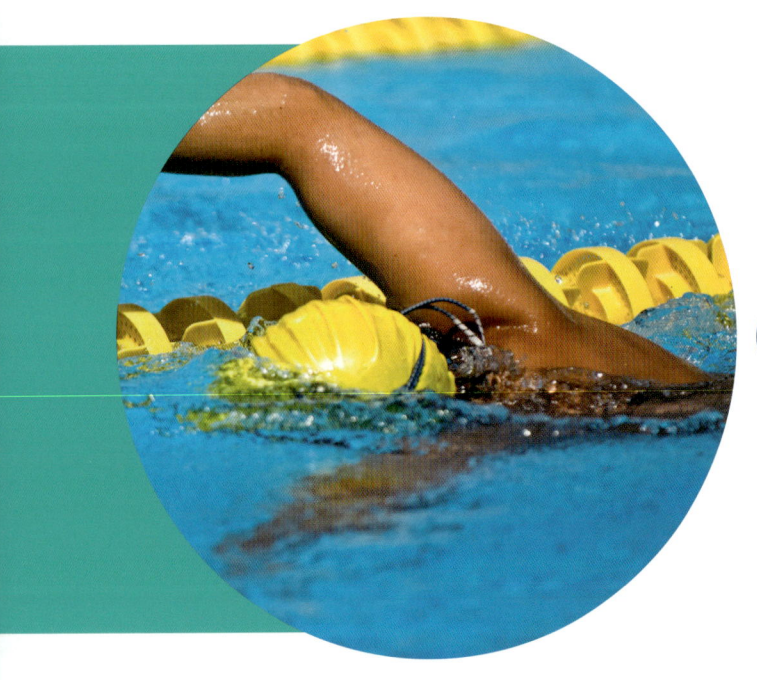

Have you used physical activity to relieve stress? If so, how did it work? If not, would you like to do this the next time you are experiencing stress?

TAKE A BREAK

Jessie, a college freshman, learned to deal with the stress of academics by thinking back to the skills she learned in her high school gym class. Whenever Jessie felt stressed out, she would run stairs like she did back in high school. "These days, every hour is sucked up with something… every time I know that a whole bunch of tests are coming up — when I'm really stressed out — I think, okay, you know how to handle this… I know that exercise will spike up my brain activity, and so I think, *Just go do it.* I wouldn't know that if it weren't for my gym class."[23]

One of the best ways to minimize the potentially damaging effects of stress is to do some physical activity. It doesn't have to take a long time either. If you are feeling stressed, try taking a short activity break. A walk outside in the fresh air, a quick bike ride or even running stairs like Jessie will rejuvenate your mind and your body.

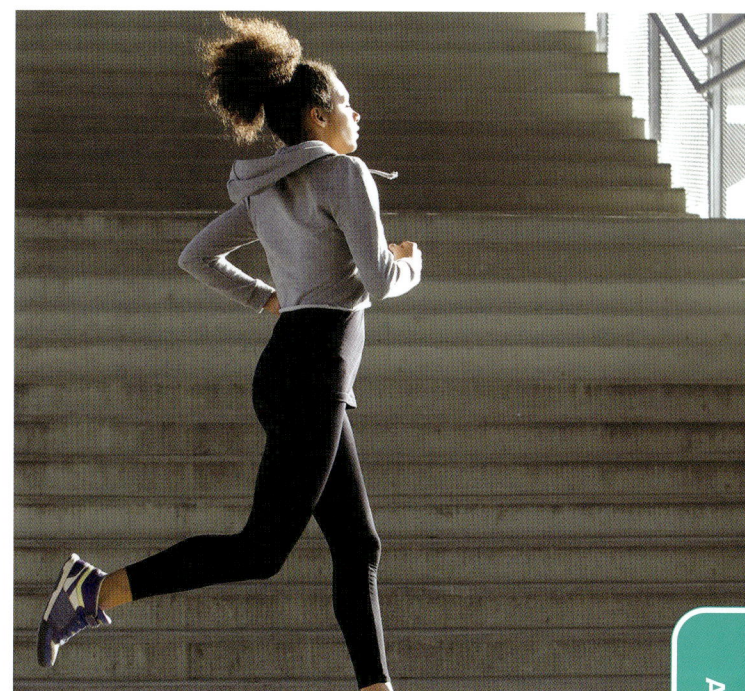

ACTIVITY

PLEASE NOTE

Always get cleared by a medical professional before beginning an exercise regimen of any intensity. Some teens may have undiagnosed health issues, which could lead to a crisis or even death if an exercise program is initiated without supervision.

HOW MUCH ACTIVITY IS ENOUGH?

So, how much exercise should you be doing on a regular basis?
The following guidelines are from the USDA (United States Department of Agriculture):

- **Teenagers (ages 13 to 17):** 60 minutes or more of physical activity each day. Most of the 60 minutes should be either moderate or vigorous intensity aerobic physical activity and should include vigorous-intensity physical activity at least three days a week. As part of their 60 or more minutes of daily physical activity, teenagers should include muscle-strengthening activities at least three days a week and bone-strengthening activities at least three days a week.[24]

- **Adults (ages 18 or older):** At least two hours and 30 minutes each week of aerobic physical activity at a moderate level or one hour and 15 minutes each week of aerobic physical activity at a vigorous level. Being active five or more hours each week can provide even more health benefits. Spreading aerobic activity out over at least three days a week is best. Also, each activity should be done for at least 10 minutes at a time. Adults should also do strengthening activities like push-ups, sit-ups and lifting weights at least two days a week.[25]

Keep in mind these are only recommendations. Your schedule may not allow you to do this much physical activity some days, or you may have time to do even more. Just realize you will still receive many health benefits by adding some type of activity to your day. Activities are considered light, moderate or vigorous in intensity depending on the extent to which they make you breathe harder and your heart beat faster. Start by choosing moderate or vigorous intensity activities, or a mix of both each week.[26]

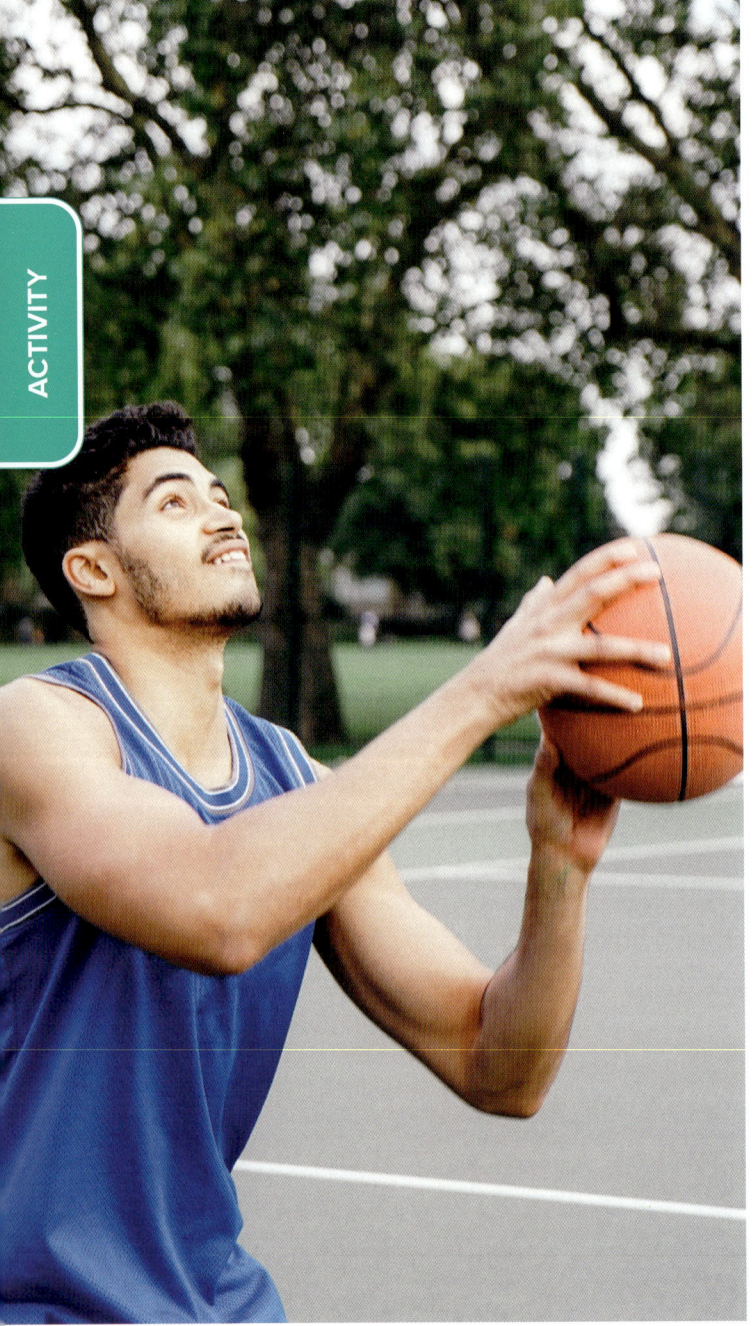

ACTIVITY

MODERATE ACTIVITY

You don't have to work yourself silly to get the benefits of an active lifestyle. Scientific evidence demonstrates that getting regular, moderate-intensive physical activity provides you with plenty of substantial health benefits. Many people can expect to receive these benefits by doing an activity that expends approximately 200 calories per day. For most people that would be equivalent to taking a brisk walk at three to four miles per hour. So, in order to meet the standard of burning approximately two hundred calories, you should walk at that speed for about two miles or approximately 30 minutes.[27] Here are some other examples of moderate-intensive physical activities (note how activity times adjust based on how physically demanding the activity is):

Common Chores

- Washing and waxing a car for 45 to 60 minutes
- Washing windows or floors for 45 to 60 minutes
- Gardening for 30 to 45 minutes
- Raking leaves for 30 minutes
- Shoveling snow for 15 minutes
- Stair walking for 15 minutes

Sporting Activities

- Playing volleyball for 45 to 60 minutes
- Playing touch football for 45 minutes
- Shooting baskets for 30 minutes
- Performing water aerobics for 30 minutes
- Swimming laps for 20 minutes
- Playing basketball for 15 to 20 minutes
- Jumping rope for 15 minutes
- Running one and a half miles in 15 minutes[28]

One study showed that changing activity patterns from "no exercise" to "moderate" exercise had greater improvements in health than changing from "moderate" to more "intense" exercise[29]

FIGHTING FATIGUE

Face it — you're a busy person. With so much to do, it's no wonder that you may be experiencing a significant amount of weariness and fatigue. This is not beneficial to your relationships, your performance in school or any other parts of your life. It may sound odd, but one of the ways you can fight feelings of fatigue is to get out and get some physical activity. In a comprehensive analysis of more than 70 studies, it was found that doing physical activity is much more effective at eliminating fatigue than taking prescription drugs commonly prescribed to help with it.[30]

VIGOROUS ACTIVITY

If you've been exercising regularly for several weeks at a moderate-intensity level, then it may be time to take things up a notch. Try going for a more vigorous workout. Vigorous-intensive activities cause rapid breathing and a substantial increase in heart rate.[31] They also provide similar health benefits as moderate activities, but in half the time.[32] Doing vigorous activities may also increase your longevity. In one study, participants were divided into five groups based on their level of exercise intensity. The researchers found that the higher the intensity of regular physical activity, the lower a subject's mortality rate.[33]

Some examples of vigorous activities include:

- Running/jogging (five miles per hour)
- Walking very fast (four and a half miles per hour)
- Bicycling (more than 10 miles per hour)
- Heavy yard work, such as chopping wood
- Swimming (freestyle laps)
- Aerobics
- Basketball (competitive)
- Tennis (singles)[34]

HOW INTENSE IS IT?

How do you know if the activity you are doing is light, moderate or vigorous? The Mayo Clinic offers the following guidelines:

Light Intensity: These activities should feel easy to do. Here are some clues that indicate you're exercising at a light level:

- No noticeable changes in your breathing pattern
- You never break a sweat (unless it's very hot or humid)
- You can carry on a conversation or even sing

Moderate Intensity: Moderate activities may feel somewhat hard to do. Here are some clues that you are exercising at a moderate level:

- Breathing quickens, but you're not out of breath
- A light sweat develops after about 10 minutes of activity
- You can carry on a conversation, but you can't sing

Vigorous Intensity: Vigorous activities are challenging. Here are some clues that you are exercising at a vigorous level:

- Deep, rapid breathing
- Sweating after a few minutes of activity
- You can't say more than a few words without pausing for breath[35]

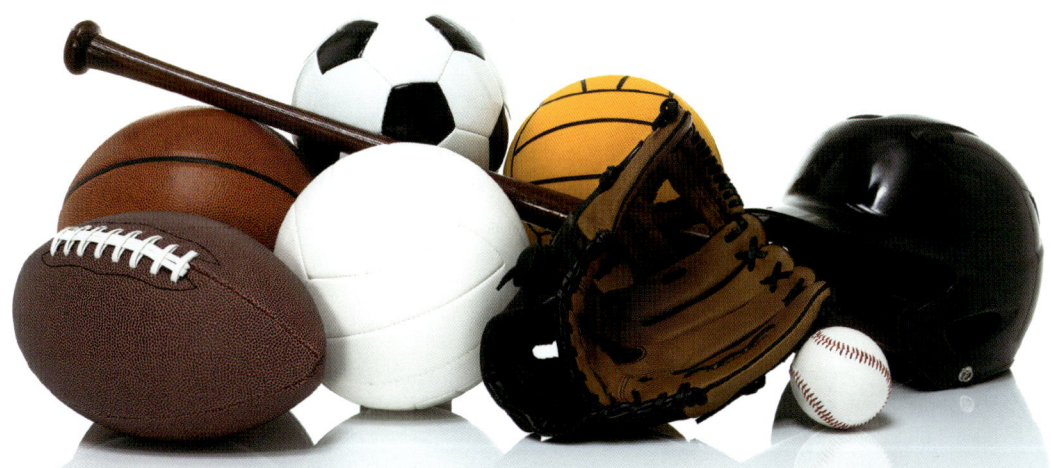

TARGET HEART RATE

A more precise way to determine the intensity of an activity is by determining whether your heart rate is in the target zone. Generally, the higher your heart rate during an activity, the higher the intensity. The following recommendations are from the Centers for Disease Control and Prevention:

First, determine your maximum heart rate.
To calculate your maximum heart rate, subtract your age from 220. For example, if you are 18, your maximum heart rate would be calculated as:

220 − 18 = 202 beats per minute (bpm)

For moderate-intensity physical activity,
your target heart rate should be 50 to 70 percent of your maximum heart rate. So if you are 18 years old, your moderate-intensity target rates would be:

50 percent level: 202 x 0.50 = 101 bpm
70 percent level: 202 x 0.70 = 141 bpm

Moderate-intensity physical activity for an 18-year-old produces a heart rate that remains between 101 and 141 bpm during physical activity.

For vigorous-intensity physical activity,
your target heart rate should be 70 to 85 percent of your maximum heart rate. For example, if you are 18 years old, your vigorous-intensity target rates would be:

70 percent level: 202 x 0.70 = 141 bpm
85 percent level: 202 x 0.85 = 171 bpm[36]

What do all these numbers mean? According to the American Heart Association, taking your heart rate during exercise can indicate how hard you need to push yourself:

- As you are doing an activity, take your pulse on the inside of your wrist, on the thumb side.

- Count your pulse for 30 seconds and multiply by two to find your beats per minute.

If your target heart rate is too high, you're straining and should slow down. If it's too low and the intensity feels light, push yourself to exercise a little harder.[37]

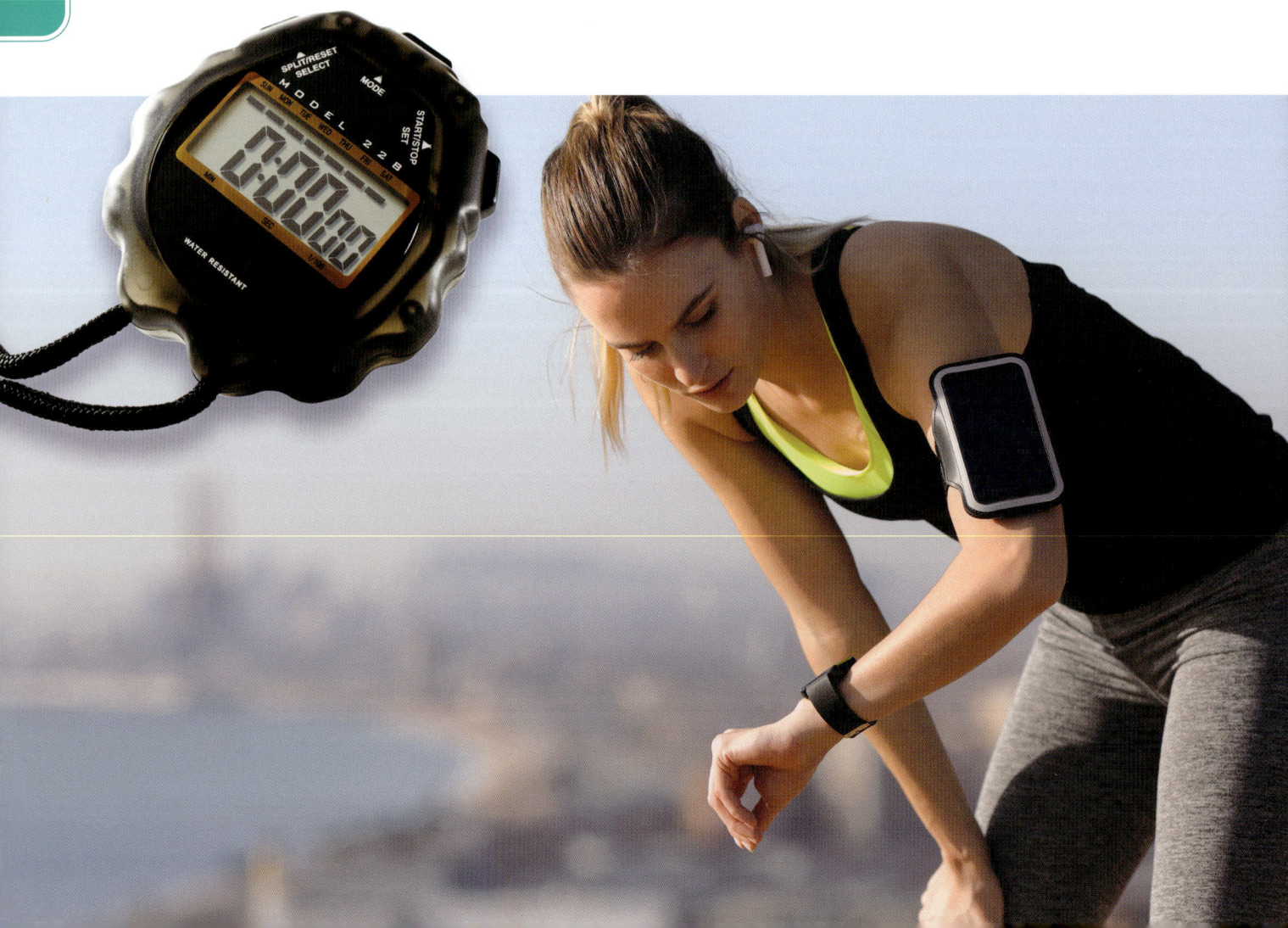

GET FITT

FITT is a model for training that helps you determine just how much exercise you need. FITT is an acronym that stands for:

Frequency refers to how many times per week you should exercise. Teenagers should get some type of physical activity every day.

Intensity refers to how hard you exercise and is best measured using your heart rate. Most of your exercise should be either moderately or vigorously intense.

Time refers to how long you perform the activity. Teenagers should get 60 minutes of activity per day. However, this can be broken up into 10 or 15 minute sessions.

Type refers to the kind of activity you perform. Teenagers should do aerobic physical activities such as walking, jogging, biking or swimming. Teens should also include muscle-strengthening activities at least three days a week and bone-strengthening activities at least three days a week.[38]

INTERVAL TRAINING

Interval training is a type of physical activity that consists of timed intervals of different intensities done in the same activity session. It involves periods of high-intensity activity alternated with low-intensity or rest. The intervals can be done at a moderate-intensity pace. Like other types of activity, interval training offers great benefits and, because of the variations, it helps to make physical activity more interesting, enjoyable and efficient.

Just how efficient is interval training? In one study, participants performed six training sessions over 14 days where two different exercise routines were compared. The interval routine was 30 seconds of "all out" cycling followed by four minutes of recovery time. This pattern was then repeated four to six times. The endurance routine was 90 to 120 minutes of continuous cycling. Over two weeks, the researchers found that both types of training induced similar improvements in muscle and exercise performance, but the time commitment for the interval group was only approximately two and a half hours compared to 10 and a half hours for the endurance group.[39]

Interval training offers the benefits of activity in less time than endurance training. If you decide to try interval training, it is important for you to increase your intensity gradually. Also, pay close attention to how you are feeling so you don't run a greater risk of injuring yourself.

Incorporating intermittent periods of lower intensity into your exercise routine can offer other benefits as well. Researchers have found that this technique of physical activity gives the same aerobic benefits as continuous aerobic exercise with the added benefits of greater loss of weight and body fat.[40-41]

ACTIVITY AND REST

There are significant benefits to taking regular periods of rest during long activity sessions. This is illustrated by long distance runners who take periods of rest in the form of walking breaks after every mile of running. Jeff Galloway, an Olympic athlete, running coach and author of *Marathon: You Can Do It,* has reported significant improvements in his finish times by using walking breaks throughout his training and races. According to Galloway, the walking break gives runners the following benefits:

- It allows people who can only run two miles to go three or four and feel fine.

- It helps beginners or heavy runners to increase their endurance to 5K, 10K or even as far as the marathon in as little as six months.

- It reduces the likelihood of injury and overtraining.

- It restores resiliency to the main running muscles before they fatigue; it's like getting a muscle strength booster shot every break.

- It speeds up post-marathon recovery.

- It helps runners of all ages to improve 10 to 40 minutes in their marathon time when compared to running continuously.[42]

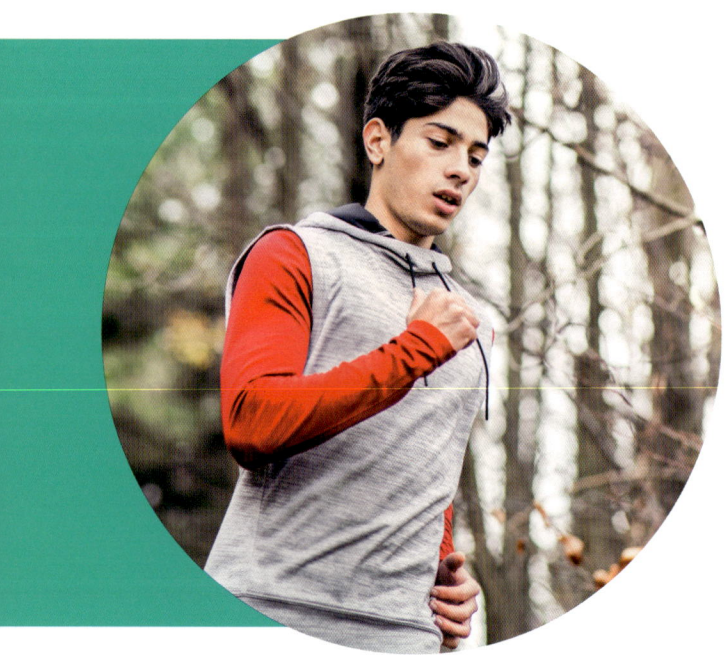

Many marathon veterans have improved their times by 10, 20, 30 or even 40 minutes by using walking breaks in a race. Ultra long-distance runner Tom Osler first tested the method of walking for himself in races lasting as long as two days. He wrote about it in his book, *Serious Runner's Handbook*. "Anyone can double the length of his or her current longest nonstop run by inserting brief walking breaks early and often."[43]

Joe Henderson, an editor for *Runner's World* for 25 years, has written more than a dozen books, countless articles and has run more than 700 races. He put Tom Osler's advice to the test by attempting a 100-mile run. His longest previous nonstop run had been 32 miles. By taking regular walking breaks, Henderson was able to more than double his previous distance by going 70 miles. Henderson said, "I failed the test in one way, by dropping out at 70 miles, but succeeded in other ways: more than doubling my longest nonstop distance; averaging only a half-minute per mile slower than usual marathon pace for the running portion; and suffering fewer after effects than if it had been a marathon. I've since inserted planned walking into most of my marathons, and it has worked every time. The running distance gained more than makes up for the walking time lost."[44]

So, maybe you aren't a long-distance, ultramarathon runner, but you can benefit from using periods of rest in your exercise routine. If you are a beginner, try alternating jogging for one minute and walking for five. As you get in better shape, you can gradually reduce your walking times until it equals your jogging time. Average runners will take one to two minute walking breaks after about three to eight minutes of running.[45]

ACCUMULATION

Evidence suggests that the amount of activity you do is more important than the specific manner in which the activity is performed. One study shows that getting 30 minutes of accumulated activity in short 10-minute sessions brings substantial benefits. Researchers evaluated two groups by using two different regimens for an eight-week training period. One group did 30 minutes of continuous activity a day, while the other group did three 10-minute exercise sessions separated by at least four hours. They found that the multiple shorter sessions of exercise produced similar and significant improvement in fitness levels when compared with the continuous exercise.[46]

It seems that your activity accumulates or builds up over time, so short sessions of exercise might fit better into your busy schedule than a single long session. Doing something as simple as using the stairs instead of taking the elevator can contribute to your 30-minute-per-day total. Some other ideas include walking instead of driving short distances, pedaling a stationary cycle while listening to a podcast, doing housework, raking leaves or even playing actively with a younger sibling.

> *"Movement is a medicine for creating change in a person's physical, emotional and mental states."*
>
> CAROL WELCH

ACTIVITY

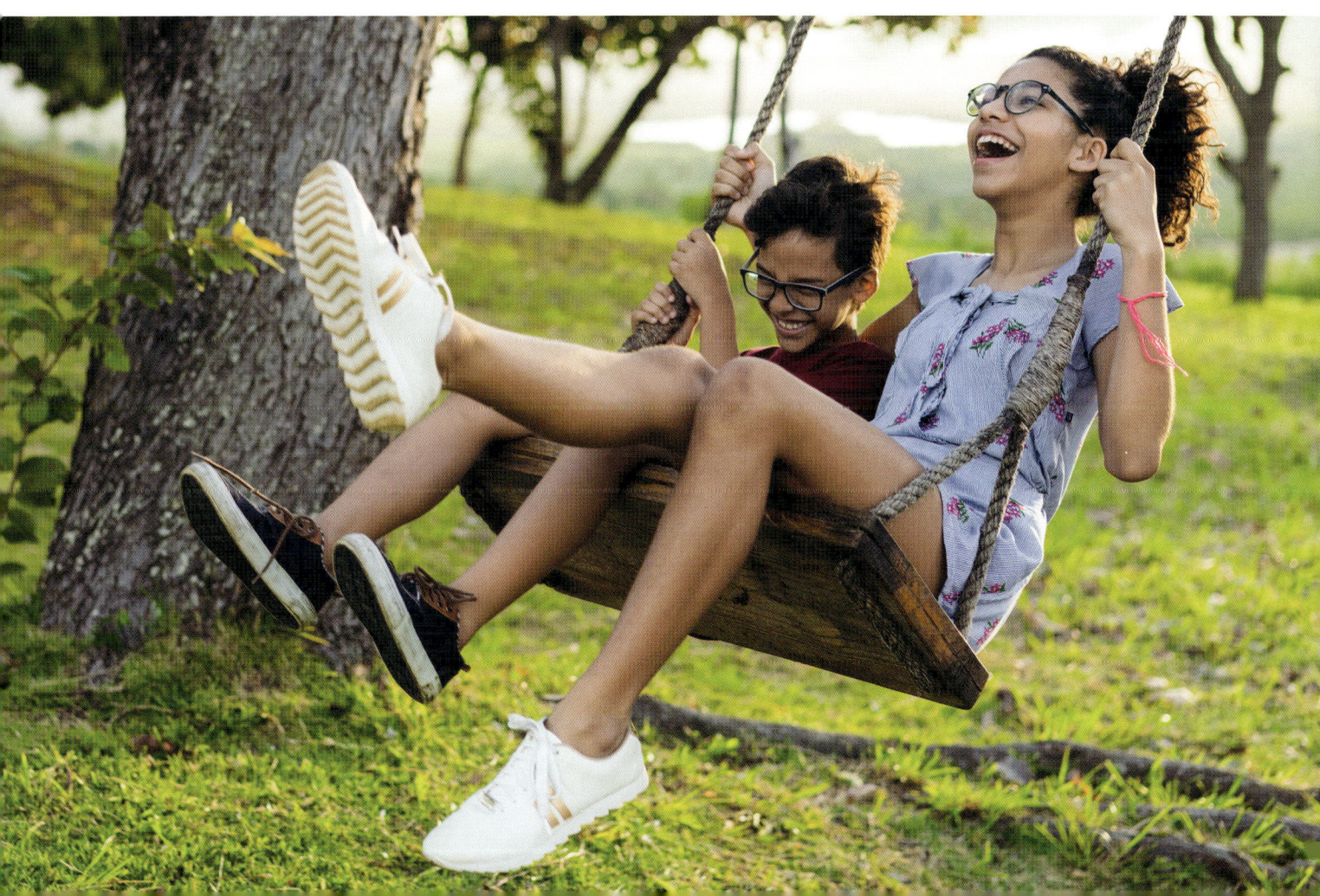

PUMP IT UP

Strength training often conjures up images of bulky, muscle-bound bodybuilders who grunt and strain to bench press the weight equivalent to a pregnant elephant. Strength training isn't just for people who want to look like professional athletes. It can provide you with a number of health benefits as well:

- Increased muscular strength, endurance and tone

- Increased ligament and tendon strength

- Increased bone density

- Better posture

- Easier acquisition of sport skills

- Greater joint stability

- Higher resting metabolic rate — this means you will burn more calories, which will also promote weight loss and maintenance. Each pound of muscle tissue gained increases your resting metabolism by 35 calories a day

- Less risk of injury and falls[47]

Some have even called strength training one of the world's greatest anti-agers. One study, published in the *Journal of the American Medical Association,* was conducted with women between the ages of 50 and 70 For one year, the women did strength-training exercises twice a week. At the end of the study, the women's bodies were 15 to 20 years more youthful. They had also regained bone density, which is helpful in preventing osteoporosis. The women became stronger, and in most cases, even stronger than when they were young. Their flexibility and balance improved, and without changing what they ate, they were leaner and trimmer. In addition, the women in this study were so energized that they became 27 percent more active.[48-49]

Try adding some type of strength training to your overall weekly activities. Even short sessions of strength training can benefit for you.

In one study, participants did a small amount of strength or resistance training for six months (specifically, one 11-minute set consisting of three to six repetitions at a high level of intensity). The participants were young adults classified as "sedentary" and "overweight," a group at high risk for developing obesity. It was found that even this small amount of exercise was enough to reprogram and boost the participants' metabolism, which led to better weight loss and weight management. Researchers concluded from this study that you could expect an increase in your daily total energy expenditures and fat oxidation if you are involved in just a small amount of high-intensity strength training.[50]

STRENGTH TRAINING: THE BASICS

Strength training (also called resistance training) should be "progressive in nature, individualized and provide a stimulus to all the major muscle groups."[51]

Frequency: Do strength training a minimum of 2 days per week.

Mode: Do 8 to 10 dynamic strength-training exercises involving the body's major muscle groups.

Resistance: Use enough weight resistance to perform 8 to 12 repetitions to near fatigue.

Sets: Do at least 1 set of repetitions.

WARM-UPS AND COOLDOWNS

Warm-ups and cooldowns are an important part of any physical activity program, but sometimes their benefits are not fully understood. Many people simply do not warm up before or cool down after exercising. This may lead to an increased risk of injury. In a 2008 review, it was found that doing warm-ups before exercising deters injuries.[52] Warm-ups have been shown to improve athletic performance as well.[53]

Typically, these activities are simple and only take three to five minutes. The principle is that you warm up or cool down the same body parts worked during the exercise session.[54] For example, if you are going to be taking a five mile jog, you could start and finish by walking for three to five minutes.

The benefits of warming up include:

- Gets blood to the muscles, which supplies necessary nutrients and oxygen

- Decreases the chance of injury

- Permits gradual changes, which in turn results in increased performance

- Helps prevent fatigue

- Provides an important increased emphasis on physical activity

- Improves coronary blood flow in the early part of exercise

The benefits of cooling down include:

- Slowly decreases the heart rate and brings the body back to a normal state

- Helps to work out the by-products that can cause muscle soreness

- Reduces the tendency for immediate post-exercise muscle spasm or cramping

- Prevents the blood from pooling in the extremities and blood pressure from rapidly dropping, thereby reducing the likelihood of light-headedness and fainting

"Since the mind and the soul find expression through the body, both mental and spiritual vigor are in great degree dependent upon physical strength and activity; whatever promotes physical health, promotes the development of a strong mind and a well-balanced character. Without health no one can as distinctly understand or as completely fulfill his obligations to himself, to his fellow beings, or to his Creator."

ELLEN WHITE

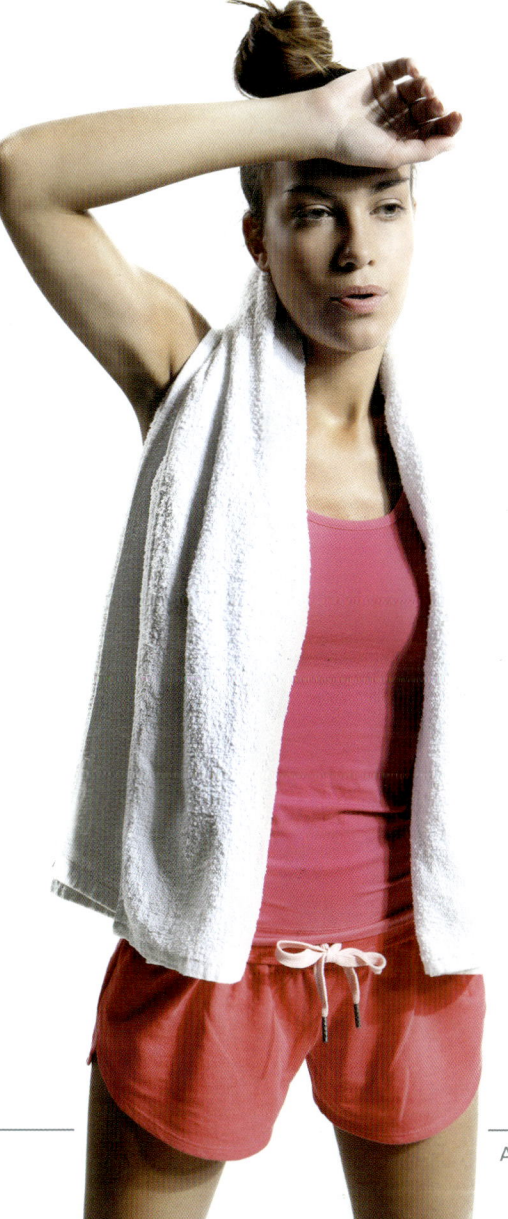

ACTIVITY

STRETCHING

Another important part of a physical activity session is stretching. You should always do stretches after your body is already warmed up. This will increase the safety and effectiveness of your stretches. In fact, the best time to stretch is right after you have done your full exercise session. This is when you are most flexible, which means you are least likely to injure yourself. The only exception to this rule is if you are doing a type of intense exercise that pushes your joints to the limit, such as sprinting. In this situation, it is best to have a long warm-up and then stretch before the activity.

Stretching is important because it can increase your performance, not only in the activity that you are doing, but in daily life. Stretching also decreases the likelihood of injuring yourself during your exercise session. Stretching after physical activity decreases soreness and tension in your muscles.

? Are you thinking of using vigorous physical activity to help boost your focus and learning power? If so, just make sure you do your studying after the activity and not during it. One research study found that college students who worked out on a treadmill or stationary bike at 70 to 80 percent of their maximum heart rate performed poorly on complex learning tests that they took while they were on the bike. The researchers found the students received the benefit of sharper thinking and analysis as a result of the physical activity after they had finished the activity.[62]

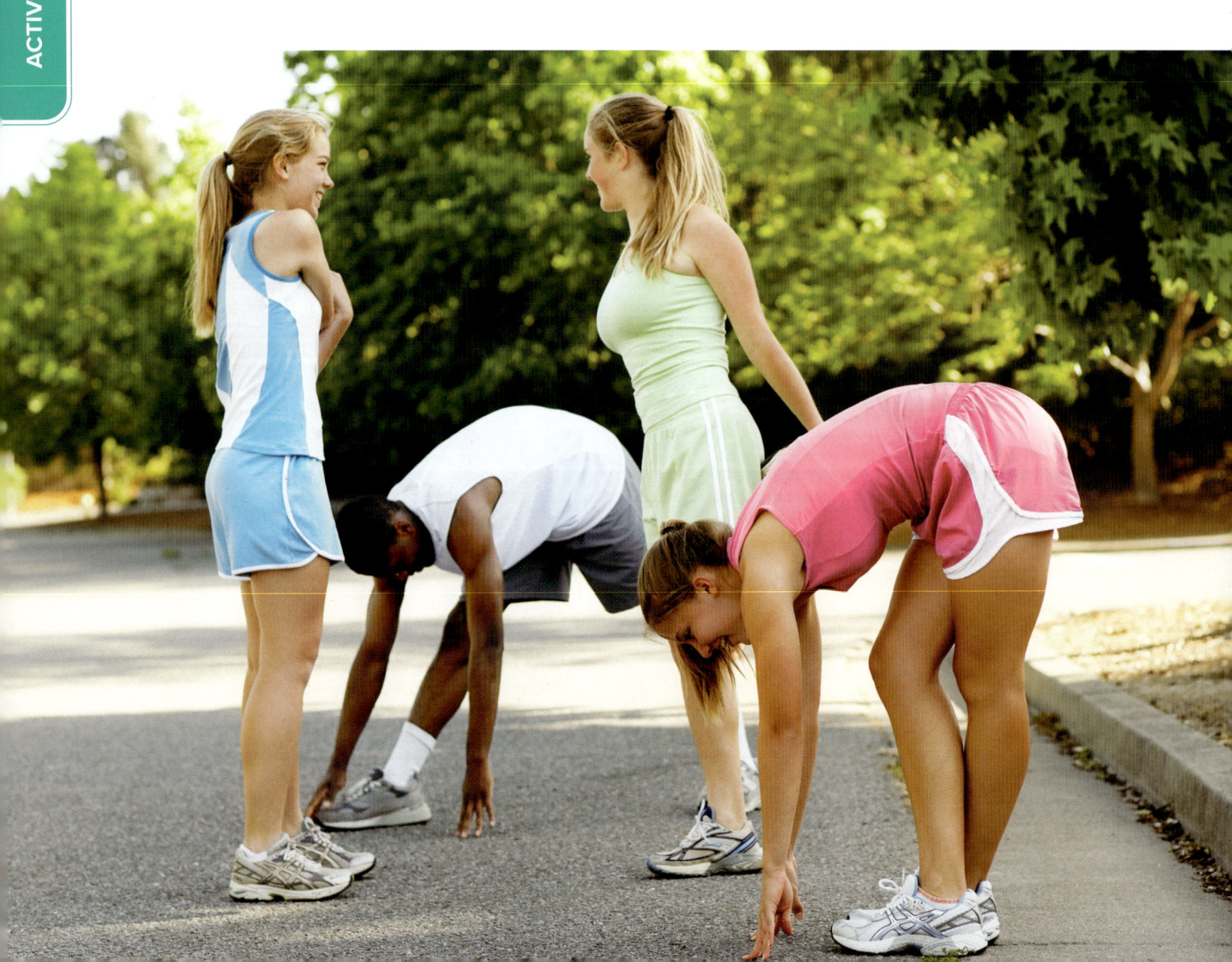

THE LINK BETWEEN

It turns out there is a strong link between mental and physical activity. For example, the best time for you to study may be right after you exercise. Activity may actually help you learn better. In one study, researchers found that test subjects learned vocabulary words 20 percent faster following a physical activity.[55] One high school decided to put the link between mental and physical activity to the test. They began what they called "Zero Hour PE," named because it was scheduled before first period. The students who participated in Zero Hour were a group of freshman who were required to take a literacy class in order to bring up their reading comprehension scores. During Zero Hour, these students were required to work out at a very high-intensity level — 80 to 90 percent of their maximum heart rate. They were then sent off to class in, what their PE teacher referred to as, "a state of heightened awareness." At the end of the semester, these students showed a 17 percent improvement in their reading and comprehension scores.[56]

The school administration was so impressed with the results of Zero Hour that they incorporated it into their curriculum as a first-period literacy class. The strategy has spread beyond freshmen who need to boost their reading scores. Guidance counselors at the school now suggest all students schedule their hardest subjects immediately after gym "to capitalize on the beneficial effects of exercise."[57]

The number of studies that support how physical activity helps with learning is growing. Activity has been found to positively impact learning in all ages, from children to adults. In one review study, a panel of researchers analyzed over 850 studies about the effects of physical activity on school-age children. The committee reported that physical activity has a positive influence on memory, concentration and classroom behavior of school children.[58] Physical activity also helps children improve their cognitive control[59] and attention.[60] And on-task behavior was improved when children participated in a 10-minute energizer session each day of the school week.[61]

YOUR BODY AND YOUR BRAIN

The link between mental and physical activity has been shown to have other benefits as well. Researchers have reported that older people who have overall greater muscle strength have a reduced likelihood of developing Alzheimer's disease.[63] Staying strong and active may do more than just help prevent cognitive impairments. It may also help to improve them. Another study examined women between the ages of 70 and 80 who had mild cognitive impairment (MCI). This means the women had memory problems that were not severe enough to interfere with their daily lives. However, MCI is often considered to be a very early stage of Alzheimer's disease. The women in the study did strength-training activities twice a week for six months. During this time, researchers also measured their memory and cognitive skills. At the end of the six months, the strength training was found to improve both their memory performance and their executive functions. This study demonstrated that strength training could help those who are already suffering from cognitive decline.[64]

By developing an active lifestyle now, you will help to prevent a number of potentially harmful diseases later on.

 **How might you plan a physical activity routine to best benefit your cognitive function?**

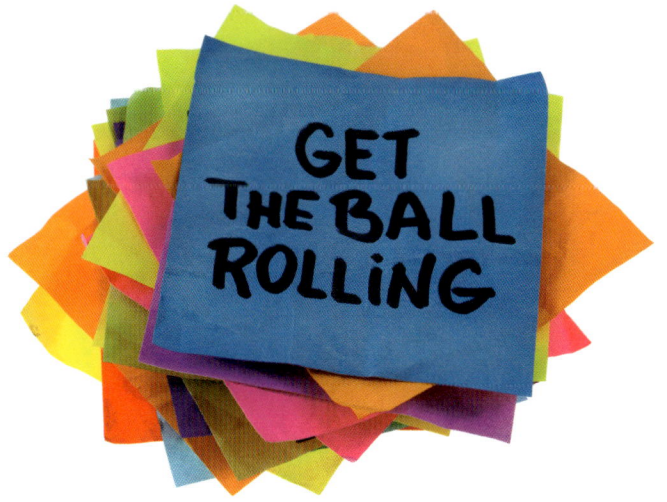

GET THE BALL ROLLING

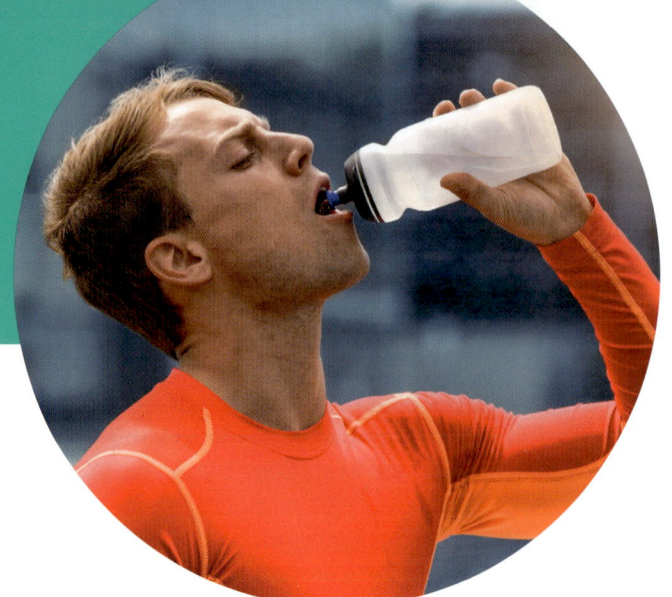

Your body needs more water when you are physically active.

FINAL THOUGHTS

God created you to be active. Mental activity improves your brain function, and regular physical activity rewards you with energy and vitality. By staying mentally and physically active you will help your mind and your body to grow, be healthy and thrive.

To see the CREATION Life active lifestyle in practice, look at Jesus as an example. First, examine His mental activity. Jesus had a perfect knowledge of Scripture, which He often quoted, most famously when He was tempted in the wilderness.[65] Because of this, Jesus was able to teach others, show them how to apply God's truth to their lives and correct those who were misinterpreting the Scriptures. In the apostle Paul's letter to the church in Rome he writes, "Do not conform to the pattern of this world, but be transformed by the renewing of your mind" (Romans 12:2). How do you renew your mind? By replacing the world's thinking with God's truth. This means regularly studying and memorizing God's Word so that you may also apply it to your life. This is an activity that provides you with great mental growth and spiritual maturity.

Second, look at Jesus' example of physical activity. In the *Journal of the American Medical Association*, an article was published entitled, "On the Physical Death of Jesus Christ." This article contained a section on the "Health of Jesus," which stated, "The rigors of Jesus' ministry (that is, traveling by foot throughout Palestine) would have precluded any major physical illness or weak general constitution. Accordingly, it is reasonable to assume that Jesus was in good physical condition."[66] By examining the places in the Bible that Jesus visited over his three-year ministry, it's possible to conclude that Jesus walked an average of 20 miles a day.[67] In order to keep up with the demands placed upon Him by His extensive ministry, it was imperative that Jesus be in good physical condition. Likewise, in order for you to best live, learn and serve others, it is important for you to get regular physical activity at a moderate or vigorous level.

Activity definitely helps you to be fit for life. Choose today to get healthy activity and become all that God wants you to be.

 **How does the example of Jesus impact your attitude toward physical and mental activity?**

ACTIVITY

14 POWER TIPS

Use these tips to get active and maintain regular physical activity:

1. **Choose activities you enjoy.** You are much more likely to follow through.

2. **Ease into it.** Gradually increase the intensity and duration of your activity.

3. **Set short-term goals.** If you've never run a mile before, don't start training for a marathon tomorrow. Keep your goals small and manageable. This will prevent you from becoming overwhelmed by larger, long-term goals.

4. **Celebrate your success.** Reward yourself each time you reach a goal.

5. **Schedule a regular time for exercise.** Make it a habit.

6. **Plan a different exercise each day.** Varying your activities will help fight boredom with your exercise routine.

7. **Remember the value of intermittent, short periods of activity.** If your schedule won't let you do an entire workout, then go for a quick walk or jog. It all adds up.

8. **Plan activity for early in the day.** You are much more likely to do it when you are less tired and have fewer interruptions or conflicts.

9. **Exercise with a friend or group.** You'll be able to encourage and hold each other accountable.

10. **Wear proper clothing.** Invest in a good pair of running shoes.

11. **Keep an exercise log.** If you want to see your improvements, write down how much you do each day. You may be surprised what you've accomplished in a short time.

12. **Add music.** It keeps you motivated and focused.

13. **Drink plenty of water.** Your body needs more when you are physically active.

14. **Energize your body with the food it needs for optimal performance.** What you eat matters, so fuel your body with the best.

ACTIVITY

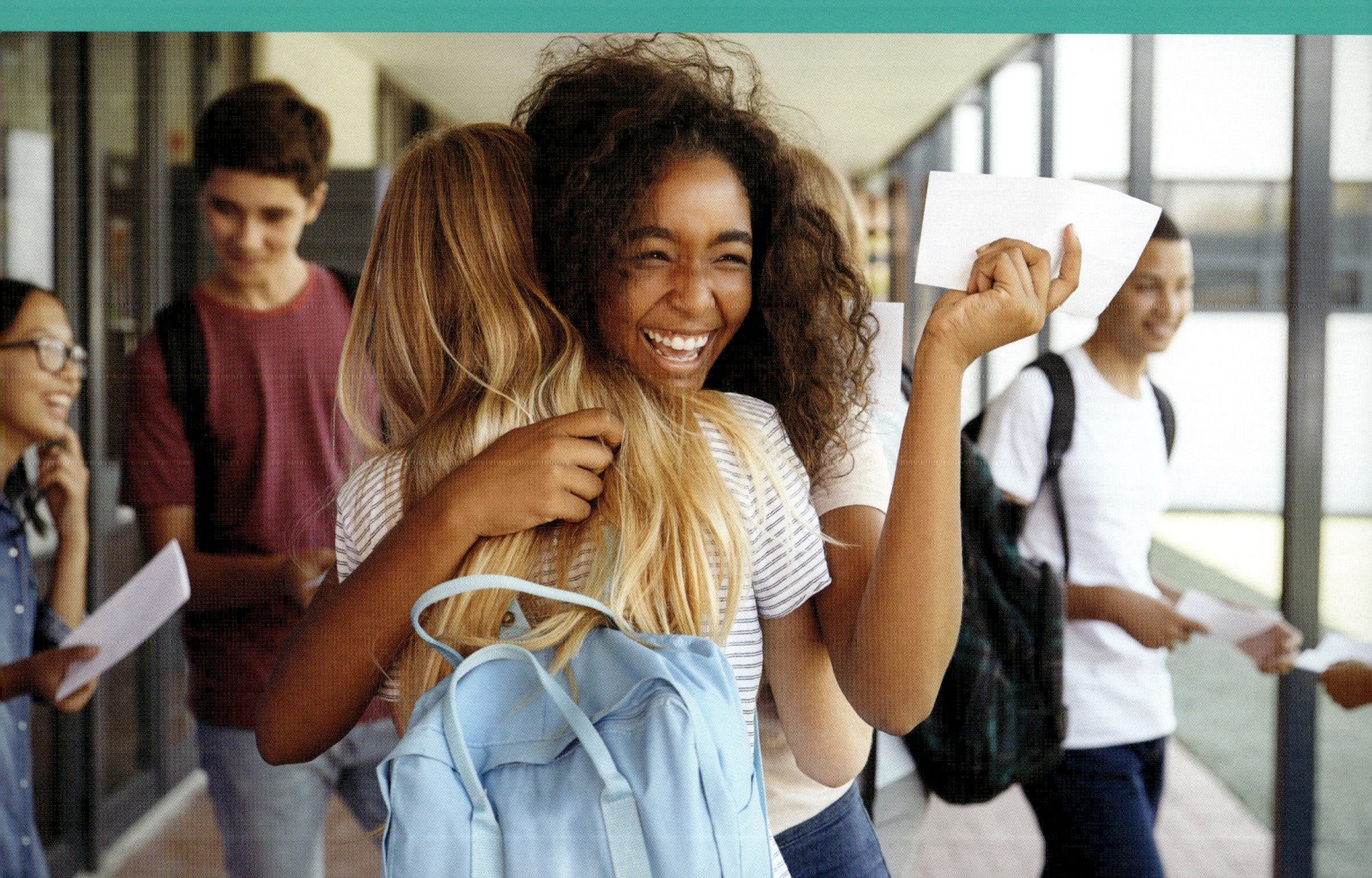

REFERENCES

1. South University. "The Shape of the Fitness Industry." Last modified May 4, 2012. https://www.southuniversity.edu/whoweare/newsroom/blog/the-shape-of-the-fitness-industry-85375.

2. Statista. "Total Number of Memberships at Fitness Center/Health Clubs in the U.S. from 2000 to 2016 (in millions)." Accessed March 1, 2018. https://www.statista.com/statistics/236123/us-fitness-center--health-club-memberships/.

3. Alliance for a Healthier Generation. "Childhood Obesity Facts." Accessed July 3, 2018. https://www.healthiergeneration.org/about_childhood_obesity/get_informed/childhood_obesity_facts/.

4. Centers for Disease Control and Prevention. "Childhood Obesity Facts." Accessed March 1, 2018. https://www.cdc.gov/healthyschools/obesity/facts.htm.

5. American Heart Association. "Cold Weather Fitness Guide." Accessed July 3, 2018. http://www.heart.org/idc/groups/heart-public/@wcm/@fc/documents/downloadable/ucm_457235.pdf.

6. Hoeger, Werner W. K, Lori Waite Turner, and Brent Q Hafen. *Wellness: Guidelines For A Healthy Lifestyle*. Belmont, CA: Thomson Learning/Wadsworth, 2007.

7. National Institute of Mental Health. "The Teen Brain: Still Under Construction." Accessed November 1, 2013. https://infocenter.nimh.nih.gov/pubstatic/NIH%2011-4929/NIH%2011-4929.pdf.

8. Hardy, Joseph and Michael Scanlon. "The Science Behind Luminosity." *Lumosity*. November 2009. http://citeseerx.ist.psu.edu/viewdoc/download?doi=10.1.1.604.651&rep=rep1&type=pdf.

9. Maguire, Eleanor A., David G. Gadian, Ingrid S. Johnsrude, Catriona D. Good, John Ashburner, Richard S. J. Frackowiak, and Christopher D. Frith. "Navigation-Related Structural Change in the Hippocampi of Taxi Drivers." Proceedings of the National *Academy of Sciences* 97, no. 8 (2000): 4398-4403. https://doi.org/10.1073/pnas.070039597.

10. Sherry, David F., Anthony L. Vaccarino, Karen Buckenham, and Rachel S. Herz. "The Hippocampal Complex of Food-Storing Birds." *Brain, Behavior and Evolution* 34, no. 5 (1989): 308-317. https://doi.org/10.1159/000116516.

11. Williams, John, Brenda Plassman, James Burke, Tracey Holsinger, and Sophiya Benjamin. *Preventing Alzheimer's Disease And Cognitive Decline*. Rockville: Agency for Healthcare Research and Quality (U.S.), 2010. http://www.ncbi.nlm.nih.gov/books/NBK47456/pdf/TOC.pdf.

12. Willis, Sherry L., Sharon L. Tennstedt, Michael Marsiske, Karlene Ball, Jeffrey Elias, Kathy Mann Koepke, John N. Morris, George W. Rebok, Frederick W. Unverzagt, Anne M. Stoddard, and Elizabeth Wright. "Long-term Effects of Cognitive Training on Everyday Functional Outcomes in Older Adults." *Journal of the American Medical Association* 296, no. 23 (2006): 2805-2814. https://doi.org/10.1001/jama.296.23.2805.

13. Verghese, Joe, Richard B. Lipton, Mindy J. Katz, Charles B. Hall, Carol A. Derby, Gail Kuslansky, Anne F. Ambrose, Martin Sliwinski, and Herman Buschke. "Leisure Activities and the Risk of Dementia in the Elderly." *New England Journal of Medicine* 348, no. 25 (2003): 2508-2516. https://doi.org/10.1056/NEJMoa022252.

14. Caspersen, Carl J., Kenneth E. Powell, and Gregory M. Christenson. "Physical Activity, Exercise, and Physical Fitness: Definitions and Distinctions for Health-related Research." *Public Health Reports* 100, no. 2 (1985): 126-131. https://www.jstor.org/stable/20056429.

15 Ibid.

16. Paffenbarger Jr., Ralph S., Robert Hyde, Alvin L. Wing, and Chung-cheng Hsieh. "Physical Activity, All-Cause Mortality, and Longevity of College Alumni." *New England Journal of Medicine* 314, no. 10 (1986): 605-613. https://doi.org/10.1056/NEJM198603063141003.

17. Pate, Russell R., Michael Pratt, Steven N. Blair, William L. Haskell, Caroline A. Macera, Claude Bouchard, David Buchner et al. "Physical Activity and Public Health: A Recommendation From the Centers for Disease Control and Prevention and the American College of Sports Medicine." *Journal of the American Medical Association* 273, no. 5 (1995): 402-407. https://doi.org/10.1001/jama.1995.03520290054029.

18. Pate, R. R., M. Pratt, S. N. Blair, W. L. Haskell, C. A. Macera, C. Bouchard, W. Ettinger, G. W. Heath, and A. C. King et al. "Physical Activity and Public Health" *Journal of the American Medical Association* 273. no 5 (1995): 403. https://www.ncbi.nlm.nih.gov/pubmed/7823386.

19. U.S. Department of Health and Human Services. *Physical Activity and Health: A Report of the Surgeon General*. Atlanta: U.S. Department of Health and Human Services, Centers for Disease Control and Prevention, National Center for Chronic Disease Prevention and Health Promotion, 1996. https://www.cdc.gov/nccdphp/sgr/pdf/chap3.pdf.

20. Blair, Steven N., Carolyn E. Barlow, Ralph S. Paffenbarger Jr., and Larry W. Gibbons. "Influences of Cardiorespiratory Fitness and Other Precursors on Cardiovascular Disease and All-Cause Mortality in Men and Women." *Journal of the American Medical Association* 276, no. 3 (1996): 205-210. https://doi.org/10.1001/jama.1996.03540030039029.

21. Rath, Tom and James K. Harter. *Wellbeing: The Five Essential Elements*. New York: Gallup Press, 2010.

ACTIVITY

22. Ratey, John J. *Spark: The Revolutionary New Science of Exercise and the Brain*. New York: Little Brown and Company, 2008: 106-108.

23. Ratey, John J. *Spark: The Revolutionary New Science of Exercise and the Brain*. New York: Little Brown and Company, 2008: 28-29.

24. Choose My Plate. "How Much Physical Activity is Needed." Accessed November 1, 2013. http://www.choosemyplate.gov/physical-activity/amount.html.

25. Ibid.

26. Choose My Plate. "What is Physical Activity." Accessed November 1, 2013, http://www.choosemyplate.gov/physical-activity/what.html.

27. Haskell, William L., I-Min Lee, Russell R. Pate, Kenneth E. Powell, Steven N. Blair, Barry A. Franklin, Caroline A. Macera, Gregory W. Heath, Paul D. Thompson, and Adrian Bauman. "Physical Activity and Public Health: Updated Recommendation for Adults from the American College of Sports Medicine and the American Heart Association." *Circulation* 116, no. 9 (2007): 1081-1093. https://doi.org/10.1249/mss.0b013e3180616b27.

28. National Heart, Lung, and Blood Institute. "Lower Your Blood Pressure by Being Active." Accessed November 1, 2013, https://www.nhlbi.nih.gov/files/docs/public/heart/hbp_low.pdf.

29. Blair, S. N., J. B. Kampert, H. W. Kohl III, C. E. Barlow, C. A. Macera, R. S. Paffenbarger Jr., and L. W. Gibbons. "Influences of Cardiorespiratory Fitness and Other Precursors on Cardiovascular Disease and All-Cause Mortality in Men and Women." *Journal of the American Medical Association* 279. no 3 (1996): 205-210. https://doi.org/10.1001/jama.1996.03540030039029.

30. Puetz, Timothy W., Patrick J. O'Connor, and Rod K. Dishman. "Effects of Chronic Exercise on Feelings of Energy and Fatigue: A Quantitative Synthesis." *Psychological Bulletin* 132, no. 6 (2006): 866-876. https://doi.org/10.1037/0033-2909.132.6.866.

31. Haskell, William L., I-Min Lee, Russell R. Pate, Kenneth E. Powell, Steven N. Blair, Barry A. Franklin, Caroline A. Macera, Gregory W. Heath, Paul D. Thompson, and Adrian Bauman. "Physical Activity and Public Health: Updated Recommendation for Adults from the American College of Sports Medicine and the American Heart Association." *Circulation* 116, no. 9 (2007): 1081-1093. https://doi.org/10.1161/CIRCULATION.107.185649.

32. Choose My Plate. "What is Physical Activity." Accessed November 1, 2013. http:// www.choosemyplate.gov/physical-activity/what.html.

33. Kujala, Urho M., Jaakko Kaprio, Seppo Sarna, and Markku Koskenvuo. "Relationship of Leisure-Time Physical Activity and Mortality: The Finnish Twin Cohort." *Journal of the American Medical Association* 279, no. 6 (1998): 440-444. https://doi.org/10.1001/jama.279.6.440.

34. Choose My Plate. "What is Physical Activity." Accessed November 1, 2013. http:// www.choosemyplate.gov/physical-activity/what.html.

35. Mayo Clinic. "Exercise Intensity: How It's Measured." Accessed June 4, 2012. http://www.mayoclinic.com/health/exercise-intensity/SM00113.

36. Centers for Disease Control and Prevention. "Target Heart Rate and Estimated Maximum Heart Rate." Accessed November 1, 2013. http://www.cdc.gov/physicalactivity/everyone/measuring/heartrate.html.

37. American Heart Association. "Know Your Target Heart Rates for Exercise, Losing Weight and Health." Accessed June 29, 2018. https://healthyforgood.heart.org/move-more/articles/target-heart-rates.

38. Choose My Plate. "How Much Physical Activity is Needed." Accessed November 1, 2013. http://www.choosemyplate.gov/physical-activity/amount.html.

39. Gibala, Martin J., Jonathan P. Little, Martin Van Essen, Geoffrey P. Wilkin, Kirsten A. Burgomaster, Adeel Safdar, Sandeep Raha, and Mark A. Tarnopolsky. "Short‐term Sprint Interval Versus Traditional Endurance Training: Similar Initial Adaptations in Human Skeletal Muscle and Exercise Performance." *The Journal of Physiology* 575, no. 3 (2006): 901-911. https://doi.org/10.1113/jphysiol.2006.112094.

40. Meyer, Katharina, Ladislaus Samek, Matthias Schwaibold, Samuel Westbrook, Ramiz Hajric, Ralph Beneke, Manfred Lehmann, and Helmut Roskamm. "Interval Training in Patients with Severe Chronic Heart Failure: Analysis and Recommendations for Exercise Procedures." *Medicine and Science in Sports and Exercise* 29, no. 3 (1997): 306-312. https://doi.org/10.1097/00005768-199703000-00004.

41. Mayer, H., D. DeRose. "A Comparison Between Intermittent Versus Continuous Aerobic Training on Cardiorespiratory & Body Composition Responses in Sedentary Adults." *Medicine & Science in Sports & Exercise* 32, no. 5 (2000): S218.

42. Galloway, Jeff. *Marathon: You Can Do It*. Bolinas: Shelter Publications Inc., 2001.

43. Osler, Tom. *The Serious Runner's Handbook*. Mountain View: World Publications, 1978.

44. Henderson, Joe. *Better Runs: 25 Years' Worth Of Lessons For Running Faster And Farther*. Champaign: Human Kinetics, 1996.

45. Galloway, Jeff. *Marathon: You Can Do It*. Bolinas: Shelter Publications Inc., 2001.

46. DeBusk, Robert F., Ulf Stenestrand, Mary Sheehan, and William L. Haskell. "Training Effects of Long versus Short Bouts of Exercise in Healthy Subjects." *American Journal of Cardiology* 65, no. 15 (1990): 1010-1013. https://doi.org/10.1016/0002-9149(90)91005-Q.

47. Pollock, M. I., Ga Gaesser, J. D. Butcher, J. P. Despres, R. K. Dishman, B. A. Franklin, and C. E. Garber. "The Recommended Quantity and Quality of Exercise for Developing and Maintaining Cardiorespiratory and Muscular Fitness, and Flexibility in Healthy Adults." *Medicine And Science In Sports And Exercise* 30, no. 6 (1998): 975-91.

48. Nelson, Miriam E., M. D. Fiatarone, and M. D. Morganti. "Effects of High-Intensity Strength Training on Multiple Risk Factors." *Journal of the American Medical Association* 272, no. 24 (1994): 1909-1914. https://doi.org/10.1001/jama.1994.03520240037038.

49. Nelson, Miriam E. and Sarah Wernick. *Strong Women Stay Young*. New York, Toronto, London, Sydney, Auckland: Bantam Books, 1997.

50. Kirk, Erik P., Joseph E. Donnelly, Bryan K. Smith, Jeff Honas, James D. LeCheminant, Bruce W. Bailey, Dennis J. Jacobsen, and Richard A. Washburn. "Minimal Resistance Training Improves Daily Energy Expenditure and Fat Oxidation." *Medicine and Science in Sports and Exercise* 41, no. 5 (2009): 1122-1129. https://doi.org/10.1249/MSS.0b013e318193c64e.

51. Pollock, Michael L., Glenn A. Gaesser, Janus D. Butcher, Jean Pierre Després, Rod K. Dishman, Barry A. Franklin, and Carol Ewing Garber. "The Recommended Quantity and Quality of Exercise." *Medicine and Science in Sport and Exercise* 30, no. 6 (1998): 975-91.

52. Woods, Krista, Phillip Bishop, and Eric Jones. "Warm-up and Stretching in the Prevention of Muscular Injury." *Sports Medicine* 37, no. 12 (2007): 1089-1099. https://doi.org/10.2165/00007256-200737120-00006.

53. Bishop, D. "Warm up II – Performance Changes to Structure the Warm following Active Warm up and How up." *Sports Medicine* 33, no. 7 (2003): 483-498.

54. Cotton, Richard. *Personal Trainer Manual: The Resource for Fitness Professionals*. San Diego: American Council on Exercise, 1996.

55. Ferris, Lee T., James S. Williams, and Chwan-Li Shen. "The Effect of Acute Exercise on Serum Brain-Derived Neurotrophic Factor Levels and Cognitive Function." *Medicine and Science in Sports and Exercise* 39, no. 4 (2007): 728-734. https://doi.org/10.1249/mss.0b013e31802f04c7.

56. Ratey, John J. *The Revolutionary New Science of Exercise and the Brain*. New York: Little, Brown and Company, 2008: 11-12, 17.

57. Ibid.

58. Ratey, John J. *The Revolutionary New Science of Exercise and the Brain*. New York: Little, Brown and Company, 2008: 22.

59. Hillman, Charles H., Matthew B. Pontifex, Lauren B. Raine, Darla M. Castelli, Eric E. Hall, and Arthur F. Kramer. "The Effect of Acute Treadmill Walking on Cognitive Control and Academic Achievement in Preadolescent Children." *Neuroscience* 159, no. 3 (2009): 1044-1054. https://doi.org/10.1016/j.neuroscience.2009.01.057.

60. Budde, Henning, Claudia Voelcker-Rehage, Sascha Pietraßyk-Kendziorra, Pedro Ribeiro, and Günter Tidow. "Acute Coordinative Exercise Improves Attentional Performance in Adolescents." *Neuroscience Letters* 441, no. 2 (2008): 219-223. https://doi.org/10.1016/j.neulet.2008.06.024.

61. Mahar, Matthew T., Sheila K. Murphy, David A. Rowe, Jeannie Golden, A. Tamlyn Shields, and Thomas D. Raedeke. "Effects of a Classroom-Based Program on Physical Activity and On-Task Behavior." *Medicine and Science in Sports and Exercise* 38, no. 12 (2006): 2086-2094. https://doi.org/10.1249/01.mss.0000235359.16685.a3.

62. Dietrich, Arne and Phillip B. Sparling. "Endurance Exercise Selectively Impairs Prefrontal-Dependent Cognition." *Brain and Cognition* 55, no. 3 (2004): 516-524. https://doi.org/10.1016/j.bandc.2004.03.002.

63. Boyle, Patricia A., Aron S. Buchman, Robert S. Wilson, Sue E. Leurgans, and David A. Bennett. "Association of Muscle Strength with the Risk of Alzheimer Disease and the Rate of Cognitive Decline in Community-Dwelling Older Persons." *Archives of Neurology* 66, no. 11 (2009): 1339-1344. https://doi.org/10.1001/archneurol.2009.240.

64. Nagamatsu, Lindsay S., Todd C. Handy, C. Liang Hsu, Michelle Voss, and Teresa Liu-Ambrose. "Resistance Training Promotes Cognitive and Functional Brain Plasticity in Seniors with Probable Mild Cognitive Impairment." *Archives of Internal Medicine* 172, no. 8 (2012): 666-668. https://doi.org/10.1001/archinternmed.2012.379.

65. Bible Gateway. "Matthew 4:1-11." Accessed August 2, 2018. https://www.biblegateway.com/passage/?search=matthew+4%3A1-11&version=NIV.

66. Edwards, William D., Wesley J. Gabel, and Floyd E. Hosmer. "On the Physical Death of Jesus Christ." *Journal of the American Medical Association* 255, no. 11 (1986): 1455-1463. https://doi.org/10.1001/jama.1986.03370110077025.

67. Holleman, Joseph. "How Many Miles Did Jesus Travel in his Life on Earth?" Last modified May 13, 2018. https://www.quora.com/How-many-miles-did-Jesus-travel-in-his-life-on-Earth.

ACTIVITY

TRUST IN GOD

Experience His love

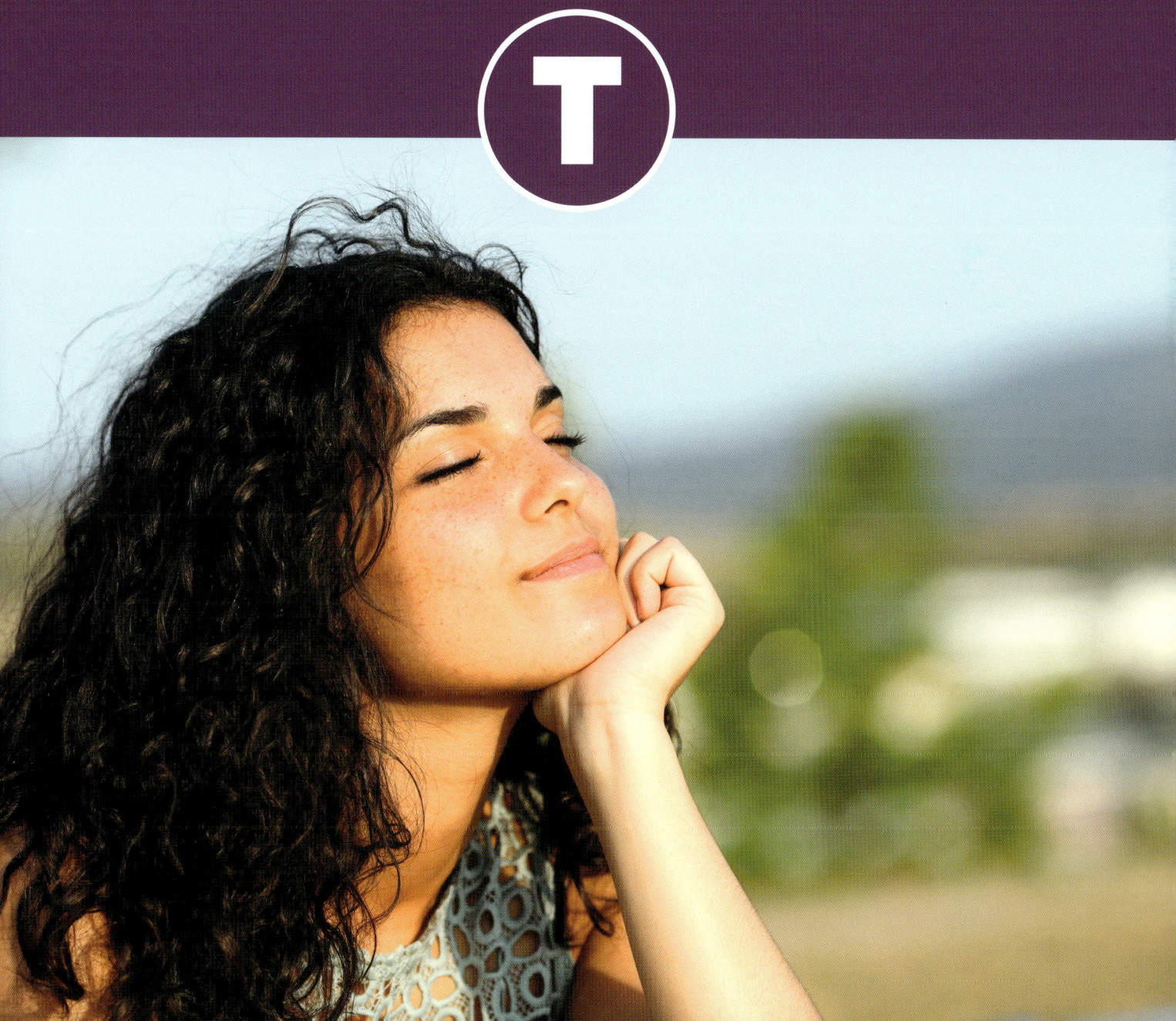

TRUST IN GOD [truhst] *verb* **1:** knowing that God loves
you unconditionally. This trusting relationship brings peace
during tough times and gives hope for the future.

THE BIG PICTURE

You've made it through half of the eight principles of CREATION Life. This brings you to the next principle — T for Trust in God. Right now you might be thinking, "What in the world does trust have to do with my health?" Quite a lot actually. In this chapter, you'll see how trust is connected not only to your health, but also to your happiness. Before you leap off the diving board into the pool of trust, it's important for you to understand one very key factor; this isn't just any kind of trust. It's trust in God.

You see, life is full of things that naturally just go together — chips and salsa, cheese and crackers, dads who wear socks with their sandals — and the same can be said for living a CREATION Life and having trust in God. After all, there wouldn't even be an option if you didn't first have a loving, all-powerful Creator. He is at the heart of everything you think and do.

God wants you to trust in Him so He can transform your life and re-create you into His own image. Understand He loves you despite your failures. Following His direction will lead you to a meaningful life full of joy and personal fulfillment. In order to have this abundant life, you first have to do one very important thing: you have to trust Him. Trust in God is the only way you can receive the power of God to transform your life.

What God desires from you more than anything is your trust. This trust manifests itself when you experience a loving relationship with your Creator. This relationship will empower and influence every aspect of your life as your Heavenly Father enables you to achieve the fullness of a CREATION Life.

TRUST is more than just having belief in another person. Trust in God is developed the same way as it is with any other person — through a close personal relationship.

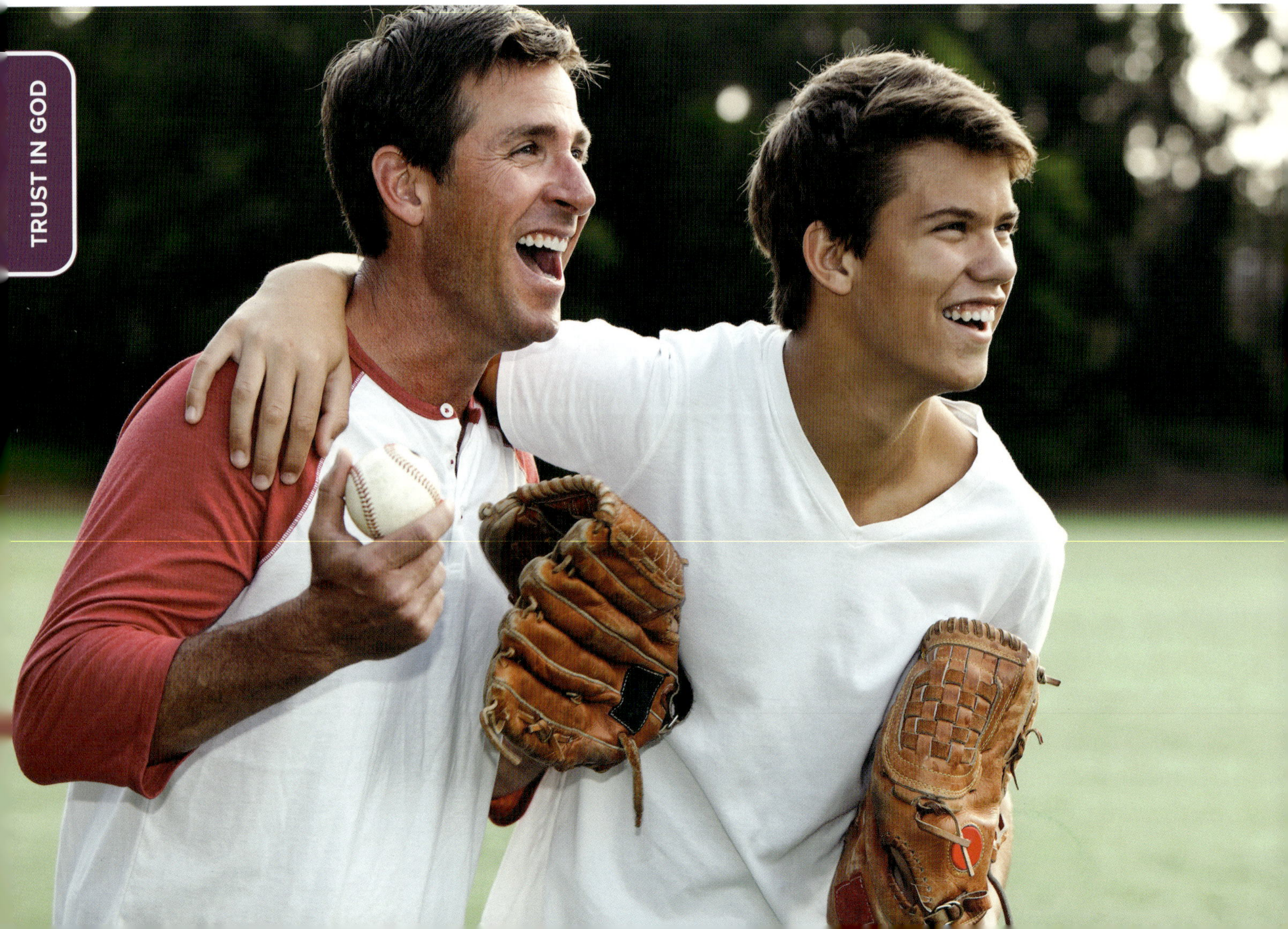

THE GIFT OF TRUST

Then the Lord God formed man of dust from the ground, and breathed into his nostrils the breath of life; and man became a living being.

GENESIS 2:7

When God created the heavens and the earth He did it *ex nihilo*, that is, "out of nothing." God spoke each element into existence, but when it came time to make the first man, He chose a completely different method. First, God formed the man from "the dust of the ground." This means He personally fashioned him to His own specifications. The word for "formed" is also used in the Bible to describe how a potter molds and shapes a piece of clay. Each vessel the potter creates has a specific function and purpose, just as God has given you a specific purpose for your life. Second, God breathed the "breath of life" into the man He created. Up until this point, the man was a lifeless form, but then God's own breath filled his lungs and he became a living, breathing soul. In the Bible, the word used for "breath" is also used for the life-giving "Spirit of God."

What does this unique creation process reveal? That to God, you are the jewel of all creation. Think about it: the Master Craftsman has formed you from the dust of the ground into His very own image. He has breathed into you His own life-giving Spirit and placed you in the world to reflect His majesty and glory. And what God asks of you in return is to lift your voice in praise along with the Psalmist who wrote:

I will give thanks to You, for I am fearfully and wonderfully made; wonderful are Your works, and my soul knows it very well.

PSALM 139:14

God created you to be in fellowship with Him. He is intimately acquainted with every aspect of your life — past, present and future. As He once revealed to the prophet Jeremiah:

"Before I formed you in the womb I knew you, and before you were born I consecrated you; I have appointed you a prophet to the nations."

JEREMIAH 1:5

God knew Jeremiah would be a prophet even before he was born. He knows what you will be as well. His knowledge of you is perfect, and that is why you can trust Him with every part of your life.

"Never be afraid to trust an unknown future to a known God."

CORRIE TEN BOOM

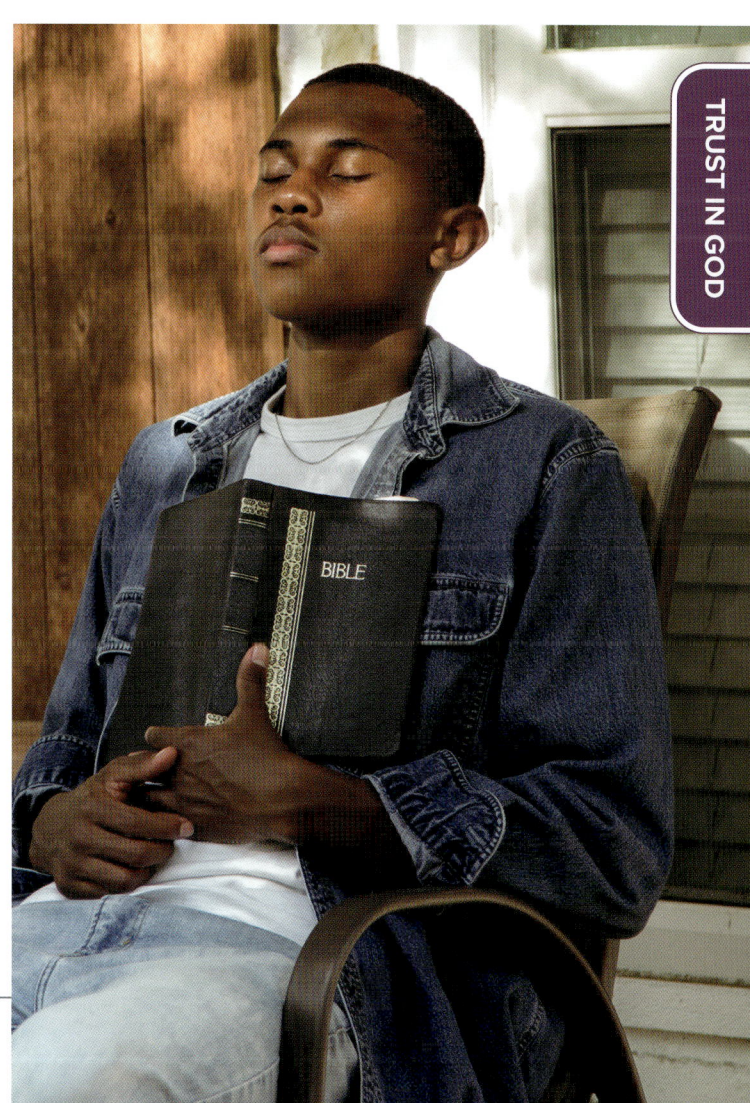

TRUST IN GOD

BROKEN TRUST

The question remains: If humanity was created for a loving relationship with its Creator, then why do so few people actually experience it? The reason has nothing to do with God. He has always remained faithful, and His Word never fails. So, if God hasn't broken His trust, the only possible explanation is that somehow humanity has broken theirs.

Now the serpent was more crafty than any of the wild animals the Lord God had made. He said to the woman, "Did God really say, 'You must not eat from any tree in the garden'?" GENESIS 3:1

You have already seen how God gave Adam and Eve the freedom to choose between life and death. In the end, their decision came down to only one thing: Whom did they trust more? God gave Adam and Eve a clear direction to follow, but it was the serpent that introduced the element of doubt. "Did God *really* say it?" "Does He *really* love you?" "Does He *really* have your best interests at heart?" At some point in your life, you may find yourself wrestling with similar questions. You will be tempted to believe that what is best for your life is to do your own thing rather than to follow the will of God. And when you make that choice, you too will sin.

Sin mutilates the image of God in your life. Like a thief, it robs you of your joy and leaves your soul bankrupt. It is the cause of all of life's problems — the great curse of the world. Disease, famine, pain, suffering, destruction and despair are all the consequences of sin, but the greatest consequence of all is that your relationship with God, your very trust, is broken by sin. You become separated from God by a chasm impossible for you to cross on your own. This leaves a vacuum in your life, what some call the "God-shaped hole," which was described by the French mathematician Blaise Pascal. Pascal wrote, "All men seek happiness,"[1] but for some reason this desire goes unmet. Humans, it seems, have an inability to fulfill their greatest desire:

(?) Have you sensed a "God-shaped hole" in your life? What have you used before to fill this hole? Did you succeed in filling it? Why or why not?

What is it then that this desire and this inability proclaim to us, but that there was once in man a true happiness of which there now remain to him only the mark and empty trace, which he in vain tries to fill from all his surroundings, seeking from things absent the help he does not obtain in things present? But these are all inadequate, because the infinite abyss can only be filled by an infinite and immutable object, that is to say, only by God Himself.

He only is our true good, and since we have forsaken Him, it is a strange thing that there is nothing in nature which has not been serviceable in taking His place... [2]

Scripture supports Pascal's observation about humanity's longing for the eternal. In the book of Ecclesiastes, the author writes of God and man, *"He (God) has made everything beautiful in its time. Also He has put eternity in their hearts, except that no one can find out the work that God does from beginning to end"* (Ecclesiastes 3:11). It makes perfect sense that if you have a thirst for eternity, it can only be quenched by the one thing that is itself eternal, namely God. Nothing else will ever completely satisfy you.

Of course, that doesn't stop many people from trying. They try to fill their "God-shaped hole" with lots of different things: money, a career, relationships, food, sex, music, drugs, entertainment, cars, sports, shopping and the list goes on. Some are doing such a good job they may not even notice the emptiness in their lives… for a short time. These feelings are always temporary. Eventually, such people get bored with what they have, so they seek new experiences and better sensations. But they will never know true contentment until they come to realize that it doesn't come from anything in this world. It comes from knowing the One who created this world.

GETTING GROUNDED

In Psalm 92:12, the Bible promises that *"The righteous shall flourish like the palm tree; he shall grow like a cedar in Lebanon."* The cedar trees of Lebanon are the stuff of legend. Their wood was strong and straight, so naturally they were God's first choice when it came to the construction of the most important building in all of Israel — the temple. Both King David and his son, Solomon, used cedar when they built their royal palaces. You can imagine a mighty cedar tree, its roots reaching deep into the ground, anchoring it to solid rock. When you anchor yourself to God, He will become your Rock. He will provide you with permanence, wisdom and strength.

God gives you everything you need in order to grow and flourish. Although there will be hard times in life, you can stand tall like a tree against the storms of life, coming out stronger than before.

TRUST IN GOD

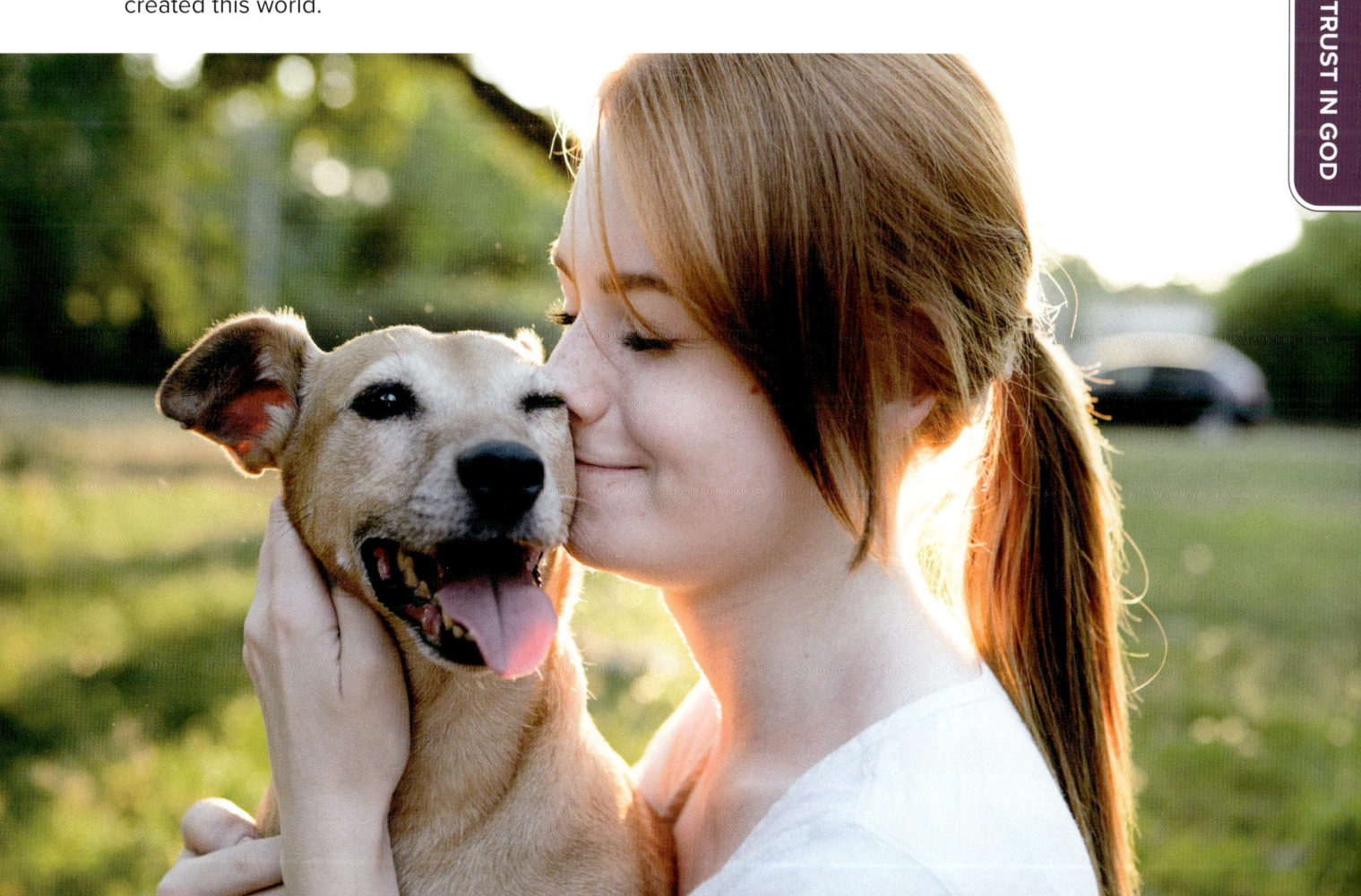

TRUST AND YOUR WELL-BEING

Let's be honest; some people have a hard time wrapping their minds around trusting in an all-knowing, all-powerful, yet unseen Creator. They prefer to remain hopeful skeptics rather than become committed believers. When you get down to it, trusting in God may not be easy for everyone, but it is absolutely essential if you are ever to receive the maximum benefits that God promises.

Trust in God has a powerful impact on your well-being. The Oxford University Press, *Handbook of Religion and Health,* offers an extensive overview of the topic through review of more than 1,600 published studies and reviews in physical, mental and social health fields. The authors state that "The majority of studies indicate that religiousness (having or showing a belief in God) is associated with less coronary artery disease, hypertension, stroke, immune system dysfunction, cancer, functional impairment and fewer negative health behaviors (e.g., smoking, drug and alcohol abuse, risky sexual behaviors).... Religiousness is also associated with increased longevity and physical activity."[3]

In a separate study published by the American Psychological Association, the relationship between religious involvement and mortality was explored in greater detail. Forty-two independent samples representing 125,826 participants examined the association between being involved religiously and all-cause mortality (all-cause mortality is the annual number of deaths in a given age group per the population in that age group). It was concluded that people with active religious involvement increased their chance of living longer by 29 percent.[4]

It makes sense that if God is the One who created you, then trusting in Him is the only way to unlock your full potential. If you do, greater health, well-being and longevity are just a few of the benefits research says will be yours.

TRUST AND ACADEMIC PERFORMANCE

Sometimes finishing high school feels harder than trying to sneeze with your eyes open. But even if you don't consider yourself to be the best student academically, you still want to give your best. One way you can do this is by building up your trust in God. Before you see the research, consider this Scripture:

For the Lord gives wisdom; from His mouth come knowledge and understanding.

PROVERBS 2:6

The Bible makes it clear that God is the source of all wisdom, knowledge and understanding. It even goes so far as to say that if anyone lacks wisdom, *"Let him ask of God, who gives to all generously... and it will be given to him"* (James 1:5). And one of the best places to find wisdom for living is in the pages of the Bible itself.

Several studies have shown that in urban areas, an increase in Bible knowledge is associated with higher levels of student academic achievement and positive behavioral patterns.[5] For example, in one of those studies it was discovered that students with the highest level of Bible literacy also had the highest average GPA. Not surprisingly, they also had the highest rankings in test scores and grades. But perhaps the most remarkable aspect of the study was that these students also demonstrated the best behavior at school. In short, they were model students. In sharp contrast, however, the students with the lowest levels of Bible literacy also had the lowest average GPA, the lowest ranking in test and grade results and the worst school behavior.[6]

This spiritual boost in academics may also be a huge factor in helping to close the achievement gap. The achievement gap refers to the difference in academic performance between different ethnic groups. It's a harsh reality, but for many school children, economic and social factors hinder their performance at school. Later in life, their lack of education will negatively affect their ability to get into college or get the job they most want. Legislators have made several attempts to close the achievement gap, but the problem persists. However, according to the

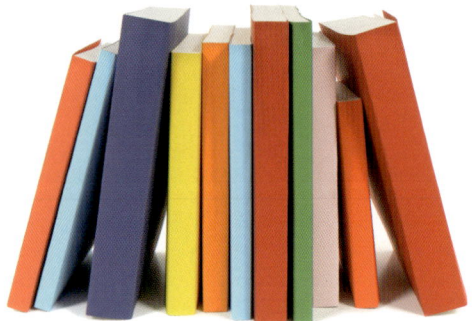

combined results from several different studies, personal religious faith was one of the two largest factors that consistently reduced the achievement gap. Personal religious commitment reduces the achievement gap by 50 percent, and attending a religious school reduces it by 25 percent. [7]

Another study including another group of students found that those who actively attended church or who saw their faith as very important to their lives also achieved higher grades in school. They also stayed on track in school, had less trouble with their teachers, other students and homework and they identified with school more strongly than students in other groups. [8]

If you attend a religious school, this will also positively impact your academic performance. Using the National Education Longitudinal Survey data set, it was found that students attending religious schools performed better academically than those who did not. These students included all private religious schools that were examined in the study. Students who did not attend religious schools included all those attending public schools and nonreligious private or nonreligious preparatory school. The results also indicated that children of low socioeconomic status, as well as African-American and Hispanic students, performed better academically in religious schools than in nonreligious schools. [9]

To put all this in perspective, consider the amazing, true story of Justin as it is told in the devotional book, *The Incredible Journey:*

"Some years ago, psychologist Dr. Elden Chalmers taught in the Seminary at Andrews University. When the new year began, a graduate student we'll call Justin, came to Dr. Chalmers to see about entering the seminary. 'I really want to be a minister,' Justin, said. 'But I'm not a good student. I heard you talk at our church last year. You said that people can become smarter. Would you show me how?' Dr. Chalmers said he would be happy to help, but he wanted to know more about Justin. Justin admitted that all through academy and college he had barely gotten by with a low C average. He knew that if he didn't improve dramatically, he'd never make it through seminary."

"Dr. Chalmers suggested that Justin first take an IQ test... the test showed that Justin was below average in intelligence. An average score is 100. Justin had scored 90. 'All right,' said Dr. Chalmers, 'here's our plan of action. I want you to study the Bible every day. Why don't you start by looking up texts on different topics, such as love, forgiveness and trust? You'll also want to begin memorizing Bible verses. Stop by my office in the next few weeks and let me know how you are doing.' 'That's all there is to do?' Justin asked. 'That's it.'"

"Justin left Dr. Chalmers' office excited about the experiment. Could Bible study raise his IQ and make him more intelligent? He couldn't wait to find out. Justin found out that studying the Bible was a whole lot more fun than he had expected it to be. He appreciated the encouragement and advice Dr. Chalmers gave him, but within a few weeks Justin decided that their visits weren't necessary anymore. He had developed a Bible study plan and he knew what he needed to do."

"In March, six months after Justin had begun the study program, Dr. Chalmers called him into his office. 'Why don't we try another IQ test to see how you are progressing?' Justin was retested. The results were astounding. In six months his IQ had gone from a 90 to 120, a 33% increase. A person's IQ usually doesn't change very much over time. But Justin proved that with God, miracles can happen. Not only did Bible study increase Justin's IQ score, but he also found that learning became much easier for him."

"He signed up for a class that was only open to the best students in the seminary. At the end of the quarter, he got the highest grade in the class. Justin continued studying his Bible during the nine quarters of his seminary training. Just before his graduation, Dr. Chalmers suggested a final IQ test. Justin's IQ had increased to 131." [10]

Perhaps, like Justin, you too could improve your performance in school by regularly studying God's Word and further developing your trust in Him.

Are you experiencing trust issues at home or at school? Pray and ask God to help you resolve those issues and to learn to trust again. This may mean repairing a broken relationship or admitting a past wrong, but trust God to give you the strength you need to rebuild.

BIBLE STUDY TIPS

Does reading the Bible feel more like you're trying to decipher a foreign language? Follow these tips to make your study times easier and more productive.

1. **Read with a prayerful spirit.** Before you start reading, pray and ask God to open your eyes to the wonders in His law (Psalm 119:18). Also, ask Him to help you understand the Scriptures as you read.

2. **Start small.** If you try to tackle an entire book of the Bible, you may get frustrated and give up. Start with just a chapter or two. Add more as you get more comfortable.

3. **Keep notes.** Underline or highlight anything that you like or have a question about. Keep a journal of your thoughts or verses that you want to study more in the future.

4. **Use online resources.** Great websites are available to help improve your study time. BibleGateway.com and BlueLetterBible.org both provide free access to several versions of the Bible as well as additional study resources and commentaries.

5. **End with prayer.** Don't just be a "hearer" of the Word but a "doer" (James 1:23). When you have finished your study time, pray and ask God to help you apply what you have learned to your spiritual walk.

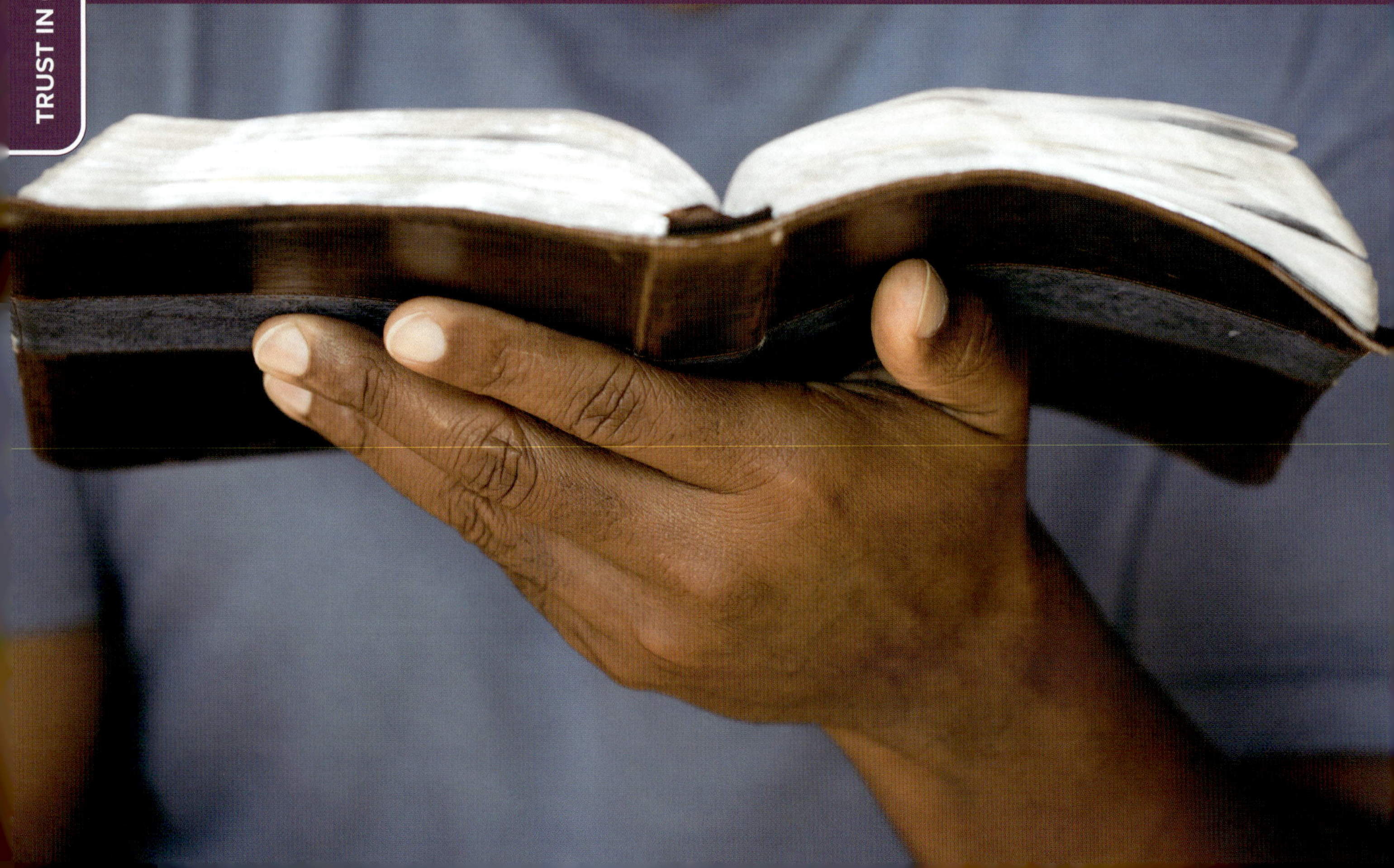

A RECIPE FOR TRUST

If you were going to whip up a batch of delicious, fluffy buttermilk pancakes you wouldn't dare leave out the eggs, the baking soda or the buttermilk, would you? All of these ingredients are crucial in order for the recipe to be a success. Tinkering with or eliminating just one means your finished product will taste less like pancakes and more like old flip-flops. Well, trust in God has basic ingredients too, and removing any of them from the equation equally spells disaster. The basic ingredients are pretty simple when you look at them individually — Bible study, prayer, fellowship with believers in a local church body and serving others — but when you add them all together you get a life that is positively bursting with flavor. After all, it was Jesus Himself who said:

"You are the salt of the earth; but if the salt has become tasteless, how can it be made salty again? It is no longer good for anything, except to be thrown out and trampled under foot by men." MATTHEW 5:13

Salt isn't just a great flavor enhancer or the world's oldest seasoning, it's also an indispensable mineral that helps all humans and animals survive. If you could somehow remove all the salt from your diet, eventually you would die. Salt was also vital to the ancient world as a way of preserving foods to eat at a later time. By comparing your life to salt, Jesus is saying that you are to be equally indispensable in the world. Your life should be full of flavor and vitality, and others should see in you the qualities they desire for their own lives.

To build trust in your life, you need to engage daily in Bible study, prayer, fellowship and service.

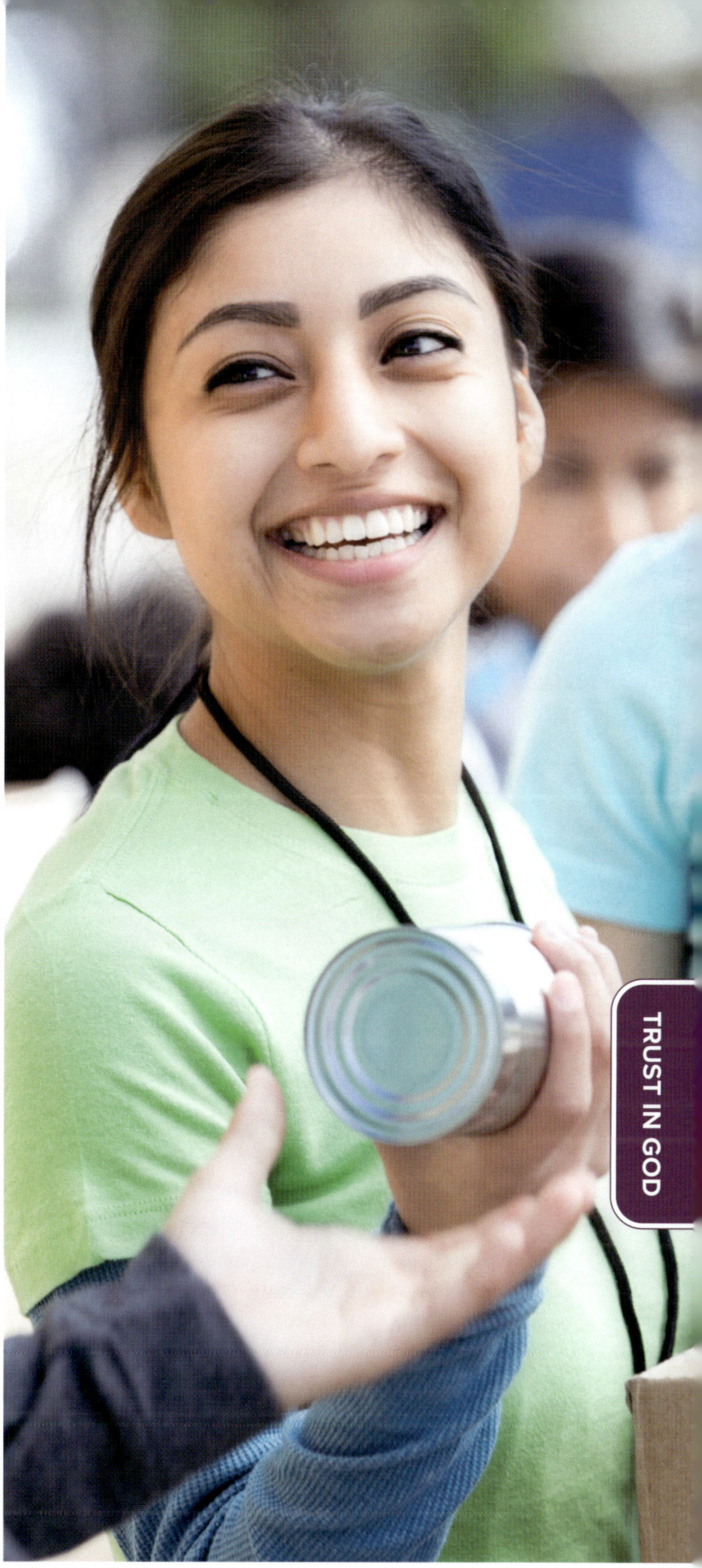

 **Do you trust in Jesus as the only way for you to be free from your sins and to have eternal life?**

TRUST IN GOD

SPIRITUAL NOURISHMENT

Do you remember how hungry you were the last time you skipped a meal? In the same way, you sustain your spiritual hunger through daily feasting on God's Word.

When He was tempted in the wilderness, Jesus said, *"It is written, 'Man shall not live on bread alone, but on every word that proceeds out of the mouth of God'"* (Matthew 4:4). The Bible is sometimes called the "Bread of Life" because bread was the primary form of sustenance in the ancient world. It is the only way you can satisfy your hunger for God.

Studying the Bible helps you develop your trust in God in several ways. First, Bible study helps you to know who God is. Its pages will vividly introduce you to His loving and trustworthy character. In each story, you will see how God always kept the promises He made. And He is the same *"yesterday and today and forever"* (Hebrews 13:8). That means He is still in the business of keeping His promises.

Reading God's Word will also help you develop a relationship with Him. As you get to know Him more intimately, you will find yourself trusting Him more and more. *"And those who know Your name will put their trust in You, for You, O Lord, have not forsaken those who seek You"* (Psalm 9:10).

In the Bible, God has given you incredible insights into living a happy and satisfying life. Naturally, the things God says to do are the best choices for you to make because He is all knowing, good and loving. God's commandments are not merely suggestions. Inside of each one you can see a cause and effect relationship. If you choose to ignore what God commands, you will have to live with the consequences, but if you choose to obey His word, you will be blessed. This can be seen in the book of Isaiah where God speaks to His people. You can almost hear the pain in His voice as He tells them:

> *"Never let your fears come above your faith."*
>
> UNKNOWN

"I am the Lord your God, who teaches you to profit, who leads you in the way you should go. If only you had paid attention to My commandments. Then your well-being would have been like a river, and your righteousness like the waves of the sea."

ISAIAH 48:17–18

If you will trust that He knows what is best for you, you will want to follow His leading. Sometimes you cannot clearly see the cause and effect relationship until after you have made the right decision, but if you know the true character of the One who tells you the way you should go, you will trust Him enough to choose to obey the principles He has revealed to you.

SPIRITUAL BREATH

Breathing has two parts, inhaling and exhaling. You are constantly breathing in and breathing out. In fact, you do it so much you don't even have to think about it. Well, prayer has been called the "breath of the soul." Like breathing, prayer has two parts as well. Of course, you speak to God, sharing with Him your needs, concerns and desires, but you also stop and let God speak to you. You let Him remind you of the wonderful things He has done so that you can respond with praise and thanksgiving. The more you practice praying, the more it will become a natural part of your life, just like breathing. Paul writes that you are to *"pray without ceasing"* (1 Thessalonians 5:17). You wouldn't try to stop breathing, would you? In the same way, prayer is designed to be a constant part of your life, forever drawing you closer to your heavenly Father.

Praying frequently, whether in public or in private, is also associated with better health, emotional well-being and lower levels of psychological distress.[11] Researchers have found this to be true regardless of your ethnic group or denomination. Think of prayer as your time to talk with God as you would a friend. You can share with Him your joys, challenges and of course, your requests. Being in communication with Him is a powerful influence on your life.[12]

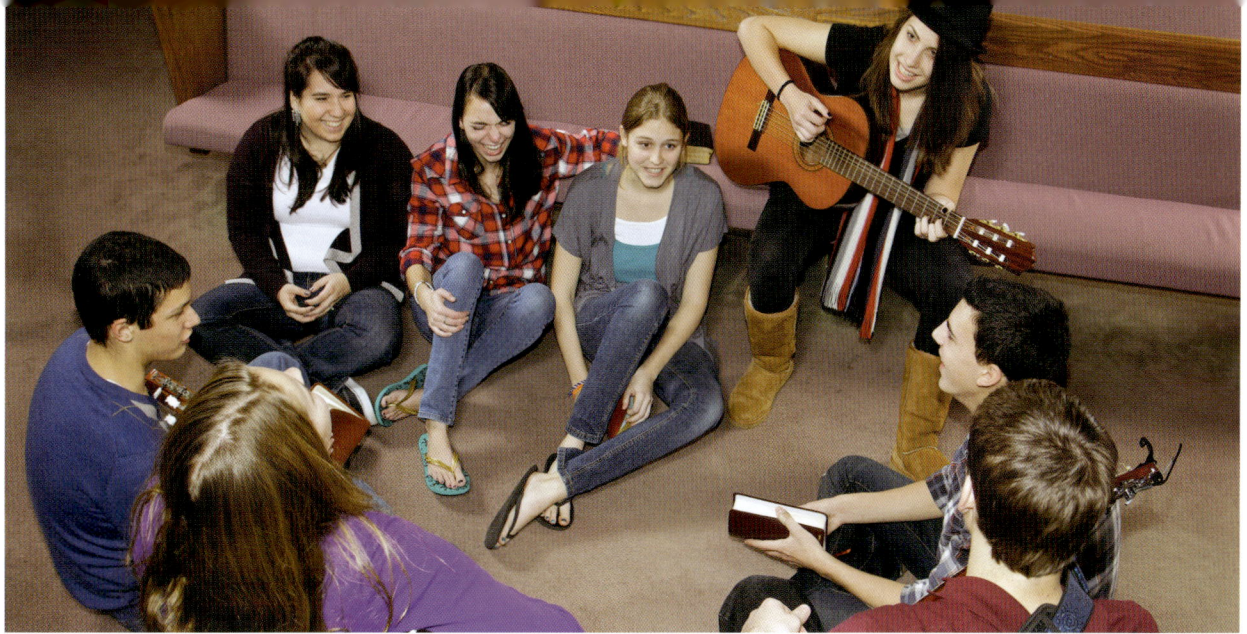

SPIRITUAL EXERCISE

It's one thing to say you have trust in God, but it's quite another to actually put your faith into action. This is what makes exercising your faith so important. Just as physical exercise keeps you healthy and strong, the spiritual exercises of the Christian life will grow you into a solid, well-rounded individual. These exercises are to fellowship with believers in a local church and participate in acts of service toward others. The Bible makes it clear that all believers need one another. In the book of Hebrews, believers are instructed, *"And let us consider how to stimulate one another to love and good deeds, not forsaking our own assembling together, as is the habit of some, but encouraging one another"* (Hebrews 10:24–25).

However, going to church can be a stumbling block for many teens. Perhaps they don't fully understand why it's important, or maybe they are discouraged by what they perceive as hypocrisy among other believers. Some may say, "I love Jesus and that's the important thing. Why do I have to go to church, too?"

Think about it this way: In the Bible, the church is pictured as the "Bride of Christ" (Ephesians 5:25–27). Imagine telling a good friend who is married, "You know, I really like hanging out with you, but I can't stand your wife." You wouldn't remain friends for long. Jesus loves His church, and if you love Jesus you will love it too. Sure, the church has its problems, but that doesn't change the fact that it is God's appointed agent for spiritual change in this world.

Going to church is one of the most common ways that people seek to enhance their relationship with God. This has also demonstrated a positive effect on health and well-being. One study found that attending religious services could increase one's lifespan by an average of seven years for Caucasians and potentially fourteen years for African-Americans.[13] Another study of over 100,000 people, performed at Johns Hopkins University, found that attending religious services on a weekly basis reduced the risk of death the following year by almost 50 percent.[14] Another group of researchers found that adults who reported weekly attendance were more likely to improve health behaviors and maintain good ones than those who did not attend church. The researchers also noted that attending religious services was associated with significantly lower smoking rates, higher levels of physical activity, less depression, more personal relationships and longer, healthier marriages.[15]

Personal and daily devotional time with God is also a powerful promoter of well-being. Time spent in worship and honest communication with God has a healing effect.[16] Just as you receive benefits from spending time with a good friend, so it is with God. Bible study, prayer and time spent in fellowship and worship are channels of direct communion with your heavenly Father, and through each of them you will be richly blessed.

TRUSTING IN THE HARD TIMES

When times get hard, where do you turn for guidance and strength? If you are like a large number of Americans, you believe in the God of the Bible and trust that He has an active presence in your life. According to a Pew Research Center study, 56 percent of Americans believe in a God as described in the Bible, while 33 percent believe in a higher power or spiritual force. The study also found that about half of Americans (48 percent) say that God, or another higher power, directly determines what happens in their lives all or most of the time. An additional 18 percent say God, or some other higher power, determines what happens to them "just some of the time."[17]

However, even though the majority of Americans realize their need for God, many fail to see how critically important it is for them to have a relationship with Him as well. Spending time with God becomes less and less a priority as other, "more important" matters take precedence. This limits God's transformative power in their lives, which is really a shame, especially when you consider how significant a role faith plays in the process of coping with stress, loss or death. One study found that faith was rated as the single most effective coping strategy in dealing with loss. Another study found 78 percent of the respondents reporting that religion was involved in helping them cope with a significant negative life event.[18]

Religion has been identified as an important coping resource for many health related challenges. Its positive effects include reducing depressive symptoms, increasing satisfaction with life, reducing length of hospital stay and reducing risk of alcohol abuse.[19] In more than 80 studies published over the last one hundred years, it was shown that religious/spiritual factors were generally linked with lower rates of depression.[20]

The research is very clear; religious beliefs and faith bring emotional and physical benefits, but is that really a surprise? After all, it's God's will for you to have an abundant life filled with health, peace, purpose and meaning. So, no matter what you may face, remember that you can always turn to God. Continue to trust in Him by praying and reading His Word. He promises, *"He will not fail you or forsake you"* (Deuteronomy 31:6), and that includes the hard times.

(?) Do you find God eternally trustworthy? What circumstances you are facing make it difficult for you to trust Him? Which of His attributes make it easy for you to trust Him?

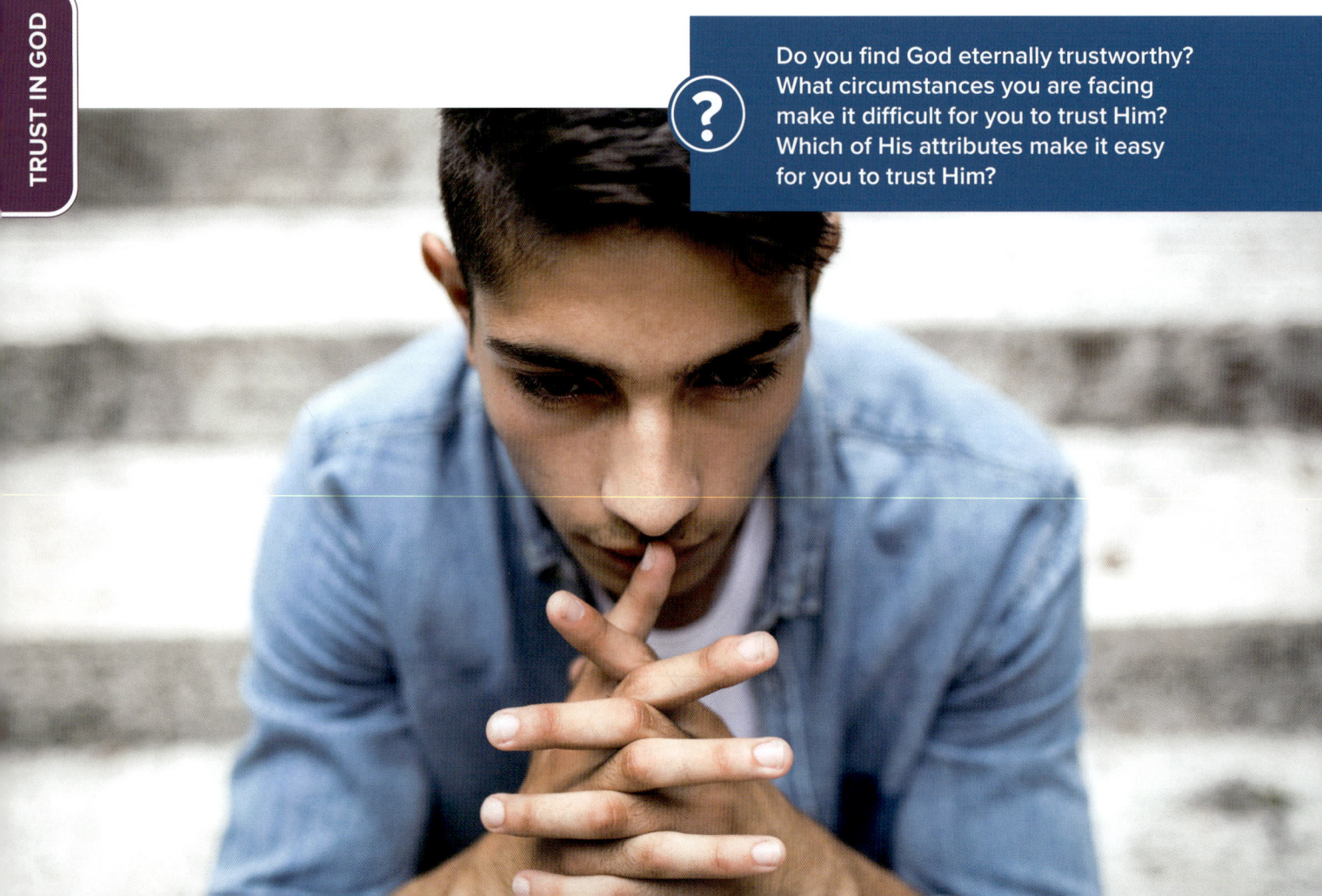

THE POWER OF GOD'S LOVE

So, where does a trusting relationship with your Creator begin? How is such an incredible thing even possible? Maybe you've heard that God loves you unconditionally, but how do you know this is true; how can you trust this claim?

The easiest way to come to believe in something is to examine the evidence surrounding it. Where is the proof? God's love for you is most clearly seen through the gift of His Son, Jesus Christ. *"For God so loved the world, that He gave His only begotten Son, that whoever believes in Him shall not perish, but have eternal life"* (John 3:16, NASB). Jesus was sent by His heavenly Father to offer His life as a sacrifice for sins. He died in your place, taking your sins into His own body on the cross. The Bible makes it clear that *"He was pierced through for our transgressions, He was crushed for our iniquities"* (Isaiah 53:5, NASB). This means Jesus suffered a horrible, agonizing death and He did it for you, but why? Why did Jesus endure such pain and suffering; what did He have to gain? The answer is so simple it's easy to miss. It was you. Jesus wanted to make a way for you and Him to be together forever. Eternal life is the free gift that is offered to whoever believes in Him. Isn't it incredible? You can access all the riches of heaven if you just put your trust in Jesus.

THE GOOD NEWS

When you come to understand the good news of Jesus Christ and His sacrificial love for you, it gives you incredible freedom to trust in Him. After all, He didn't wait for you to come to Him. He took the first step, gave the greatest gift and paid the ultimate price. He loves you and desires for you to prosper. *"'For I know the plans that I have for you,' declares the Lord, 'plans for welfare and not for calamity to give you a future and a hope'"* (Jeremiah 29:11). God truly has your best interests at heart, and with His help you can be empowered to rise above any challenges you may face. You can place your past, present and future entirely in His hands.

The Bible assures you that *"God is love"* (1 John 4:8). God's love is a powerful force that unlocks your full potential. Just consider the dynamic impact positive emotions have on your health. "Experts have singled out love as foremost among the human emotions capable of promoting and maintaining health and achieving healing."[21]

"It seems something deep inside our cells responds positively when we feel love. Love appears capable of sparking healthy biological reactions in much the same way as good food and fitness."[22]

Dr. Bernie Siegel, a Yale physician and the author of the best-selling book *Love, Medicine and Miracles,* affirms the power of love. "Unconditional love is the most powerful stimulant of the immune system. The truth is love heals."[23]

This healing power of love can be seen in another study, where it was found that receiving love could reduce the risk of coronary artery disease, hypertension, cancer[24] and alcoholism.[25] Yet another study reports that feeling loved is the strongest predictor of an individual's sense of positive self-esteem.[26] It seems that knowing you are loved and accepted by someone else helps you to love and accept yourself. Other benefits of being loved include increased levels of immunoglobulin A (an antibody that is an important part of your immune system) and smoother, more regular heart rhythms.[27-28] By contrast, another study found that a lack of love shown to parents by their children was associated with higher levels of psychological distress.[29] Loss of love was among the most common reasons given for suicide or suicidal behavior.[30]

What you believe about God affects your well-being. In order to receive the most benefits, you must start by placing your trust in God's unconditional love for you. Love will even motivate you to make the healthiest choices, to rest in His peace, to surround yourself with a healing environment, to be active physically and mentally, to trust fully in Him, to serve others, to have a positive outlook and to eat nutritious foods for strength and health. You will be motivated to live the abundant life because you long to make His love known to others.

INEFFABLE LOVE

In the hymn *O Worship the King*, the hymn writer uses a certain word to describe God's love, "ineffable love." Ineffable is a peculiar word in that it symbolizes something that cannot be described in words. This means that God's love is beyond comprehension, impossible to put into words; there is no language or idea to fully define it.

It's hard to wrap your head around this idea. It's a bit like going to the ocean and trying to hold the water in your hands. The tighter your grasp, the more it drips away. There is only one response when you are in the presence of such great, ineffable love — *wonder*. The word may conjure in your mind the natural breathtaking sights of the world — standing at the majestic Grand Canyon, exploring the splendors of the Great Barrier Reef, the mind-blowing view from atop Mt. Everest — but nothing is more wondrous, more deserving of praise and adoration than the love of God.

Another great hymn puts it like this:

Could we with ink the ocean fill,
and were the skies of parchment made,
were every stalk on earth a quill,
and every man a scribe by trade;
to write the love of God above
would drain the ocean dry;
nor could the scroll contain the whole,
though stretched from sky to sky.[31]

You can see these claims affirmed in Scripture in the last verse of John, *"And there are also many other things which Jesus did, which if they were written in detail, I suppose that even the world itself would not contain the books that would be written"* (John 21:25). Think of that; there are not enough books in the world that can contain all the wonderful things that Jesus has done. All the libraries aren't big enough to hold the volumes. Even all the world's computers, with their billions and billions of gigabytes of information are just one drop in an ocean so vast and immeasurable — the ocean of God's ineffable love.

TRUSTING OTHERS

Trusting and loving other people also plays a big part in helping your body to heal. Consider this study published in the *Journal of the American Medical Association*. The *Journal* reviewed pain medications over the previous 25 plus years. It seems they found an interesting connection between a patient's pain level and their trust in their physician. Their conclusion was, "The quality of interaction or trust between the patient and the physician can be extremely influential in patient outcomes, and in some (perhaps many) cases, patient and provider expectations and interactions may be more important than the specific treatments."[32] In other words, patients who trusted their physicians more experienced less pain and greater results from their medication than patients who trusted less.

There is more than just a psychological reason for this effect. When you see a person whom you have a trusting relationship, your brain releases a chemical called oxytocin. Research suggests this amazing hormone is responsible for the feelings of well-being associated with interacting with close friends. It's even been called the "trust hormone" because this feeling of well-being helps you to interact and open up with others. Apparently it also inhibits the stress hormone cortisol.[33]

Healthy, trusting relationships give a sense of love and belonging that are essential to the enjoyment of life. You often try to meet or exceed the expectation of your close friends and family because you value the sense of belonging. This means that trusting others will help you to be the best you can be.

How would you describe that which is indescribable? What words or images does the love of God bring to your mind?

THE POWER OF FORGIVENESS

For if you forgive others for their transgressions, your heavenly Father will also forgive you.

MATTHEW 6:14

How should you respond when someone you trust at school mistreats you? What about when they talk about you behind your back or try to intimidate or bully you? In high school, you might experience behavior like this and more all before lunchtime. How should you respond? The best choice you can make for yourself and the other person is to offer forgiveness.

You probably know that forgiveness is a foundational principle of your spiritual well-being. After all, your ability to trust God comes from the fact that He has first forgiven you. But did you know that research now suggests the benefits of forgiveness extend far beyond the spiritual realm? By learning to forgive others you'll actually be doing your health a big favor. In the book, *Forgive for Good,* Dr. Fred Luskin, Director of the Stanford University Forgiveness Project says, "The practice of forgiveness has been shown to reduce anger, hurt, depression and stress and leads to greater feelings of hope, peace, compassion and self-confidence."

People who are able to forgive and move away from past hurts are freeing themselves from carrying the heavy burdens of hatred, resentment and bitterness. You can imagine the amount of stress and anxiety created when you harbor these feelings for an extended period of time. This is why it is so important to learn to forgive. Researchers have found that when subjects were encouraged to think forgiving thoughts, their stress response was diminished. Another study found that forgiveness is directly related to fewer problems with substance abuse. It only makes sense that you are less likely to turn to alcohol or drugs as a coping mechanism when you have forgiven the hurt and pain caused by another person.

Still, some people are resistant to forgive. They feel they are entitled to bear a grudge. Some even go so far as to seek revenge for the wrongs done to them. This creates a vicious cycle best reputed by a famous quote (often attributed to Mahatma Gandhi), *"An eye for an eye leaves the whole world blind."* However, the Bible's instruction to forgive remains, and science now supports the powerful, positive impact this can have on your life. Of course, this doesn't mean forgiveness is easy. In fact, it may be one of the hardest things you ever have to do in your entire life, but it's worth it. You will not only improve your relationships and your physical health, but you will demonstrate a true trust in your heavenly Father who tells you to, *"Be kind to one another, tender-hearted, forgiving each other, just as God in Christ also has forgiven you"* (Ephesians 4:32).

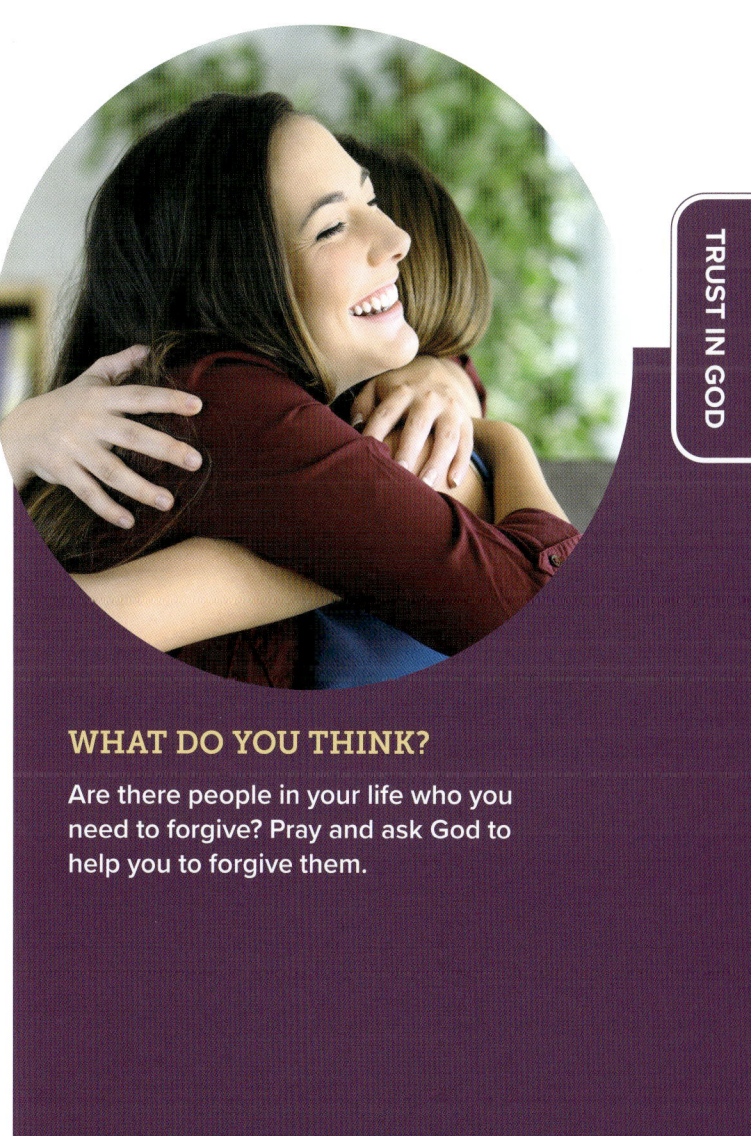

WHAT DO YOU THINK?

Are there people in your life who you need to forgive? Pray and ask God to help you to forgive them.

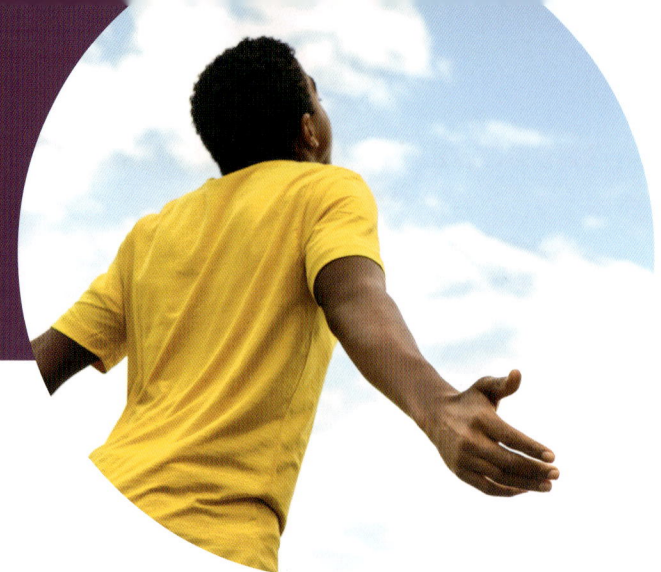

"Faith begins as an experiment and ends as an experience."

WILLIAM INGE

Do you see the benefits of trusting God's method of healthful living enough to do it?

THE POWER OF TRUST IN GOD

It's easy to see how relationships built on trust can create a sense of security. It's also true that relationships can quickly turn sour as feelings get hurt and emotions run wild. While you may often experience limitations and difficulties in your human relationships, God has promised to always be there for you for whatever you need, no matter how big or small.

It's not surprising that one study found that belief in God gave one an overall increase in life satisfaction, as well as a greater satisfaction with one's community, job and even marriage.[37] A study conducted at UCLA revealed that people who were most likely to perceive God as a remedy, as a being or force that releases them from or resolves the problems of living, reported the highest levels of marital satisfaction and satisfaction with personal health.[38] These studies support the biblical truth that a positive, loving view of God is a powerful healing force in your life.

How you view God is important. Belief in a loving God contributes to positive outcomes in your life, while a perspective that emphasizes obedience to a vengeful, punishing God contributes to negative ones.[39]

WHEN COGNITIVE DISSONANCE STRIKES

In the acclaimed novel *Catcher in the Rye,* 16-year-old protagonist Holden Caulfield expresses his disgust at all the so-called "phonies" of the world. Over the years, Holden's feelings have resonated especially with young readers who share his frustrations with those people they perceive as less than genuine. Maybe you feel the same, lashing out at hypocrites and frauds wherever you may find them, but take a good, long look in the mirror. Do you always practice what you preach?

How you answer this question is important, not only to your reputation, but also to your health. Research has shown that if you don't practice what you preach, it can lead to increased anxiety, depression, guilt and stress.[40] This is "cognitive dissonance." Merriam-Webster's dictionary defines cognitive dissonance as psychological conflict resulting from incongruous beliefs and attitudes held simultaneously.[41] One example of cognitive dissonance would be dating someone who does not share your values or beliefs. On one hand, you are attracted and drawn to the person physically or emotionally, but at the same time you are frustrated and repulsed by their opinions and beliefs that go against your own. When talking about God's law and your obedience to it, you might also experience cognitive dissonance between your beliefs and your behaviors. If you claim to be a Christian, but are not living the way you believe is right, then you will experience cognitive dissonance. The only way to stop this is to try to harmonize your beliefs with your actions. When you do, the dissonance goes away, your relationship with God is strengthened and so is your health.

GET IN THE WHEELBARROW

On June 30, 1859, performer Charles Blondin became the first person to ever cross Niagara Falls by walking across on a tightrope. The feat was incredible, and Blondin became a sensation. In the years that followed, he repeated the stunt many times, adding more and more daring elements to his act. One on occasion, he even crossed the falls while pushing a wheelbarrow. The crowd was enchanted; they wanted to see more, and so Blondin asked, "Who thinks I can do it again?"

The crowd cheered their approval.

"Who thinks I can do it with someone in the wheelbarrow?" Blondin said.

The crowd erupted in applause. "We believe in you." they shouted.

"Very well," Blondin said. "Then who will be first to volunteer to sit in the wheelbarrow?"

No one ever accepted Blondin's invitation. Sure, the crowd was happy to watch him risk his own life, but when it came down to it, they were much more content to stay where they were than to climb into the wheelbarrow.

What about you? You've now made it more than halfway through the CREATION Life principles. You've learned how following God's plans for your life will provide you with greater health and well-being. You've heard how God has promised you an abundant life, if you will only choose to live in obedience to His commands.

But will you get in the wheelbarrow?

In other words, do you actually trust God enough to put your words into action? The entire crowd said they *believed* that Blondin could push a person across the tightrope, but no one had the trust to get into that wheelbarrow. Like the inside of a dead tree, their trust was empty and hollow.

Commit your way to the Lord, trust also in Him, and He will do it.

PSALM 37:5

Trust in God is more than just saying, "I believe in You." It means you have to do the things God commands. When you commit yourself to Him, completely, He doesn't just guarantee results; He is the one who brings them to fruition. Of course, it is highly possible to know the truth and yet to never trust it, that is to never let what you have learned bring about a change in your life (just think about the countless smokers aware of the undeniable fact that cigarettes cause lung cancer). The Bible is clear that "*Faith without works is dead*" (James 2:26), or to put it another way, without action, trust doesn't exist.

Don't let the abundant life pass you by. Keep your trust in the Creator of Heaven and Earth, and follow His plan to live your life to the fullest.

TRUST IN GOD

> *"Trust in God is like a gyroscope. It keeps you stable even if life puts you on a precarious angle."*
> CUMMINGS AND REED, CREATION Life

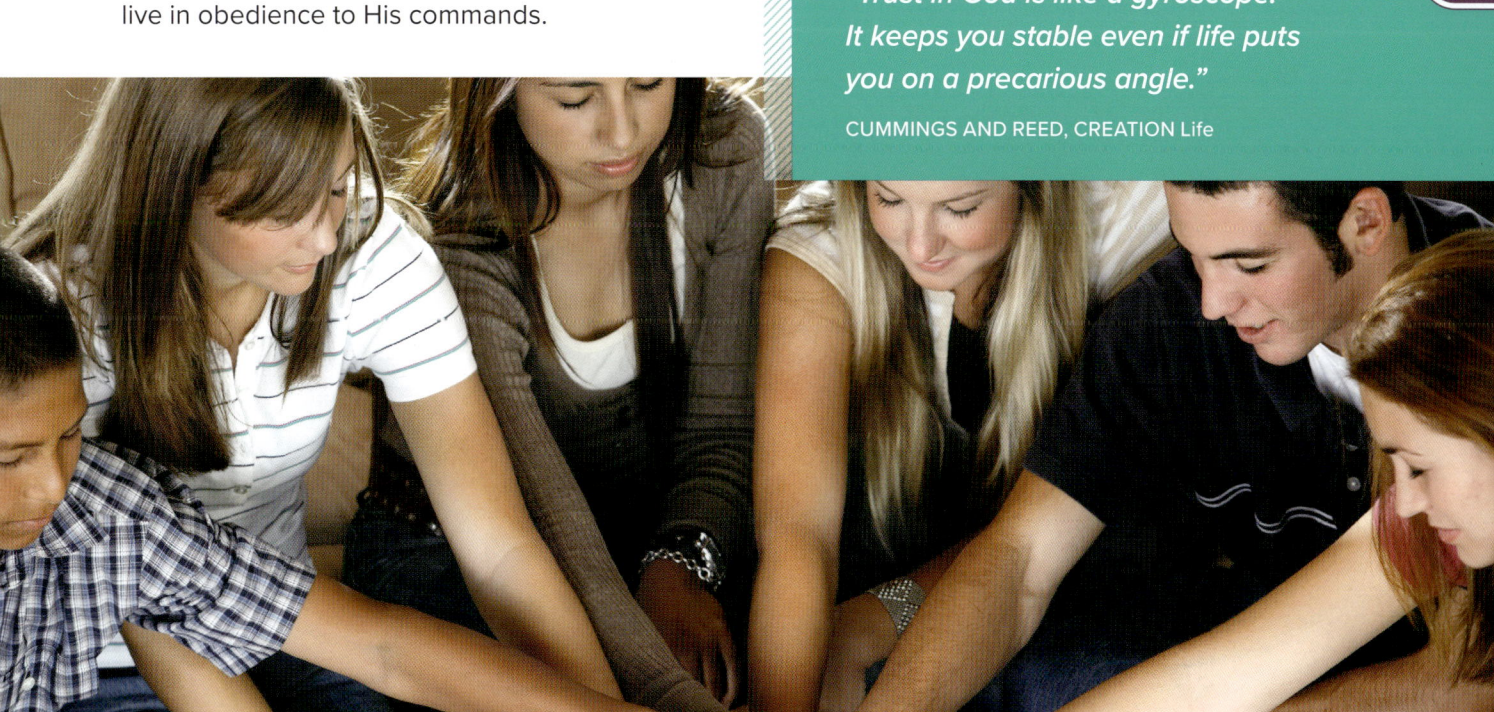

21 DAYS OF TRUST

Follow these daily tips to increase your trust in God:

Day 1
Live by the principles of integrity outlined in the Bible.

Day 2
Recognize that your inability to trust may come from negative experiences in your past. Try to move beyond the past and learn to trust people in the here and now.

Day 3
Become trustworthy at school by showing up on time, turning in your assignments on time, meeting your teacher's expectations and being honest in all your dealings.

Day 4
Find someone whose trust you betrayed in the past. Make it right today by asking for their forgiveness.

Day 5
Stay true to yourself. Don't pretend to be someone you're not.

Day 6
Build trust with God or another person by spending time with them. Set aside a special time each day to be with God and your family.

Day 7
Listen to positive Christian music. It can have a great impact on your mood as well as build your trust in God.

Day 8
Give back by volunteering at your church or charity.

Day 9
Sign-up for a daily devotional text message. Read and reflect on it every day.

Day 10
Make a list of your prayer needs. Categorize your requests under different topics like, work, home, church, etc. Share the list with a friend you can trust and ask them to pray with you.

Day 11
Follow the "Lord's Prayer." This prayer Jesus gave to His disciples in Matthew 6:9–13 is really a model of how we should pray every day, as it includes praise and confession.

Day 12
Keep a prayer journal to remember what you've prayed for and how God answers your prayers.

Day 13
Pray for your parents, family, teachers, friends and nation.

Day 14
Commit to praying even if you feel like you don't have time. Try praying short sentence prayers that are sincere. God knows your heart, and He will reward you for your faithfulness.

Day 15
Trust in God to meet your needs even when you are stressed about finances, a job or other essentials.

Day 16
Be honest in all your dealings, no matter how desperate you may feel.

Day 17
Put your trust in God when you get the "bad" news. He is always with you.

Day 18
Show yourself as trustworthy by keeping secrets to yourself and avoiding gossip.

Day 19
Be an encouragement to someone today by sharing your faith and trust in God.

Day 20
Set some goals for your future that depend on your trust in God. Trusting God is not something you just do once. It's a lifelong endeavor.

Day 21
Read the Bible to find God's direction for your life. God's Word is "a lamp" to your feet and "a light" to your path (Psalm 119:105).

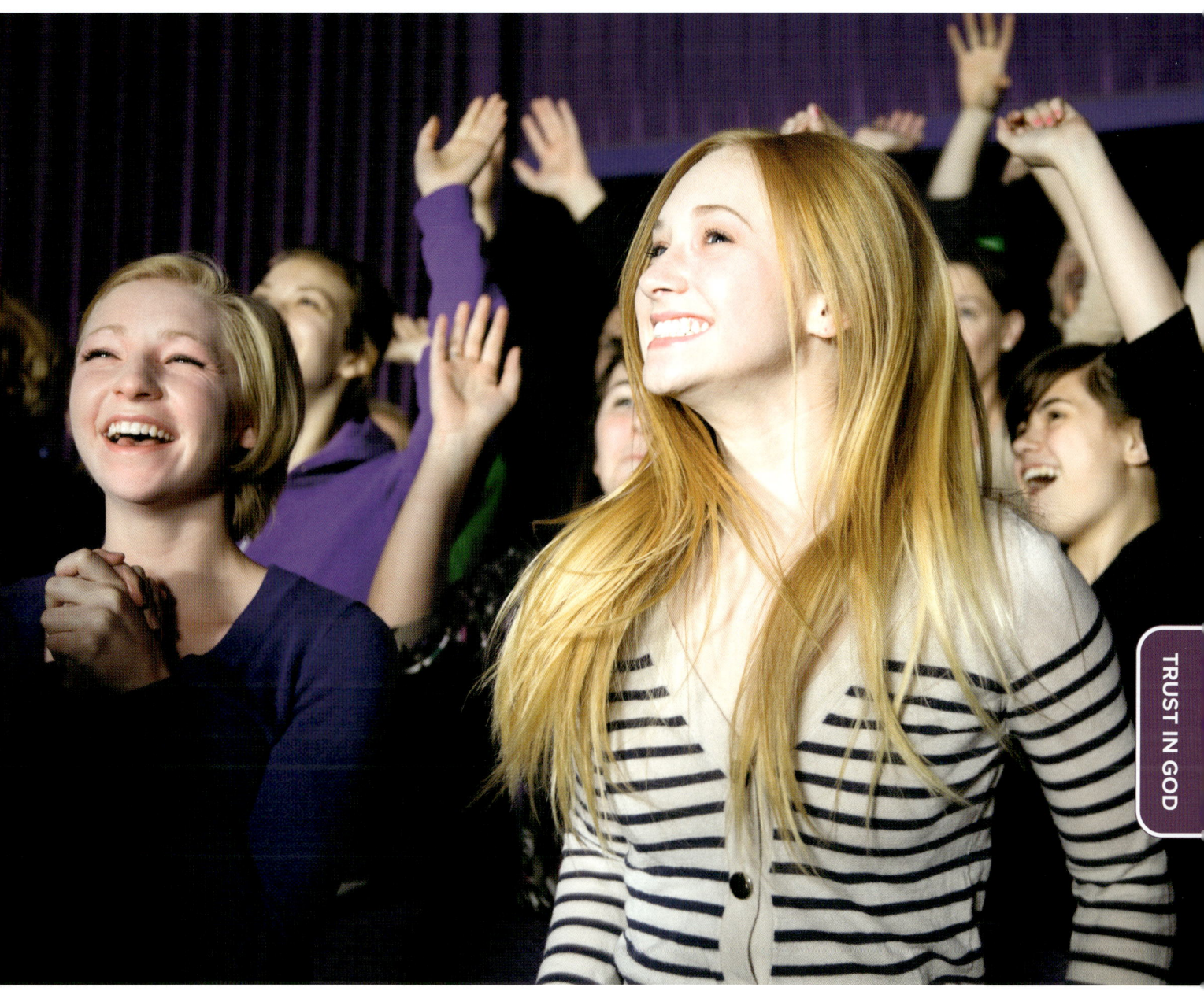

REFERENCES

1. It's interesting to note that God called the man's name "Adam." This is closely related to the Hebrew word "adamah," which means "the earth" or "the ground."

2. Pascal, *Pensées*, Section VII, 425, accessed August 19, 2013, http://www.gutenberg.org/files/18269/18269-h/18269-h.htm #SECTION_IV.

3. Ibid.

4. H. Koenig, M. McCullough, et al., *Handbook of Religion and Health* (New York: Oxford University Press, 2001), 6, 394.

5. M. McCullough, W. Hoyt, et al., "Religious Involvement and Mortality: A Meta Analytic Review," *Health Psychology* 19, no. 3 (2000): 211–222.

6. W. Jeynes, "The Relationship Between Bible Literacy and Behavioral and Academic Outcomes in Urban Areas: A Meta-Analysis," *Education and Urban Society* 42, no. 5 (July 2010): 522–544.

7. W. Jeynes, "The Relationship Between Bible Literacy and Academic Achievement and School Behavior," Education and Urban Society 41, no. 4 (May 2009): 419–436.

8. W. Jeynes, "Religiosity, Religious Schools, and Their Relationship with the Achievement Gap: A Research Synthesis and Meta-Analysis," *Journal of Negro Education* 79, no. 3 (2010): 263–279.

9. "Religion Matters: Predicting Schooling Success among Latino Youth. Interim Reports," D. Sikkink and E. Hernandez, Institute for Latino Studies, University of Notre Dame, retrieved May 10, 2012, http://latinostudies.nd.edu/cslr/research/pubs/Sikkink_paper.pdf.

10. W. Jeynes, "Educational Policy and the Effects of Attending a Religious School on the Academic Achievement of Children," *Educational Policy* 16, no. 3 (July 2002): 406–425.

11. R. Coffee, *The Incredible Journey a Daily Devotional* (Coldwater, Michigan: Remnant Publications, 2005), 20–21.

12. Thankfully salt occurs naturally in many foods, so this really isn't an issue. In fact, most people have the opposite problem — overindulging in salty foods.

13. J. Levin, *God, Faith, And Health* (Canada: John Wiley & Sons, Inc., 2001), 77.

14. J. Levin and R. Taylor, "Panel Analyses of Religious Involvement and Well-Being in African Americans: Contemporaneous vs. Longitudinal Effects," *Journal for the Scientific Study of Religion* 37 (1998): 695–709.

15. M. Musick, "Religion and Subjective Health Among Black and White Elders," *Journal of Health and Social Behavior* 37 (1996): 221–237.

16. RA Hummer, et al., "Religious Involvement and U.S. Adult Mortality," *Demography* 36, no.2 (May 1999): 273–85.

17. G. Comstock, et al., "Education and Mortality in Washington County, Maryland," *Journal of Health and Social Behavior* 18 (1977): 54–61.

18. DB Larson & SS Larson, "Religious Commitment and Health: Valuing the Relationship," *Second Opinion: Health, Faith, and Ethics* 17, no. 1 (1991), 26–40.

19. "Center for Research on Religion and Urban Civil Society," CRRUCS/Gallup Spiritual State of the Union: Center for Research on Religion and Urban Civil Society, University of Pennsylvania, 2003.

20. K. Pargament, DS Ensing, et al., "God Help Me: I. Religious Coping Efforts as Predictors of The Outcomes to Significant Life Events," *American Journal of Community Psychology* 19 (1990): 793–824.

21. M. Beatz, D. Larson, et al., "Canadian Psychiatric Impatient Religious Commitment: An Association with Mental Health," *Canadian Journal of Psychiatry* 47, no. 2 (2002): 159–165.

22. M. McCullough, D. Larson, "Religion and Depression: A Review of the Literature," *Twin Research* 2 (1999), 126–136.

23. B. Siegel, *Love, Medicine and Miracles: Lessons Learned About Self-Healing from a Surgeon's Experience with Exceptional Patients* (New York: Harper Perennial, 1986), 181.

24. E. Padus, *The Complete Guide to Your Emotions and Your Health: New Dimensions in Mind/ Body Healing* (Emmaus, PA: Rodale Press, 1986), 648.

25. B. Siegel, *Love, Medicine and Miracles*, 181.

26. C. Thomas, "Precursors of Premature Disease and Death: The Predictive Potential of Habits and Family Attitudes," *Annals of Internal Medicine* 85: 653–658.

27. L. Russek, G. Schwartz, et al., "Feelings of Parental Caring Predict Health Status in Midlife: A 35-Year Follow-up of the Harvard Mastery of Stress Study," *Journal of Behavioral Medicine* 20, no. 1 (Feb. 1997): 1–13.

28. A. Walsh and P. Walsh, "Love, Self-esteem, and Multiple Sclerosis," *Social Science and Medicine* 29 (1989): 793–798.

29. D. McClelland and C. Kirshnit, "The Effect of Motivational Arousal through Films on Salivary Immunoglobulin A," *Psychology and Health* 2 (1988): 31–52.

30. J. Levine, "A Prolegomenon to Epidemiology of Love: Theory, Measurement, and Health Outcomes," *Journal of Social Psychology* 19, no. 1 (Spring 2000): 117–27.

31. A. Marinoni, A. Degrate, et al., "Psychological Distress and its Correlates in Secondary School Students in Pavia, Italy," *European Journal of Epidemiology* 13, no. 7 (1997): 779–786.

32. T. Hattori, K. Taketani, et al., "Suicide and Suicide Attempts in General Hospital Psychiatry: Clinical and Statistical Study," *Psychiatry and Clinical Neurosciences* 49 (1995): 43–48.

33. F. Lehman, "The Love of God," Public Domain.

34. J. Turner, R. Deyo, J. Loeser, et al., "The Importance of Placebo Effects in Pain Treatment and Research," *Journal of the American Medical Association* 271, no. 20 (May 25, 1994): 1609–1614.

35. G. Kreutz, S. Bongard, et al., "Effects of Choir Singing or Listening on Secretory Immunoglobulin A, Cortisol, and Emotional State," *Journal of Behavioral Medicine* 27, no. 6 (2004): 623–635.

36. F. Luskin, *Forgive for Good: A Proven Prescription for Health and Happiness* (New York: HarperCollins Publishers, Inc., 2002).

37. C. Witvliet, T. Ludwig, et al., "Granting Forgiveness or Harboring Grudges: Implications for Emotion, Physiology, and Health," *Psychological Science* 12, no. 2 (2001): 117–123.

38. J. Webb, "Spiritual Factors and Adjustment in Medical Rehabilitation: Understanding Forgiveness as a Means of Coping," *Journal of Applied Rehabilitation Counseling* 34, no. 3 (2003), 16–24.

39. FK Willits, DW Crider, et al., "Religion and Well Being: Men and Women in the Middle Years," *Journal of Health and Social Behavior* 29 (1988): 281–294.

40. M. Pollner, "Divine Relations, Social Relations, and Well-Being," *Journal of Health and Social Behavior* 30 (1989): 92–104.

41. K. Pargament, H. Koenig, et. al., "Religious Struggle as a Predictor of Mortality among Medically Ill Elderly Patients: A Two-Year Longitudinal Study," *Archives of Internal Medicine* 161 (2001): 1881–1885.

42. J. Stone, N. Fernandez, "To Practice What We Preach: The Use of Hypocrisy and Cognitive Dissonance to Motivate Behavior Change," *Social and Personality Psychology Compass* 2, no. 2 (2008): 1024–1051.

43. Merriam-Webster's Online dictionary, retrieved August 23, 2013, http://www.merriam-webster.com/dictionary/%20cognitive%20dissonance.

TRUST IN GOD

NOTES

INTERPERSONAL
RELATIONSHIPS
Connect, belong and support

I

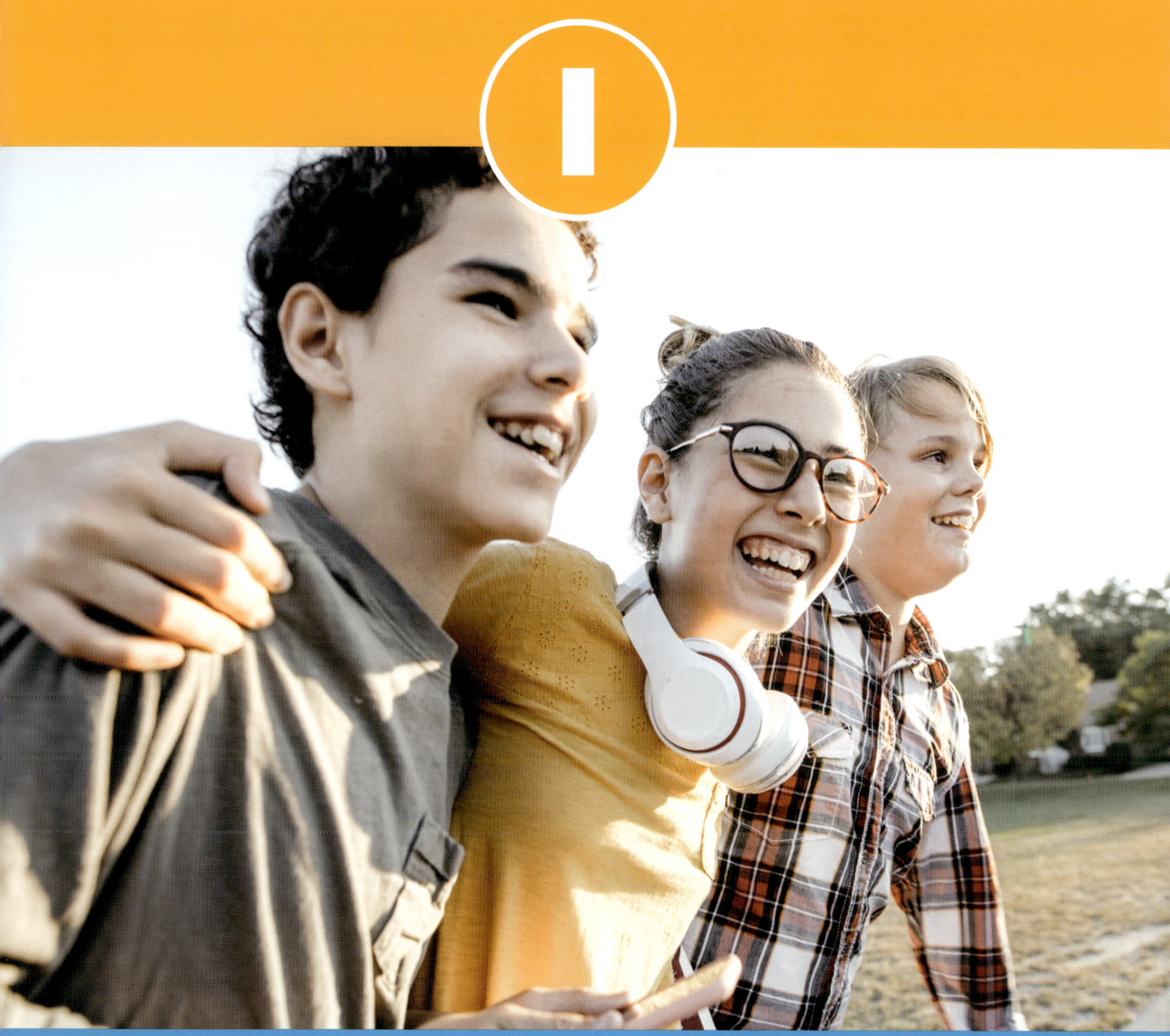

INTERPERSONAL [in-ter-pur-suh-nl] *nown* **1:** the social connections you have with others. Healthy relationships bring happiness and make life better.

THE BIG PICTURE

In the classic movie *It's a Wonderful Life*, a distraught George Bailey receives a remarkable gift one Christmas Eve. Thanks to the help of an angel named Clarence, George gets to see what the world would be like if he had never been born. George is overwhelmed at how different the small town of Bedford Falls is without him. Though he considered his life insignificant, he comes to realize he made a tremendous impact on the people around him. At the end of the film, George receives a book from Clarence, inscribed with the following words to remind him of his worth to others: "Remember, no man is a failure who has friends."

Friends and family are important parts of Interpersonal Relationships, the sixth principle in CREATION Life. "Inter" is a prefix that means "between," "among" or "together."[1] For example, the interstate highway system is a series of roads that run between states, connecting them to each other. In a similar way, interpersonal relationships connect you to other people. While the nature of these connections varies, they should ideally generate a similar sense of openness, generosity and goodwill between the participants. That's because an interpersonal relationship is more than just a social connection. It also fulfills a physical or emotional need in you and the other person. Interpersonal relationships provide you with a number of health benefits as well.

To better understand some of these benefits, ask yourself these questions: do I have someone who really cares for me? How about someone who feels close to me, loves me and wants to help me? Is there someone in my life in whom I can confide? If so, then according to some studies, you may have three to five times lower risk of premature death and disease from all causes than those who don't have these kinds of relationships.[2] But greater longevity is just one of the many benefits provided to you through interpersonal relationships.

Dr. Dean Ornish is a well-known physician and author, known for his lifestyle-driven approach to the prevention and control of heart disease. When most people think about avoiding heart disease, they tend to think of eating a low-fat diet, exercising regularly and avoiding stress. While these are all important parts of preventing a heart attack, if you ask Dr. Ornish about the most important part of his program, his answer might come as a surprise. He identifies it as interpersonal relationships.[3]

In his book *Love and Survival: The Scientific Basis for the Healing Power of Intimacy*, Dr. Ornish writes, "I'm not aware of any other factor in medicine — not diet, not smoking, not exercise, not stress, not genetics, not drugs, not surgery — that has a greater impact on our quality of life, incidence of illness and premature death from all causes than does love and intimacy."[4]

In this section, you'll see how your interpersonal relationships have an incredible impact on your life, your health and your well-being.

INTERPERSONAL RELATIONSHIPS are the connections and associations that exist between two people, which also fulfill their emotional and physical needs. Interpersonal relationships occur in a variety of forms, from family and friends to professional and even romantic.

INTERPERSONAL

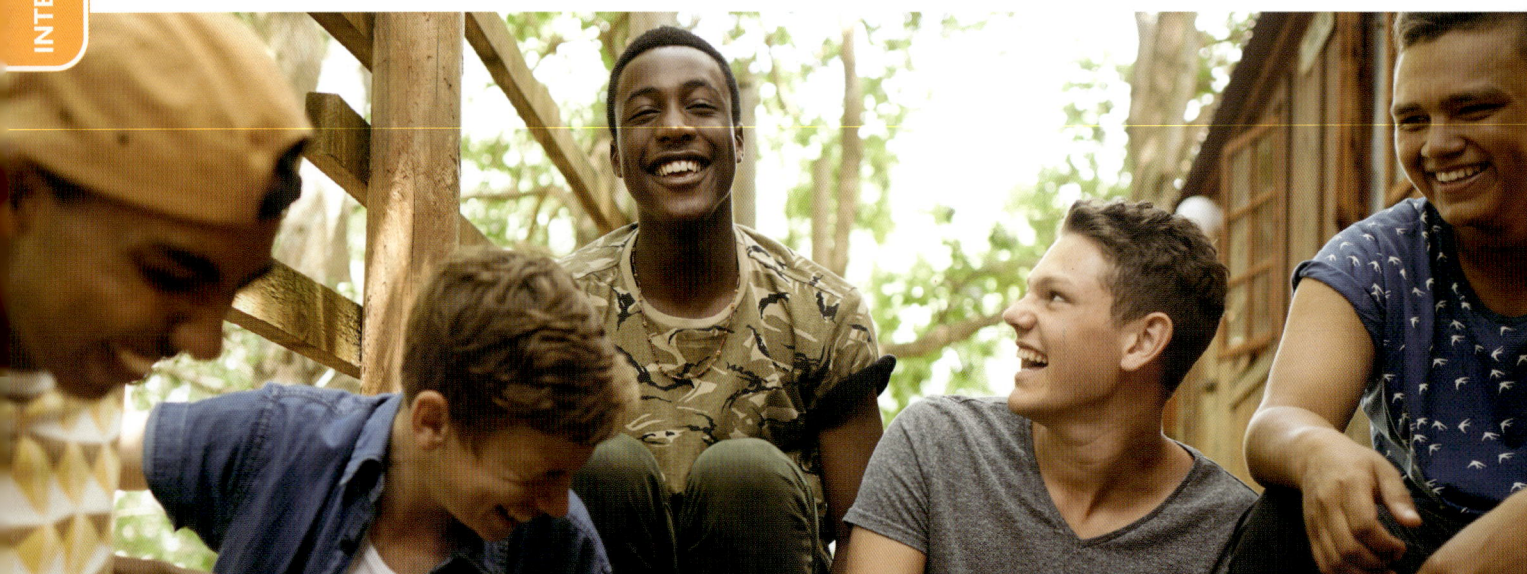

THE GIFT OF RELATIONSHIP

Then the Lord God said, "It is not good that the man should be alone; I will make him a helper fit for him." GENESIS 2:18

When God created the world, He made everything perfectly. But there was one thing God saw that did not please Him, that He knew He must change. It was the only time in the whole story of creation that God said something was "not good." It was the fact that Adam was all alone.

Adam had a perfect environment, nutritious food to eat and a God-given mission to fulfill. Yet something was still missing. He had no one to help him, no one with whom to share his experiences. His life was unbalanced.

So, God decided to do something about it. First, He caused all the animals to parade themselves in front of Adam. Adam named each and every one of them, but it became clear that none were to be his special counterpart. If God was going to give him a helper, it would have to be something

unique — something that had never been seen before. So, God caused Adam to fall into a deep sleep. He then took a rib from Adam's side, and out of this God fashioned the ideal helper suitable for Adam in every way. Adam would not know loneliness again in the garden. God had attended to every detail and made sure that everything He created was good.

When Adam saw God's creation, his heart was overwhelmed:

"This is now bone of my bones, and flesh of my flesh." GENESIS 2:23

Adam waited a long time to meet this new creation, this helper who would work alongside him. Now, at last, the wait was over. Finally he had someone he could share his life with.

From the very beginning, God created you to be in relationship, not just with Himself but also with the people around you. You can find true fulfillment and joy in life by sharing in interpersonal relationships.

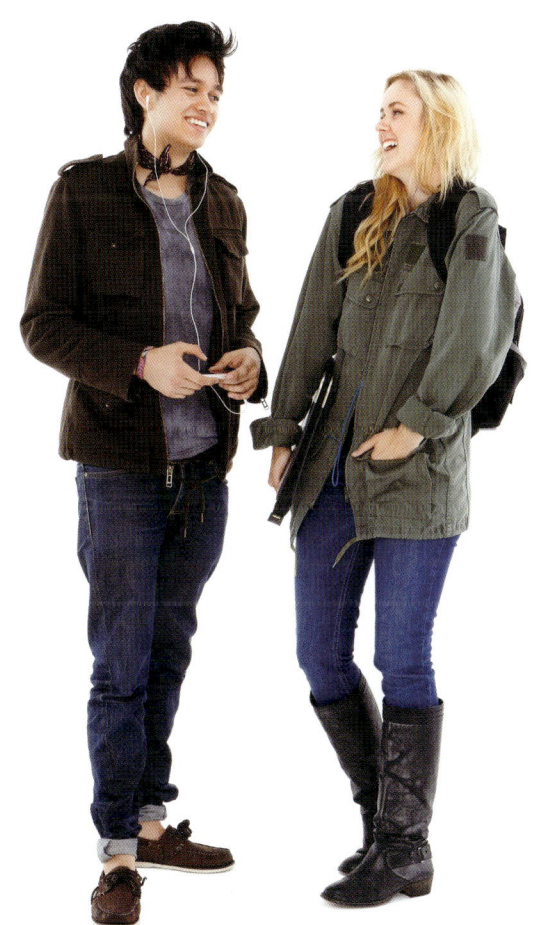

 **What attributes do you especially appreciate in your relationships? What attributes would you like to have in your life and share with others?**

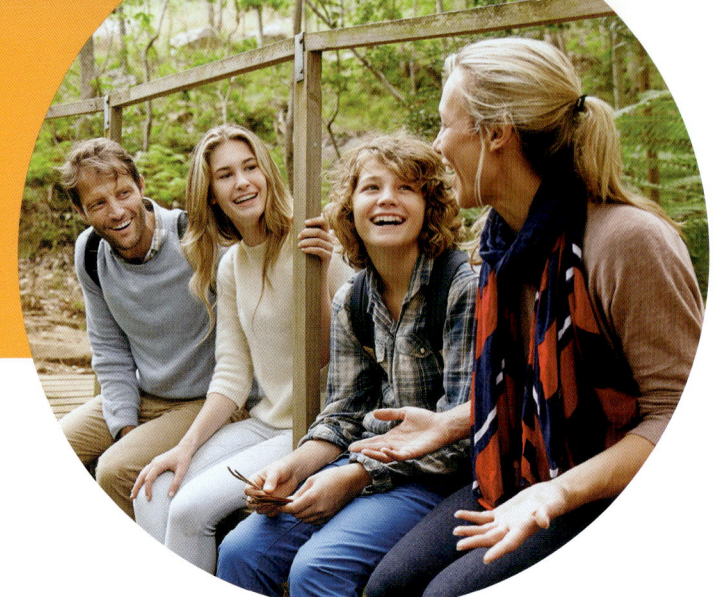

THE ROSETO EFFECT

In 1962, the typically quiet town of Roseto was abuzz with scientists and researchers. They came for one reason — to discover the town's "fountain of youth." For some reason, the inhabitants of the small eastern Pennsylvanian village had a heart attack mortality rate that was roughly half the rate of every neighboring community. It didn't make sense; the people of Roseto had the same risk factors as their neighbors, drank the same water, even worked at the same jobs. What was their secret?

It certainly wasn't their diet. The people of Roseto ate foods loaded in fat and cholesterol. But as the researchers looked deeper, they discovered one thing that made the Rosetans stand out from among the others, one factor that made all the difference.

"What made Rosetans die less from heart disease than identical towns elsewhere? Family ties… it turns out that Roseto was peopled by strongly knit Italian-American families who lived right and consequently lived longer. In short, Rosetans were nourished by people."[5]

A high level of social connectedness characterized the Rosetans. This included strong family ties and a supportive, nurturing community. The researchers hypothesized that this might be the key factor that was buffering residents from heart disease and early death.

The study on the town lasted 50 years, but by the end something had changed. Heart disease in Roseto had risen to the same levels as the other towns. It was discovered that over time the cohesiveness of the community began to weaken. The people in Roseto gradually became more Americanized, and their strong family ties disintegrated. With their social support weakened, their health was also affected as much as their neighboring communities.[6]

The people of Roseto showed the world the strong link between social support and health. This link has even been termed the Roseto effect.[7] What you should take away from the people of Roseto is that your social support system does have an impact on your health, for good or for bad. By surrounding yourself with friends and family in positive interpersonal relationships, you can get the greatest benefits.

INTERPERSONAL

"FRIENDLY" IMMUNE BOOSTERS

Could having more friends keep you healthier and boost your immune system? Several studies seem to indicate this is a possibility. According to one study published in the *Journal of the American Medical Association*, having more friends may even help keep away the common cold. In the study, volunteers were exposed to the virus that causes the common cold. Almost all of the people exposed to the virus were infected by it, but the study found that those people who had more friends were less likely to develop the signs and symptoms of a cold.[8] Another study showed increased immune function in elderly people, both in terms of natural killer cells and antibodies, after weekly visitations by friends or relatives.[9]

Close friends may even be a valuable advantage when it comes to battling medical conditions such as heart disease and cancer. A study of 2,230 breast cancer patients in China found that supportive relationships was the most important predictor of both cancer recurrence and survival. The women with the highest relationship scores had a 38 percent higher survival rate compared with those with the lowest score. In addition, they had a 48 percent decreased risk of breast cancer recurrence.[10]

Another study on heart disease examined 2,320 men who had survived a heart attack. After researchers statistically controlled for genetics, exercise, diet, weight, smoking, alcohol and so on, the men who were socially isolated and had high stress had more than four times the risk of dying sooner than those who had a stronger social network.[11]

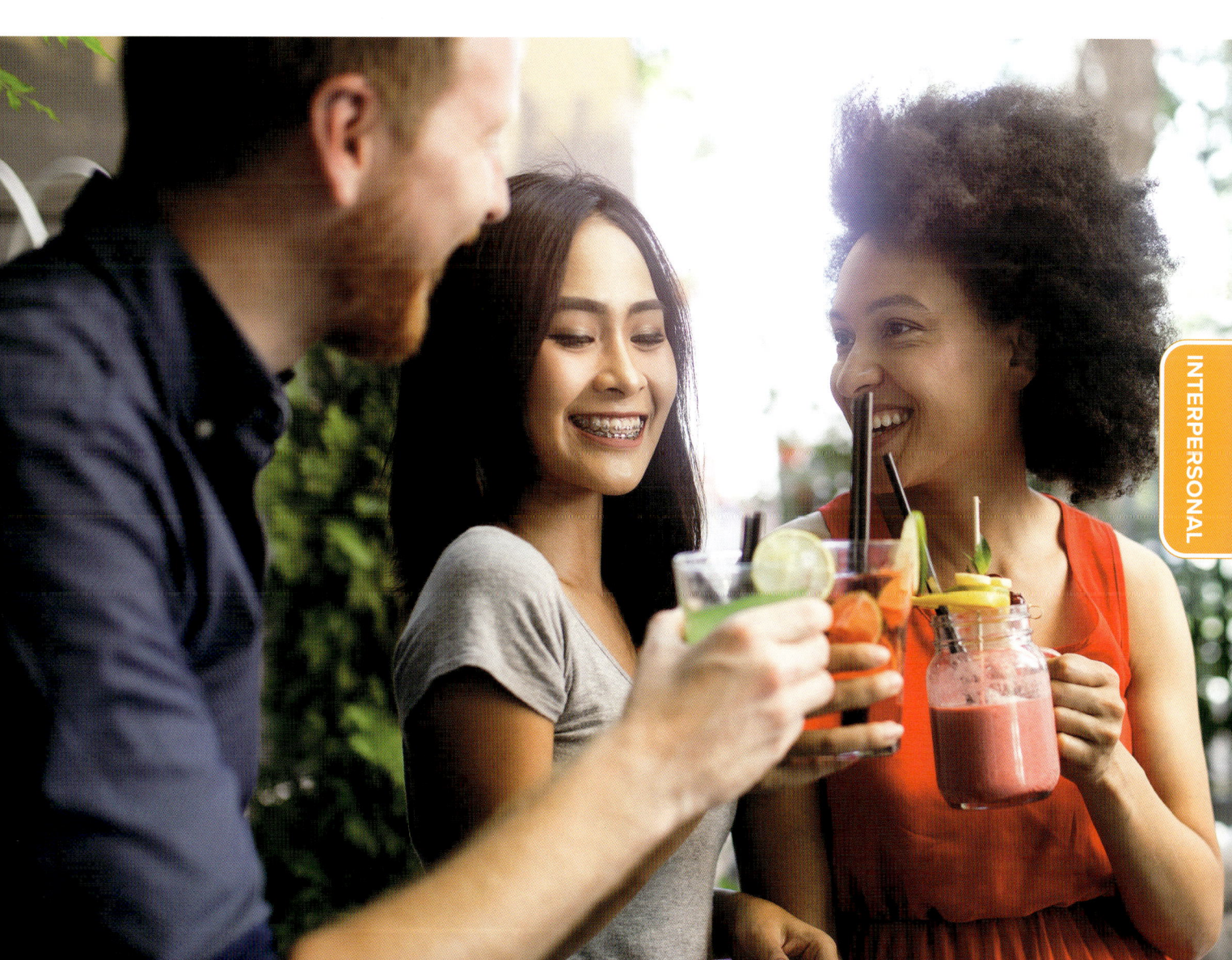

RELATIONSHIPS AND HAPPINESS

Depression is a worldwide problem that affects millions of people.[12] Dr. Martin Seligman, a physician and author who is known for his work studying optimism, contends that today's epidemic levels of depression stem partly from "impoverished social connections." These are quite evident in Western societies, which Dr. Seligman describes as "individualistic." On one hand, they offer personal control and an opportunity to express one's feelings and talents. However, on the other side is the risk of a less connected, more detached self. For example, America is one of the wealthiest nations in the world; it is also one of the most depressed.[13]

Compare that with Bangladesh, "known as one of the poorest and most densely populated countries in the world."[14] One study found the people of Bangladesh reported "levels of happiness that are higher than those found in many other countries. This includes 'developed' countries where people have higher per capita incomes and can access a wider range of public services and goods."[15] The researchers also discovered a significant link between the "construction of their happiness" and their "networks of relationships."[16] The researchers concluded, "Our findings highlight the centrality of relationships to people's subjective well-being…. Relationships determine individuals' values, choices, actions and indeed the construction of self. More than any other factor, they determine what people are able to do or be, and what they actually achieve or become."[17]

If you want to experience happiness in your life, then it's important to have good interpersonal relationships. In a worldwide study, participants in Australia, Croatia, Germany, Italy, Portugal, Spain and South Africa described happiness as a state of emotional balance and harmony with family and other interpersonal relationships.[18] Many other studies have found that people report more positive feelings when they are with others,[19] and "people who can name several intimate friends with whom they share their concerns freely are healthier, less likely to die prematurely and happier than people who have few or no such friends."[20] "Compared with depressed people, happy people are less self-focused, less hostile and abusive and less vulnerable to disease. They also are more loving, forgiving, trusting, energetic, decisive, creative, helpful and sociable."[21]

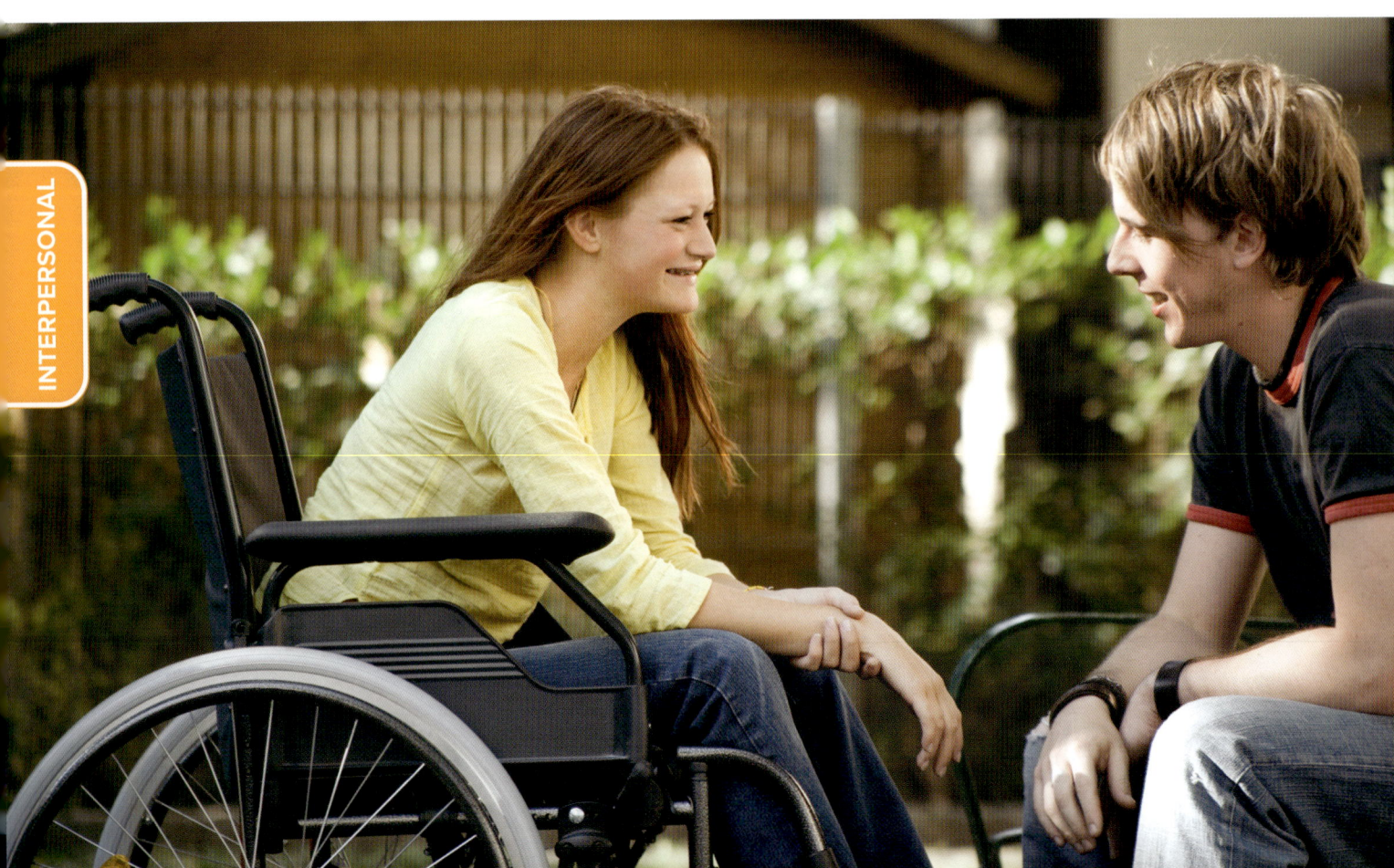

INTERPERSONAL

RELATIONSHIPS AND LONGEVITY

The quality and quantity of an individual's interpersonal relationships has been linked not only to happiness, but also to longer life. Researchers in Alameda County, California, studied more than 7,000 people for 40 years, looking closely at their medical history and current health practices. Two epidemiologists, Dr. Lisa Camfield and Dr. S. Leonard Syme, wrote one of the studies that came from this data. "Their study found that individuals with strong social ties, including membership in a church or synagogue, had significantly lower death rates than those without such connections."[22]

The study, one of the most quoted in the field of health, also revealed:

- People classified as lonely and isolated had three times higher mortality rates.

- People with many social contacts had the lowest mortality rates.

- The amount of social support was the best predictor of good health.[23]

> *"Don't ever let somebody tell you you can't do something."*
>
> WILL SMITH

SEVENTY TIMES SEVEN

Then Peter came and said to Him, "Lord, how often shall my brother sin against me and I forgive him? Up to seven times?" Jesus said to him, "I do not say to you, up to seven times, but up to seventy times seven."

MATTHEW 18:21–22

In the section on Trust in God, you learned about the positive impact forgiveness can have on your overall health. But the power of forgiveness can also heal your relationships and give you greater emotional health and happiness. A cross-sectional survey of 30 divorced or permanently separated mothers with children ages 10 to 13 found that mothers who had forgiven the fathers for previous transgressions committed against them were more likely to report a greater sense of self-acceptance and purpose in life, as well as less anxiety and depressive symptoms.[24] Another study found people who were more forgiving enjoyed greater satisfaction with life, compared to less forgiving people.[25] When faced with interpersonal conflict, individuals cope in a variety of ways. Some may retaliate directly, such as taking revenge. Others may avoid the situation or offender. However, both the expression and the avoidance of anger and aggression can have negative consequences.[26] The good news is that an alternative exists, and that alternative is forgiveness. Forgiveness leads to an increase in optimistic thinking and hopefulness, higher levels of social and emotional support and connection and greater communion with God — all of which promote good health and lasting happiness.[27] When you forgive, you choose a more compassionate understanding of the transgressor, you let go of negative thoughts, feelings and behaviors and you humbly recognize your own flaws and shortcomings. It is not a one-time word, action or feeling, but "an embodied way of life."[28]

Developing a forgiving spirit is vital to your health and happiness. By learning to respond positively when others have hurt you, you can grow in all your relationships, not just with your friends or family, but also with God.

INTERPERSONAL

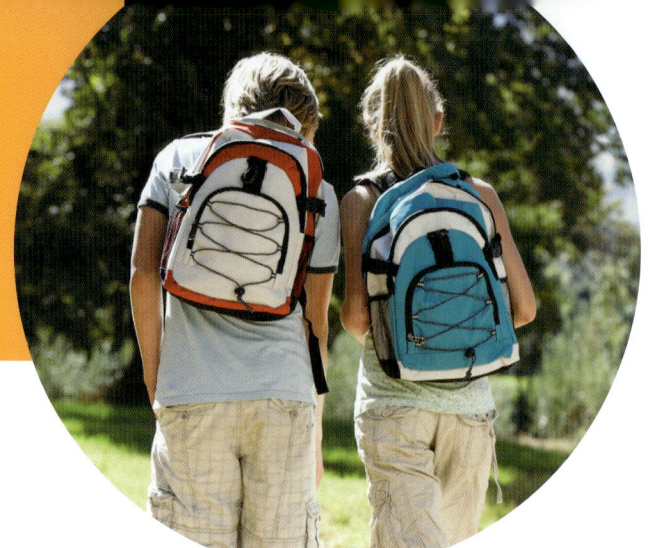

*"As iron sharpens iron,
so a friend sharpens a friend."*

PROVERBS 27:17

PRAY TO FORGIVE

*"And forgive us our debts, as we
also have forgiven our debtors."*

MATTHEW 6:12

Included in the Lord's Prayer is a spiritual check-up of sorts. When you ask God to forgive you as you have forgiven others, it causes you to examine your relationships and see if there is any bitterness or resentment you may be harboring. It also causes you to reflect on how great a debt of sin you have been freely forgiven in Christ. Let this be your greatest motivation for forgiveness, and let prayer be the fuel that feeds the fire of your faith.

University studies have shown that praying for a relationship partner increases their willingness to forgive. In addition, prayer over time has been shown to decrease an individual's selfish concerns, thus mitigating the conflict in the relationship.[29]

Christian author, Jack Zavada says, "For our own good, and the good of the person who hurt us, we simply must forgive. Just as we trust God for our salvation, we have to trust Him to make things right when we forgive. He will heal our wounds so we can move on."[30]

FRIENDSHIP

Friends come in all different shapes and sizes and have a tremendous impact on your life. On one level, a friend is someone you enjoy doing things with, but is also someone you can count on to support you in times of need. Friends are the people you share your life with. They listen to your problems, your concerns and your ideas and they provide you with valuable feedback that is both positive and constructive. Friendship is an important relationship that is cherished by practically everyone. In this section, you will explore how friendship influences your happiness and your health.

When it comes to being happy, research shows it's not quantity of friends that matters as much as quality. One study found that a person might have several friendships; however, it is the strong connections in those friendships, not the number of friends they have, that adds something extra to their lives and has the potential to increase their happiness level.[31] In another study, researchers investigated "perceived mattering" to friends and its effect on happiness. "Perceived mattering" refers to the feeling that one counts and makes a difference in another person's life. This study conclusively showed that greater feelings of perceived mattering increase your happiness.[32] On the other hand, being rejected and isolated from your peers can result in increased feelings of sadness and depression. Another study examined the connection between childhood friendship and depression levels. Over time, children who tended to avoid friendships or who were rejected by their peers showed increasing high levels of sadness.[33]

MAKING FRIENDS

The following is a list of qualities, skills and attitudes to help you to develop friendships that will last:

- **Know yourself.** In order to create a lasting friendship, "you must first understand what kind of person you are and who would want to be your friend in return." For example, "if you are the kind of person who loves to be the center of attention... then you probably won't be capable of forming a lasting friendship with somebody else who likes being the topic of most conversations."[34]

- **Consider your interests.** Personal interest sharing is often the main reason two friends begin to spend time with one another. This makes your interests and hobbies important factors to consider when determining who would make a good friend.[35] For example, if you are into sports you may try reaching out to a fellow teammate.

- **Be yourself.** There is no point in creating a friendship that is not based on truth, so don't pretend to be someone you are not. "Lasting friendships are built on more than just superficial activities... true friends will accept each other for who they are and not just on what they do together."[36]

- **Be faithful and true.** "A major cause for most friendships ending or not advancing beyond the initial stage is that one party leaves the other one hanging at a critical moment."[37] Know that there may come a time in your relationship in which your friend needs you to step up. If you can tell your friend is struggling with something, be willing to make "small sacrifices" to help. This will help build trust and show that you care.[38]

- **Reach out.** "Every time you walk down the street... you are passing hundreds of potential friends. The reason most of us don't consider reaching out to prospective friends is that we are worried they don't share the same interests and won't enjoy spending time with us. Sometimes people with opposite personalities and interests make the best friends and are able to commit to lasting relationships. These types of personalities tend to complement one another, and they don't steal each other's thunder because they have different interests and concerns."[39]

- **Be positive with everyone.** Many people rely on sarcasm because they think it makes them come across as "funny," but never doubt the power of the positive. "People like to hear good things about themselves and always enjoy a compliment."[40]

- **Be willing to admit when you are wrong.** "We all make mistakes, and it is important to recognize that neither you nor your friend is perfect... these are the times when friendships are truly challenged and tried. If you happen to have hurt a friend, you need to be willing to offer an apology and ask for forgiveness. These times will cause tension in a friendship, but you can't assume the tension will just disappear... always admit to any mistakes and be willing to forgive your friend if they are the one who has messed up."[41]

- **Know that all friendships will not last forever.** "Some friendships only exist because they are convenient or to fulfill some purpose at a specific time in your life. Understand that not all of your friendships will last forever. When you have created a long-lasting friendship, you will be able to recognize it. When you recognize that you have made one of these friends, you should be willing to do the things necessary in order for that friendship to last, even during difficult times."[42]

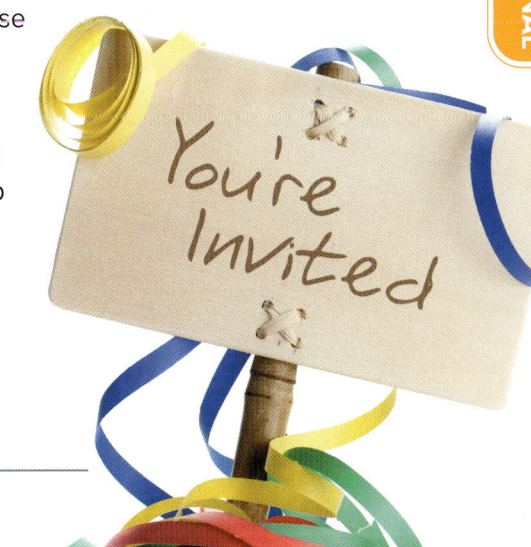

PEER PRESSURE

Peer pressure is a strong force that exists in more places than just middle and high schools. As you get older, there is a pronounced shift in influence from parents to peers as students seek to establish a friend network that will be a source of support and intimacy. The truth is that no matter how old you get, peer pressure will always be a part of life, so learning how to deal with it now by making decisions independently of what others think is an important part of growing up.

Peer pressure is generally referred to as the influence exerted by a peer group, encouraging individuals to change their attitudes, values or behaviors in order to conform to group norms.[43] A person affected by peer pressure may or may not want to belong to these groups, but conforms to avoid the negativity that can come toward those who are not members of their peer groups. Many studies have confirmed the impact peer pressure has on influencing students to drink alcohol, experiment with drug usage and participate in risky sexual encounters. Researchers have observed that young adults with conforming personalities, who were seeking social status, reported feeling more controlled by peers and showed a much higher use of drugs and alcohol and engagement in premarital sex.[44] Other studies have found that young adults with fortitude and strength of character reported not feeling influenced by peer pressure and did not participate in unhealthy, immoral behaviors.[45] One study looked at the factors that influenced students to resist peer pressure to drink alcohol. They found that students who were more socially secure — meaning they felt safe and comfortable in specific social situations — had a high resistance to social pressure and resisted alcohol usage.[46]

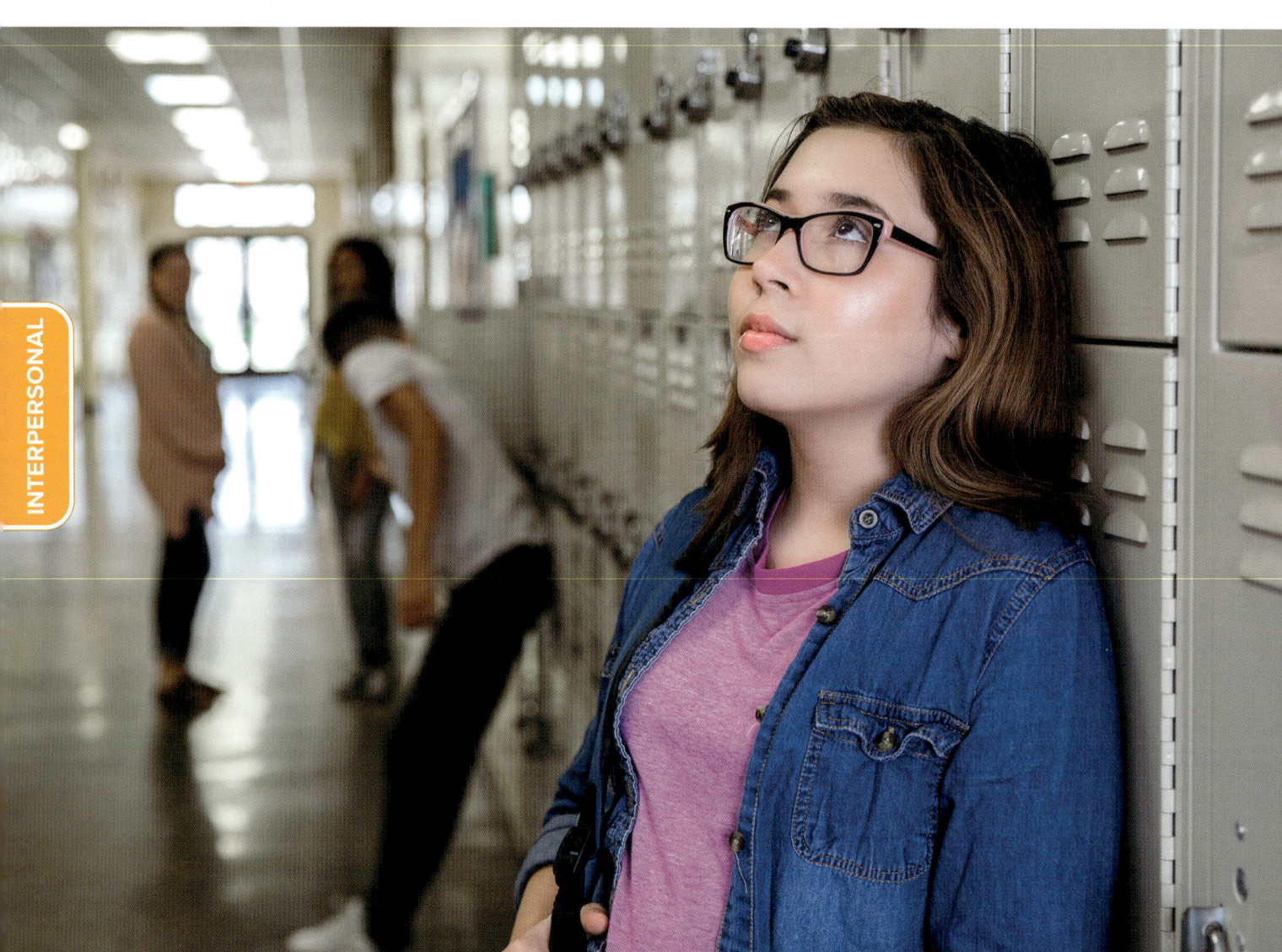

OVERCOMING PEER PRESSURE

If you are experiencing negative peer pressure in school, here are some pointers to help guide you through it:

- **Know your own values.** Do you like or dislike something simply because of a friend's opinion? Carefully decide what you value and believe before giving in to peer pressure. Be open to new experiences but stay true to yourself.

- **Seek positive support.** If your friends are pressuring you to do things that are harmful or dangerous, then it's probably time to find new friends. People who don't like you as you are are not the best choice in friends.

- **Remove yourself from negative situations.** If people are participating in activities that are unhealthy, immoral or not in alignment with your values, then it's time to move on. Leaving a situation that makes you uncomfortable also leaves you free to pursue your own healthy activities and relationships.

- **Be yourself.** Don't waste your time comparing yourself to others or trying to be like someone else. God has created you unique and special. Be happy to be the person God made you to be.

- **Become a force for good.** Peer pressure works both ways. While others might try to influence you for bad, you can also work to influence them for good. Be a positive resource for your friends and encourage them to do better, to work harder and to stay out of trouble.

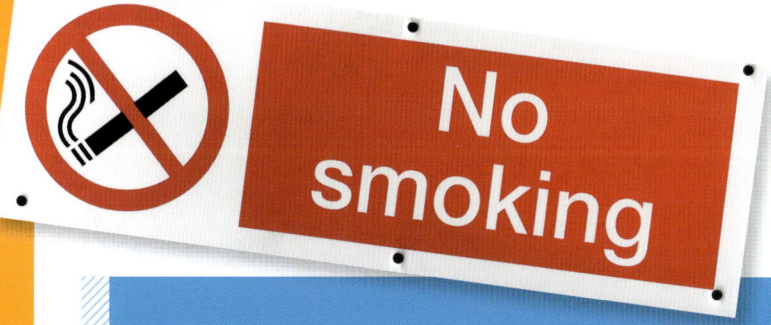

"No one can make you feel inferior without your consent."

ELEANOR ROOSEVELT

INTERPERSONAL

CLIQUES

You don't have to watch too many teen movies to know that high school is famous for having cliques. Jocks, nerds, preps and cheerleaders are just some of the stereotypes populating the landscape. The main reason cliques seem to exist is that people tend to stick with those with whom they have something in common. Sociology professor Suzanne Hudd says this about the phenomenon of cliques: "It seems that there is some 'security' in a clique of other people like oneself who affirm that whatever I've chosen is acceptable to a group of people. I also think many people seek to avoid differences. Dealing with differences in other people stretches (and matures) us. A clique — a group of people who believes and acts in similar ways to you — enables you to avoid analysis of your own thoughts and (potentially harmful) behavior. It is just easier to be with people like you who affirm, rather than question what you do."[47]

There is a big difference between a clique and a supportive group of friends. A clique is exclusive. They don't let just anyone in. People from a different background, race, social class or religion are not allowed to join. But a supportive group of friends is inclusive and open. It encourages diversity and allows anyone to be a part of the group, regardless of their differences.[48]

Spend more time with friends who are a positive influence in your life, and do your best to be a positive influence in theirs. Remember that in a supportive group, your friends will not only appreciate your willingness to support them, but they'll also refuse to take advantage of you. To help you determine if your friends are an exclusive clique or a supportive group, ask yourself the following questions:

- Does time spent with this group of friends cause me to turn gossipy and judgmental toward others?

- Does this group seem to have developed a negative attitude toward anyone outside of the circle?

- Do my friends put me down if I behave differently or express different opinions from them?

- Do my friends pressure me to conform to a way of thinking that's against what I really believe?

- Do members of this group pressure me to shun other friends and family members?

- Do they listen and offer empathy when someone has a problem or simply wants to talk about what is going on in their life?

- Do they offer encouragement and positive reinforcement to help me and others overcome obstacles?[49]

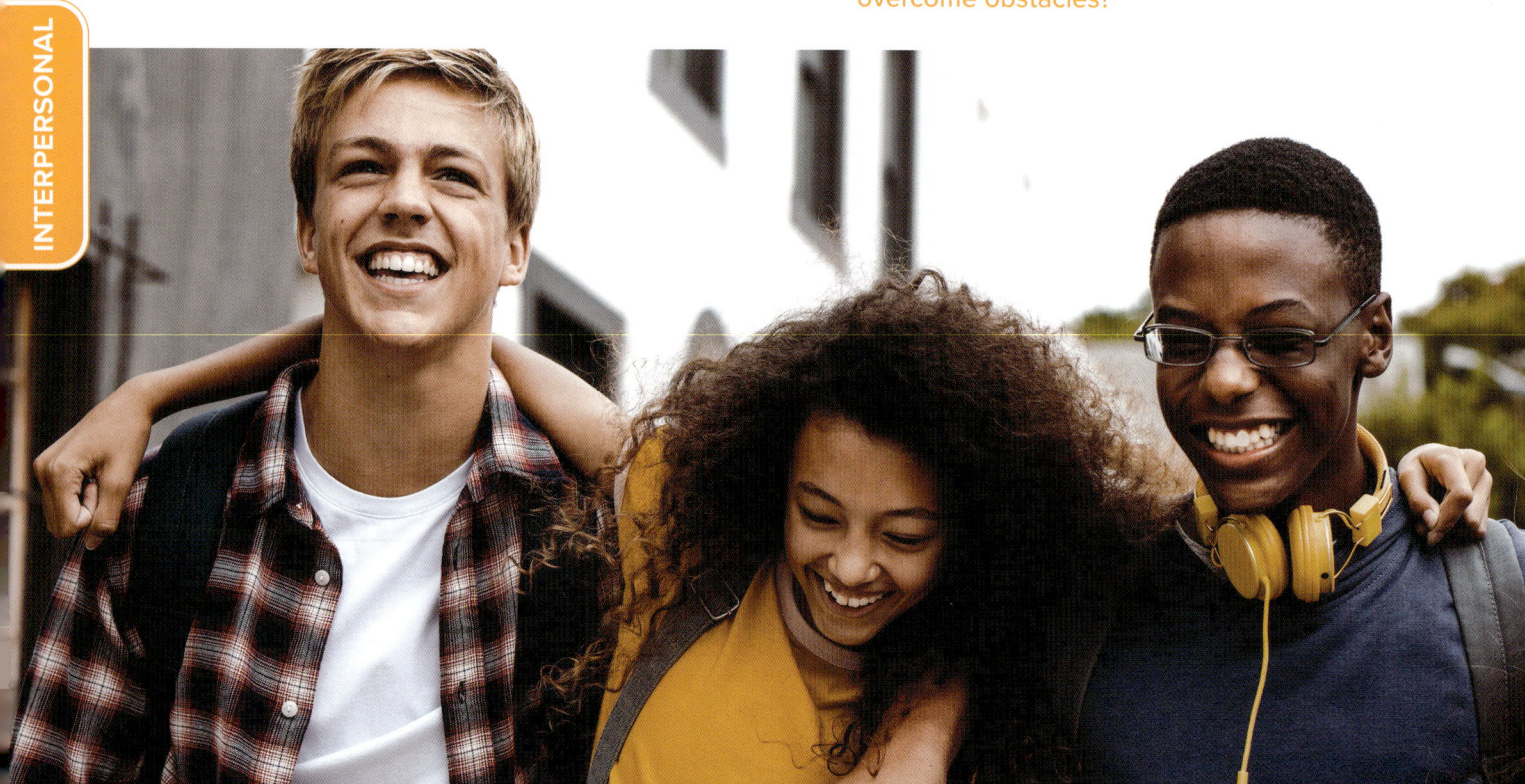

THE DANGERS OF SEXTING

Sexting is when teens send sexually suggestive, nude or nearly nude photos to each other. Although many teens see sexting as harmless, this form of communication can have severe consequences. Imagine your photos showing up online for anyone in the world to see. Imagine them showing up years after the fact, only to further damage your reputation. The humiliation caused by sexting has even brought some students to the brink of suicide.[60] "There are also legal implications: when a person under 18 takes or sends a nude or sexually suggestive photo, even of him or herself, the act constitutes a crime."[61] But the problem of sexting is not going away anytime soon. A recent survey revealed that one in every five teens has sent or received a sexually suggestive, nude or nearly nude photo, and of the teens who do sext, 80 percent are under the age of 18.[62] Even though many teens recognize the dangers of sexting, they do it anyway. According to David Walsh of the National Institute on Media and the Family, teenagers simply underestimate the risks they take online. "The part of their brain that puts the brakes on things is under major construction," Walsh says.[63] Recognize the inherent dangers of sexting, and don't think you're immune to the consequences. Take it seriously for the good of yourself and others.

In what ways do you think sexting is dangerous? What advice would you give to your fellow students about the consequences of sexting?

THE VIRTUAL WORLD

You've seen how relationships are critical to your health and happiness, but it seems today more teens prefer a virtual world to the real one. Teens have more ways of connecting than ever before, including instant messaging, email, social media, blogging and microblogging and texting. In its first year, the social media website Facebook had just one million users, and in just a few years that number has grown to nearly three billion.[50] In addition, data gathered by the Nielson Company reveals that teenagers ages 13 to 17 exchange an average of 3,295 text messages per month, or approximately 110 messages per day.[51] Because these virtual connections have such an impact on your life, it's important to examine the potential consequences of their misuse and learn how to use these resources in a way that enhances and strengthens your connections with others.

One consequence to consider is that time previously spent connecting face-to-face is now being replaced with social networking. Some studies have found that when Internet use increases it is also associated with "declines in communication with family members in the household, declines in the size of their social circle and increases in their depression and loneliness."[52] The researchers conclude that the ease of online communication encourages people to spend more time alone, to talk online with strangers or to form superficial relationships at the expense of deeper discussion and companionship with friends and family. These findings offer support for the "displacement" theory of Internet use — time online is largely an asocial activity that competes with, rather than complements, face-to-face social time.[53] In other words, you cannot spend time in face-to-face relationships when you are using the Internet instead.

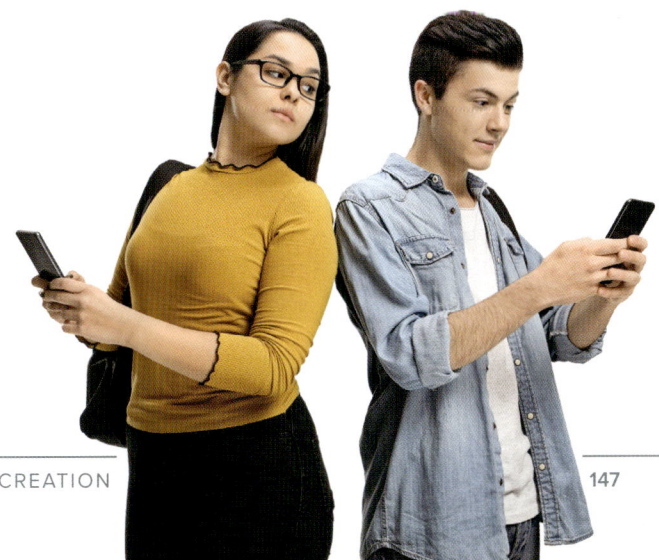

Have you ever experienced problems in your relationships caused by using technology for communication?

Long-term exposure to electronic environments could diminish your interpersonal skills. One study indicated that social interaction time drops by nearly 30 minutes for every hour a person spends using a computer. "The rapid proliferation of electronic media is now making private space available in almost every sphere of the individual's life. Yet this is now the most significant contributing factor to society's growing physical estrangement. Whether in or out of the home, more people... are physically and socially disengaged from the people around... "[54] Another similar study found that after long periods of time on the Internet, students display poor eye contact and a reluctance to interact socially.[55]

The challenge with social media sites is that they give you the ability to post only what you want other people to see and know. You choose the best pictures and the funniest status updates; your profile is the picture of success. The problem is you may find it hard to live up to the way you portray yourself. Plus, you may start to gauge how other people view you through their comments. Instead of being who you truly are or sharing how you really feel, you become used to thinking and doing everything in front of an audience. Pretty soon it's other people's opinions that determine your own level of value and importance. This may lead to stress and anxiety as you constantly seek approval from others.

For example, one study found that the more social media friends you have, the more likely you are to feel stressed out. Forty-two percent of the individuals in the study said that social media made them feel anxious, and 32 percent said rejecting friend requests led to feelings of guilt and discomfort.[56] Study leader Dr. Kathy Charles said, "Our data suggests that there is a significant number of users who experience considerable social media-related anxiety, with only very modest or tenuous rewards. Those with more

friends are the most likely to be more stressed because they have invested the most time in the site. Other causes of tension include 'unfriending' unwanted contacts, the pressure to be inventive and entertaining, using appropriate etiquette for different types of friends, feelings of exclusion, paranoia, as well as envy of others' lifestyles."[57]

A report from the American Academy of Pediatrics describes a phenomenon called "social media depression," in which children and teenagers who spend an inordinate amount of time on social networking sites develop symptoms of depression. The researchers note that relationships with peers become critical during adolescence and that social media facilitates engagement with friends. Teens become very competitive and want to be chosen. Since social media allows adolescents to see the number of friends their peers have, some youth may perceive that they are not as popular if they have fewer. They may also perceive that they are not having as much fun as their peers, resulting in jealousy.[58]

Another consequence is that people communicating online seem more willing to be extreme than they would be in face-to-face communication. A study conducted in a social psychology class found that people behave differently online than they behave in person. Students were asked to rate how strongly they agreed or disagreed with a series of statements made on a questionnaire. Half of the students were asked to write the answers on a sheet of paper that was handed to the questioner, and the other half were asked to fill out the questionnaire online. The results showed that people expressed more hostile and extreme views when the questionnaire was filled out online. The researchers concluded online interaction provides anonymity and an ability to present yourself differently than you might ordinarily.[59]

Do you have the necessary interpersonal skills for the job you want to do? Could a lack of interpersonal skills make it more difficult for you to get hired?

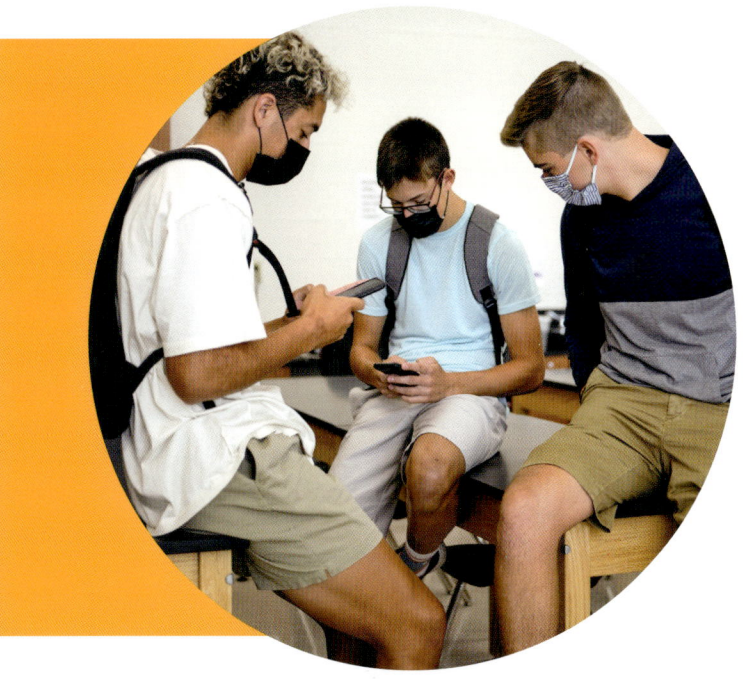

TECH AT SCHOOL

Many schools have tried to curb student use of cell phones by banning them in class. Sixty-five percent of students who attend schools that ban cell phones still bring them every day, and 43 percent of students reported that they text in class at least once per day.[64] Numerous studies have shown that cell phone use frequency may have a negative effect on academic performance. For instance, one study found that frequent cell phone use was related to school failure among high school students.[65] Another study revealed that text messaging on cell phones during class caused lower academic test scores among undergraduate students.[66] An additional study found that students who experienced a cell phone intrusion were often unable to identify the lecture material being discussed during the disruption and suggested that these intrusions could potentially impair the learning process.[67]

Have cell phone or social media interruptions at school affected your grades?

?

CYBERBULLYING

According to StopBullying.gov, not all bullying occurs in person. "Cyberbullying is a type of bullying that happens online or through text messages or emails."[68] They recommend taking the following steps to protect yourself:

- **Think about what you post.** You never know what someone will forward. Being kind to others online will help to keep you safe. Do not share anything that could hurt or embarrass anyone.

- **Keep your password a secret.** Even kids that seem like friends could give your password away or use it in ways you don't want.

- **Think about who sees what you post online.** Complete strangers? Friends? Friends of friends? Privacy settings let you control who sees what.

- **Keep your parents in the loop.** Let your parents have your passwords. Tell them what you're doing online and who you're doing it with. Let them "friend" or follow you. Listen to what they have to say about what is and isn't okay to do. They care about you and want you to be safe.

- **Talk to an adult you trust.** Discuss any messages you get or things you see online that make you sad or scared. If it is cyberbullying, report it.[69]

- **Report It.** Cyberbullying often violates the terms of service established by social media sites and Internet service providers. Report cyberbullying to the social media site so they can take action against users abusing the terms of service.[70]

HOW TO USE TECHNOLOGY

Use technology more responsibly by following these guidelines:

Use as a Supplement

Connecting with others is critical to your well-being and happiness, and technology works well as a supplement to these connections. Don't replace real, face-to-face relationships with technology-based ones. Balance the benefits and challenges of technology by using it in moderation. Make sure the time you spend with technology isn't crowding out other social activities.

Remember Your Digital Footprint

Everything you do online leaves a permanent record. This is called your digital footprint, which is "a map of everywhere you've been with your technology — everyone you've spoken to, every image, chat or comment you've posted and every file you've downloaded."[71] Your digital footprint is almost impossible to erase, especially when other people may easily share what you are trying to get rid of. Your digital footprint is a permanent map of the journey you take to becoming your adult self, so think carefully about how much of what you're experimenting with you want made public in a month, a year or even five or 10 years down the road.[72]

Think About the Future

Are you hoping to get into a good college? You might want to think twice about what you are posting online. According to a recent survey, "schools are increasingly discovering information on social media and the Internet that negatively impacts applicants' acceptance chances."[73] But it's not just colleges and universities. Potential employers are also looking closely at your presence on social media sites.[74] Think about that the next time you're tempted to post an embarrassing photo.

Be Careful

Sending and downloading images and videos is easier than ever before; the hard part is not knowing what another person might do with it. If you wouldn't want something displayed in public, then think twice before you post, email or text it to anyone. Also, be respectful of other people's privacy. Don't take pictures of someone unless they know you are taking them — especially if they are doing something that might get them or you into trouble.[75]

INTERPERSONAL

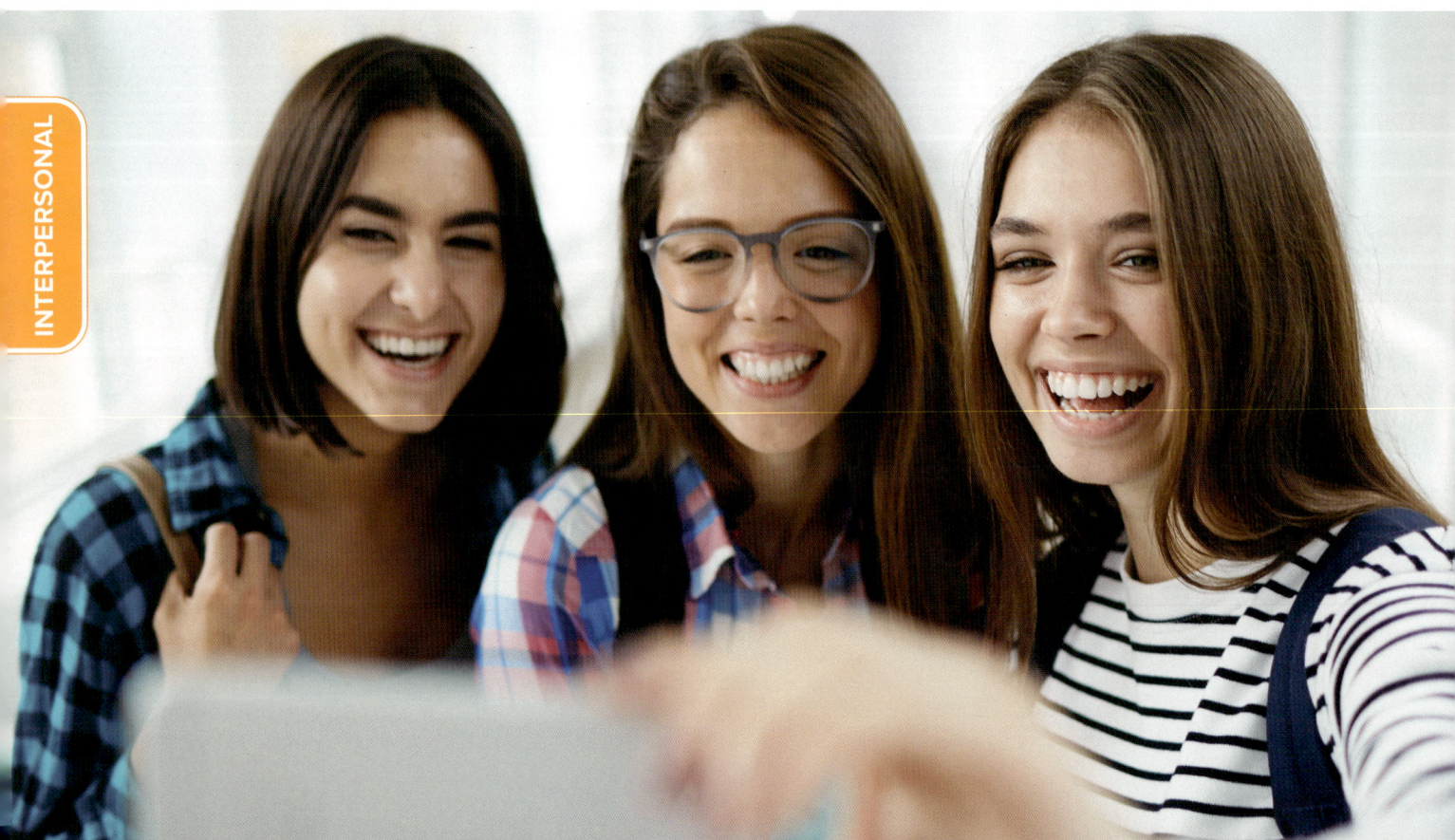

FACE-TO-FACE

God created you to be in the presence of others, and connecting with people provides a great sense of unity and common purpose. Face-to-face contact involves nonverbal communication and demonstrating physical touch such as shaking hands or hugging. There are many reasons why face-to-face communication is still important and vital for you to function at your best.

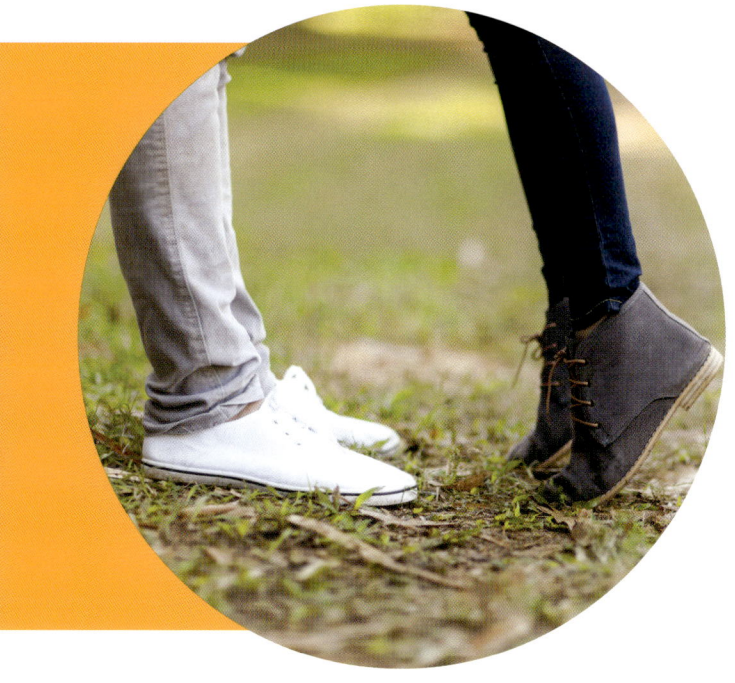

NONVERBALS

Dr. Albert Mehrabian, professor emeritus of psychology at UCLA, conducted extensive research on the effectiveness of communication. He determined that humans gain seven percent of meaning from words that are spoken, 38 percent from the way that the words are said and 55 percent from the facial expression and body language of the person speaking. This means 93 percent of your communication is completely nonverbal. When you communicate in a purely digital realm your communication context is stripped away. This means you are trying to forge a relationship and make decisions entirely based on words completely devoid of nonverbal communication.[76]

The human face and body communicate huge amounts of information that can't be received any other way. Nonverbal communication is the act of communicating without using any spoken words. This includes things like gestures, eye contact, touch, signs and symbols, body language, facial expressions, postures, proximity, color, appearance, habits and even handwriting style.[77] Words are only part of the message.

When the words being said don't match the nonverbal cues a person is sending, you will tend to put more trust in what is not being said. And when you use only words, such as in an email or text, it is all too easy to misunderstand the emotion behind the words.[78]

INTERPERSONAL

"Alone we can do so little, together we can do so much."

HELEN KELLER

Do you notice a difference between the words a person says and their nonverbal communication? Which are you more likely to believe?

PHYSICAL TOUCH

Physical touch is one of the most basic expressions of social connectedness,[79] and hundreds of studies have shown its benefits. In one study of preterm infants, researchers found that touching or stimulation for three 15-minute periods a day for 10 days produced an average of 47 percent greater weight gain per day. The infants were also more active and alert during sleep/wake behavior observations. Those infants who experienced the human touch and movement had a hospital stay six days shorter than those who weren't touched in the same manner.[80]

Physical touch is very important to your health, and it doesn't have to be dramatic or uncomfortable to make a difference. One study conducted in a university library stopped students who were leaving and asked how satisfied they were with the service they had received. What the students didn't know was that the study wasn't about the library — it was about touch. The library clerk had received specific instructions that half the people checking out were to have their hands touched as they received their library cards back. They were touched just lightly, almost imperceptibly, but the researchers found that the students who had been touched had much higher opinions of the library service than those who were not touched.[81]

Many studies have shown that physical touch lowers stress levels and improves your mood. A study at the University of North Carolina found that levels of cortisol, the hormone produced when you're under stress, were significantly lowered when subjects hugged partners for at least 20 seconds. The researchers also found that hugging instigated an elevated release of oxytocin and prompted loving and caring feelings.[82]

 **What are you missing by only spending virtual time with friends? How might getting more face-to-face time benefit you in the long run?**

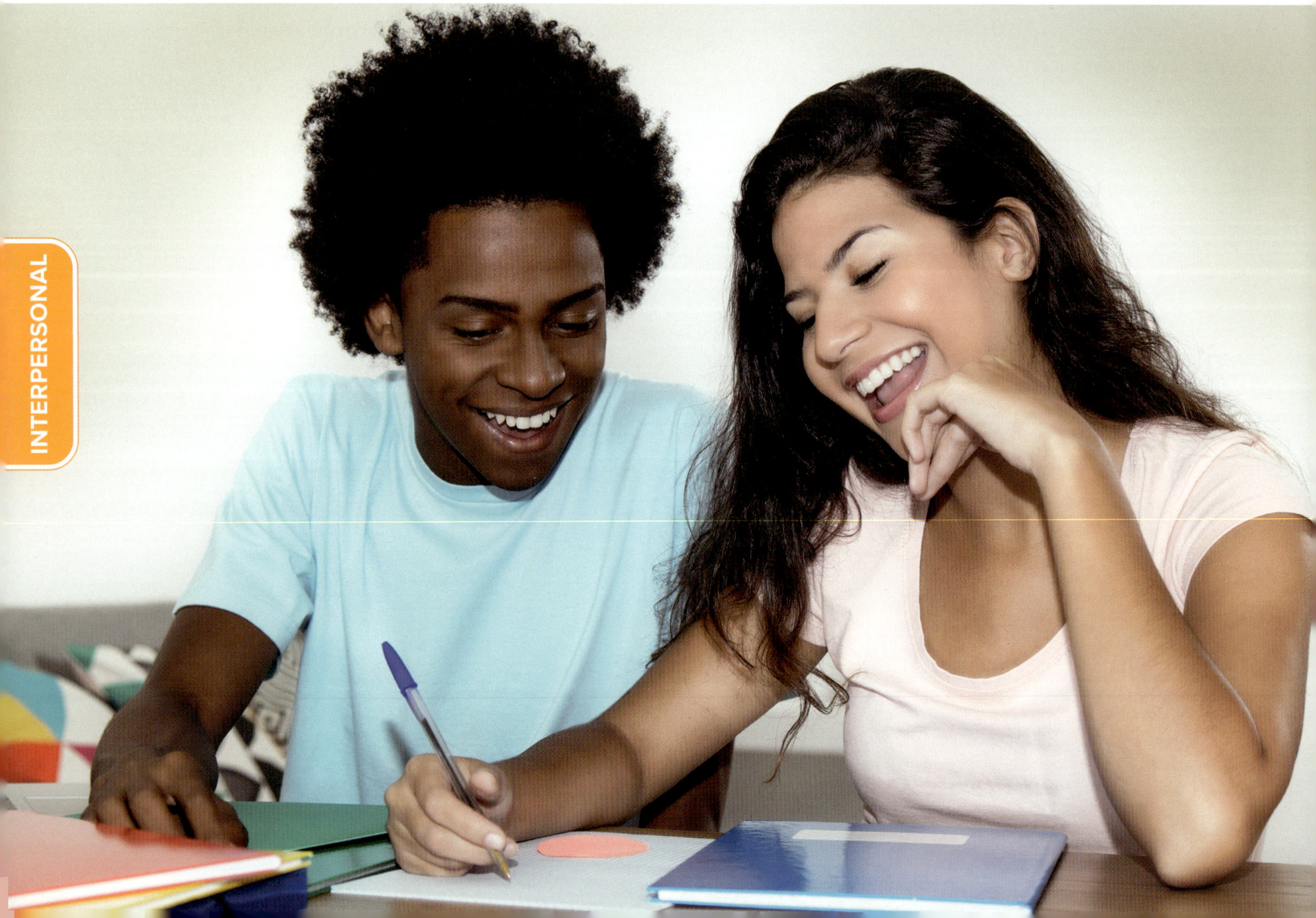

INTERPERSONAL

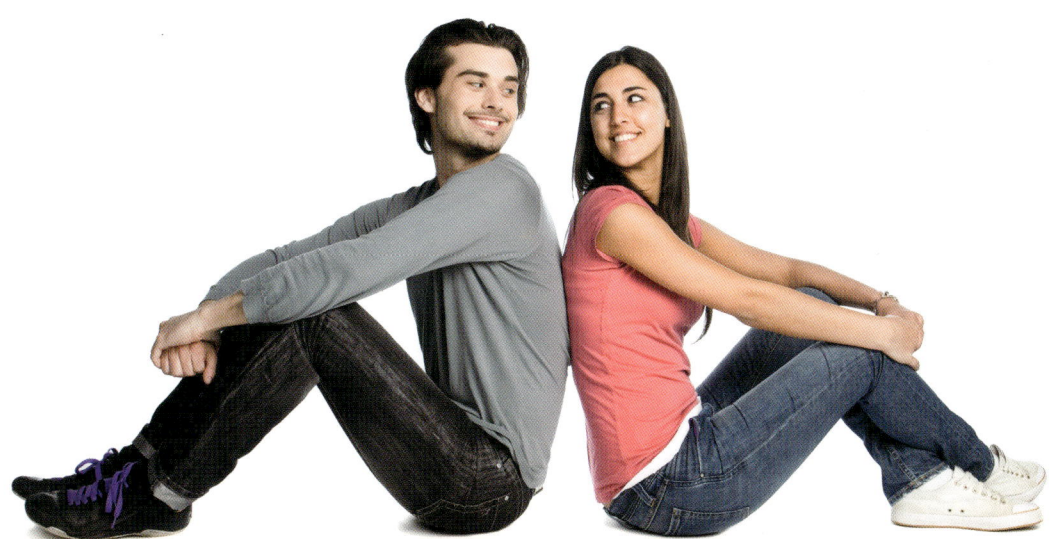

INCREASE YOUR FACE-TO-FACE TIME

Face-to-face communication does not come naturally to everyone. You may have to work hard to improve. Here are four actions you can take to get more comfortable with your face-to-face communication skills:

1. **Learn to listen.** Listening is hard work that involves an active, present mind. Think about the times you've spoken to someone who wasn't listening to you. It's easy to tell when they're distracted. To listen well, you must focus on the other person more than yourself, but listening is more than just using your ears. Watch the speaker's body language as well for nonverbal communication.[83]

2. **Ask the right questions.** Learning how to ask the right questions will help keep your conversation on the right track. And asking good questions gives people the feeling that you are genuinely interested in what they have to say. Try to avoid general questions like, "How are you?" and opt for more personal questions. You may ask about a friend's family, their pets or hobbies. Often a simple question relating to one of these topics, along with a genuine show of interest, will lead to deeper and more relevant topics.[84]

3. **Make consistent eye contact.** Maybe you've heard how the eye is the window to the soul? Well, how can you expect to communicate your "soul" to another person if your windows have the blinds drawn? Making eye contact may feel uncomfortable at first, but it communicates how much you genuinely care for a person. It also shows you are listening, and it expresses interest in what they have to say.[85]

4. **Use facial expressions.** An expressive face shows thoughts and feelings that enhance and verify the words coming out of your mouth. If your face doesn't agree with the words you say, no one is likely to believe your words. However, a smile in both the eyes and the mouth, along with a friendly greeting, increases the effectiveness of what you have to say. The best way to practice an expressive countenance is to observe the faces of others as they speak, especially if their faces vary dramatically from moment to moment depending on what they are saying. Try to match their expression and understand what causes it.[86]

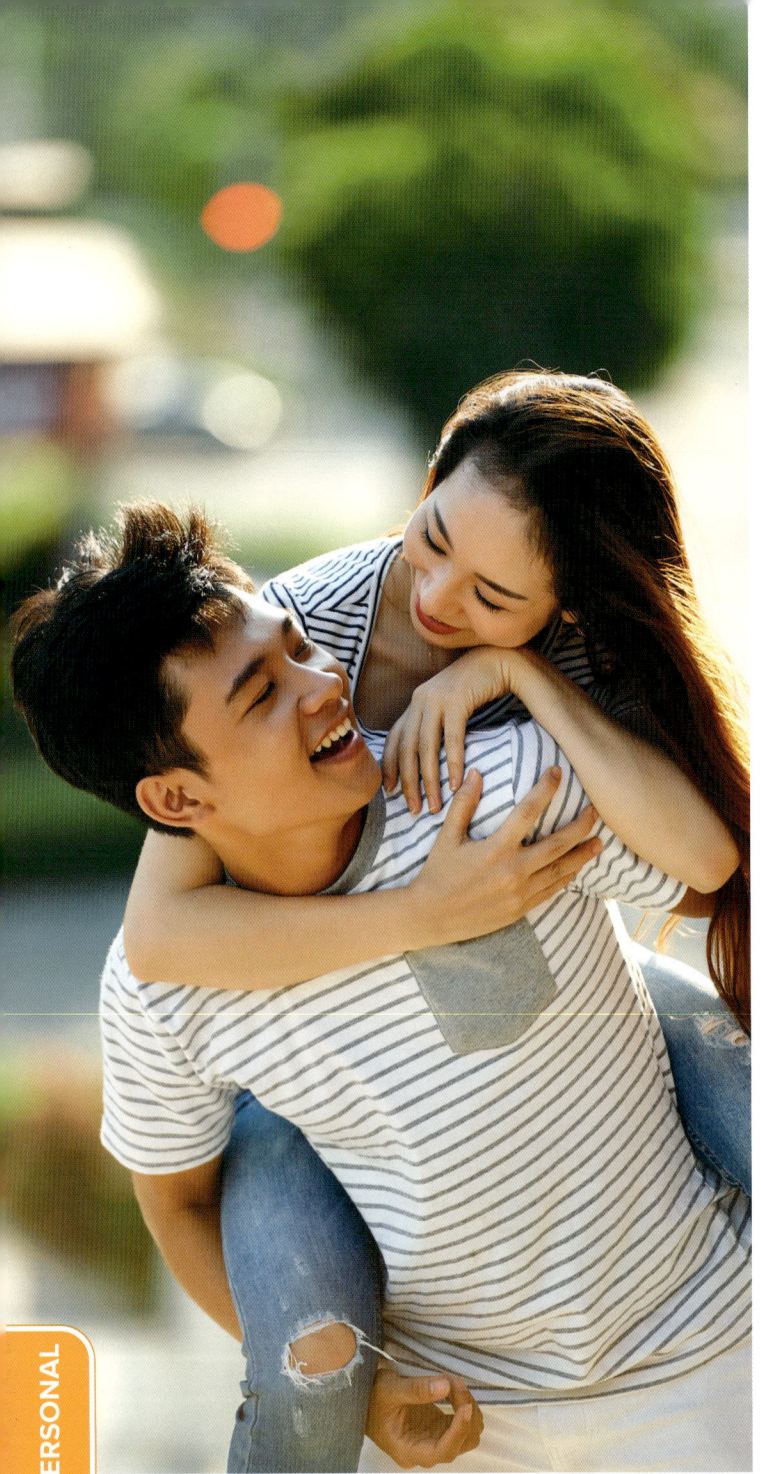

DATING

Dating can be a great experience as long as you balance it within God's boundaries of what is right and good. Dating is not a game to play with another person's emotions, and it is never right to date someone just to satisfy your ego or fulfill your sexual desires. In God's plan, dating is an opportunity for you to spend time with another person, as you consider whether or not they are the person you will marry. In his book *Waiting and Dating*, author Myles Munroe says that dating is where a couple learns about each other's interests, life purpose, personal and professional goals, education, intellect and emotional makeup, stability and boundaries.[87]

Today, many teens have a different idea about the purpose of dating. Movies, commercials and TV have portrayed dating as an activity solely for meeting one's sexual and short-term companionship needs. The idea that dating is an activity for finding a lifetime partner has all but disappeared from society's view.[88]

Dating God's way is still the best way, and it has many benefits as well. For starters, it gives you the opportunity to learn, not just about someone else, but also about yourself and what you want out of a relationship. Dating also provides opportunities for you to mature before making a marriage commitment. Dating will help you build your relationship skills and learn how to function within a relationship. And dating gives you a context to meet and spend time with a wide variety of people. You can find out what you like, what you need and what is good for you. The purpose of dating God's way is to choose the most compatible marriage partner for you.[89]

> *"The mandate to 'Love your neighbor as you love yourself' is not just a moral mandate. It is a physiological mandate. Caring is biological. One thing you get from caring for others is you are not lonely; and the more connected you are to life, the healthier you are."* DR. JAMES LYNCH

 **What is your view of dating? Do you see it as a short-term commitment or as a way to find your potential marriage partner?**

LIVING TOGETHER

Another major change in dating practices is society's acceptance of unmarried couples living together prior to, or instead of, marriage. One study found that 60 percent of Americans believe that the best way to establish a successful marriage is to cohabit prior to marriage.[90] Another study found almost 69 percent of high school senior boys agreed or mostly agreed with the statement, "It is usually a good idea for a couple to live together before getting married in order to find out whether they really get along." Estimates are that as many as 50 percent of Americans cohabit at one time or another prior to marriage.[91]

Is living together before getting married the best way to prepare for a strong marriage? According to many studies, the answer is a resounding "No." Researchers have found that unmarried couples who live together prior to marriage have a greater risk of divorce than traditionally married couples. Research has also shown that one of the major reasons for the high divorce rate is because couples who live together are not as committed in their dedication to the continuation of the relationship.[92]

One review, published by the National Marriage Project, found that men who enter into cohabitation do so with less intention to marry than women. "Women tend to see it as a step toward eventual marriage, while men regard it more as a sexual opportunity without the ties of long-term commitment. A woman's willingness to cohabit runs the risk of sending men precisely the wrong signal."[93] So, while women may believe they are headed for marriage, men are often entertaining a different future.

The authors of the book *The Case for Marriage: Why Married People Are Happier, Healthier, and Better off Financially* discuss that "test driving" a partner is dehumanizing to a potential marriage partner, treating them as if they were a product. This mindset can have significant emotional consequences. In fact, one study shows that partners who cohabit before marriage are less happy and scored lower on well-being measures, including sexual satisfaction, following their actually becoming married. It was also found that couples who cohabit for an extended period of time have less financial resources than married couples, particularly because of employment and tax benefits offered to married couples.[94]

Do you think living together before you are married is a good way to prepare for a lasting marriage?

INTERPERSONAL

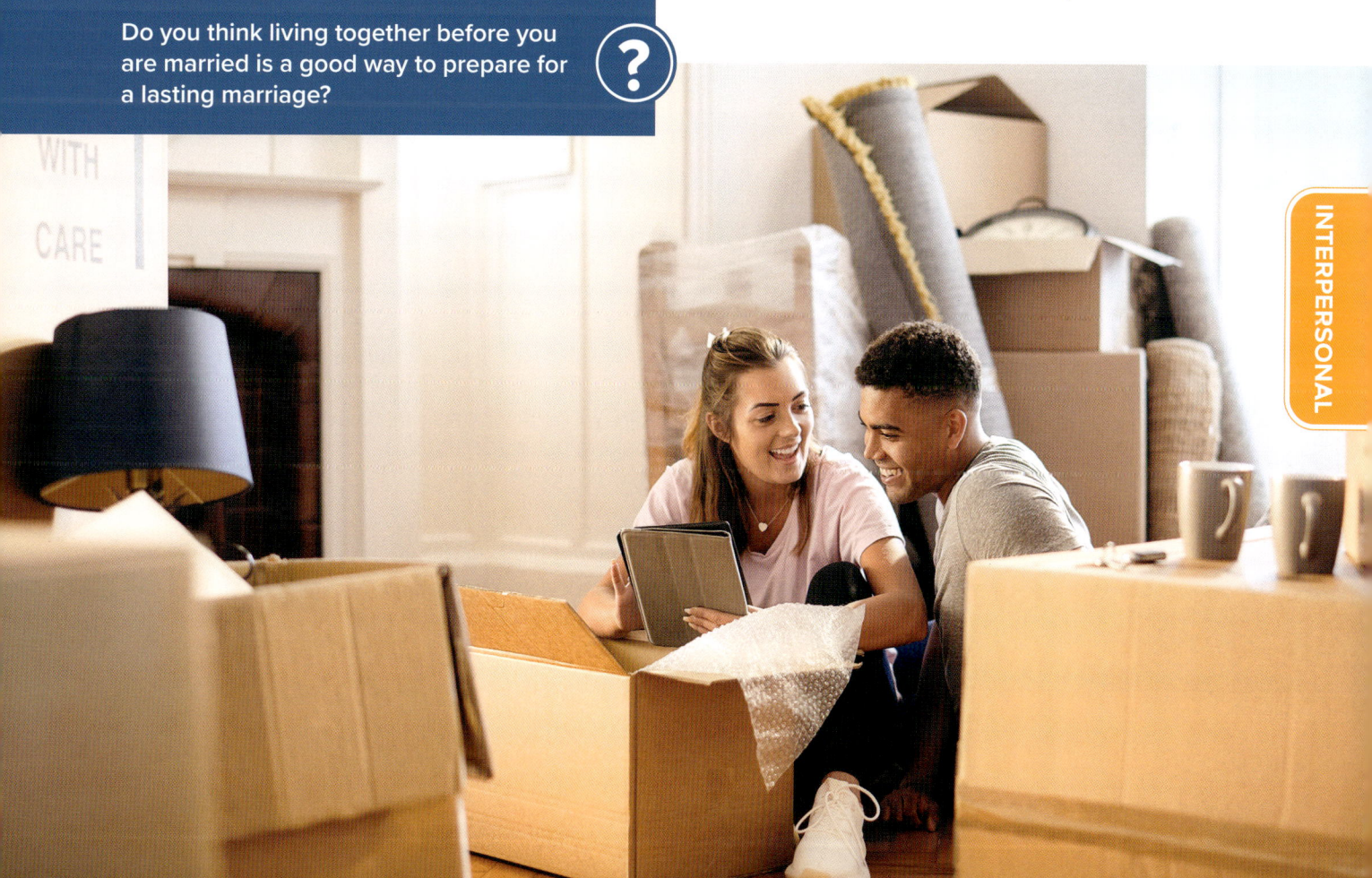

SEXUALITY

As a couple grows in their relationship, passing from friendship to dating to deciding whether they want to spend the rest of their lives together, questions will arise about physical attraction and sexuality. This is a natural part of dating because God created sex for your pleasure and enjoyment, but He also intended it to be experienced within the boundaries of a committed marriage.[95] If you are going to honor God with your dating life, you will abstain from sex and focus on getting to know the other person spiritually and emotionally. This delayed gratification will require self-control, but following God's way is truly best for you and the other person.

Your sexual desires are not bad or dirty, but they can be misplaced. In marriage, sex is good and even wonderful. On the other hand, sexual activity outside of marriage can hurt oneself and others.

If we confess our sins, He is faithful and righteous to forgive us our sins and to cleanse us from all unrighteousness.

1 JOHN 1:9

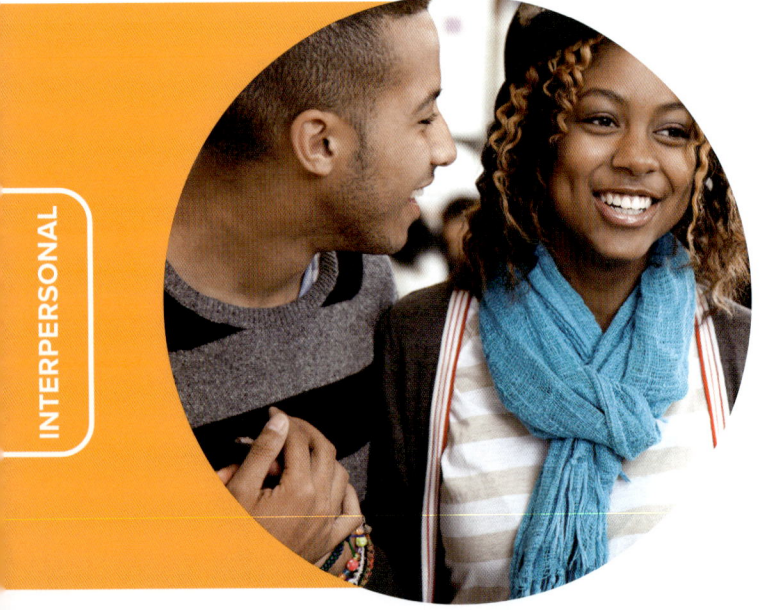

Have you experienced the pressure to have sex? How have you handled this?

LEARNING TO WAIT

The facts are clear. Premarital sex with one or multiple partners will increase your risk for unplanned pregnancy and sexually transmitted diseases (STDs). According to the Department of Health and Human Services, there were 305,420 babies born to females ages 15 to 19 in 2012, and nearly 89 percent of these births occurred outside of marriage.[96] Data reported by the Centers for Disease Control shows that sexually active adolescents and young adults, ages 15 to 24, are also at an increased risk for STDs. Young people now represent 25 percent of the sexually experienced population in the United States, but they account for nearly half of new STDs. The long-lasting health effects are particularly serious for young people. For example, untreated chlamydia can steal a woman's chance to have her own children later in life.[97] By choosing to wait to have sex until after marriage, you will save yourself from the devastating effects of both of these issues.

How can you postpone sex until marriage? One way is to stay connected in your relationship to God. This has been confirmed by numerous studies, which have found that individuals with no religious beliefs have more sex partners than those who have a strong religious affiliation.[98] It's also important to stay connected to other people. Scientific evidence continues to reveal how connectedness protects against risky behaviors. One study collected data from 90,000 teens and 18,000 of their parents across the United States. The one word that encapsulated all this research was connectedness. In short, teens who felt connected to family, church, school and community were far less likely to participate in risky behaviors than those who didn't have tight connections.[99] In other words, having strong interpersonal relationships with God, friends and family members may help to protect you from making risky decisions.

A NEW START

Have you already engaged in premarital sex? Are you experiencing feelings of regret or guilt? The good news is you can have a fresh start. Don't let the past destroy your future. Confess your sins to God and ask Him to help you to live a pure life.

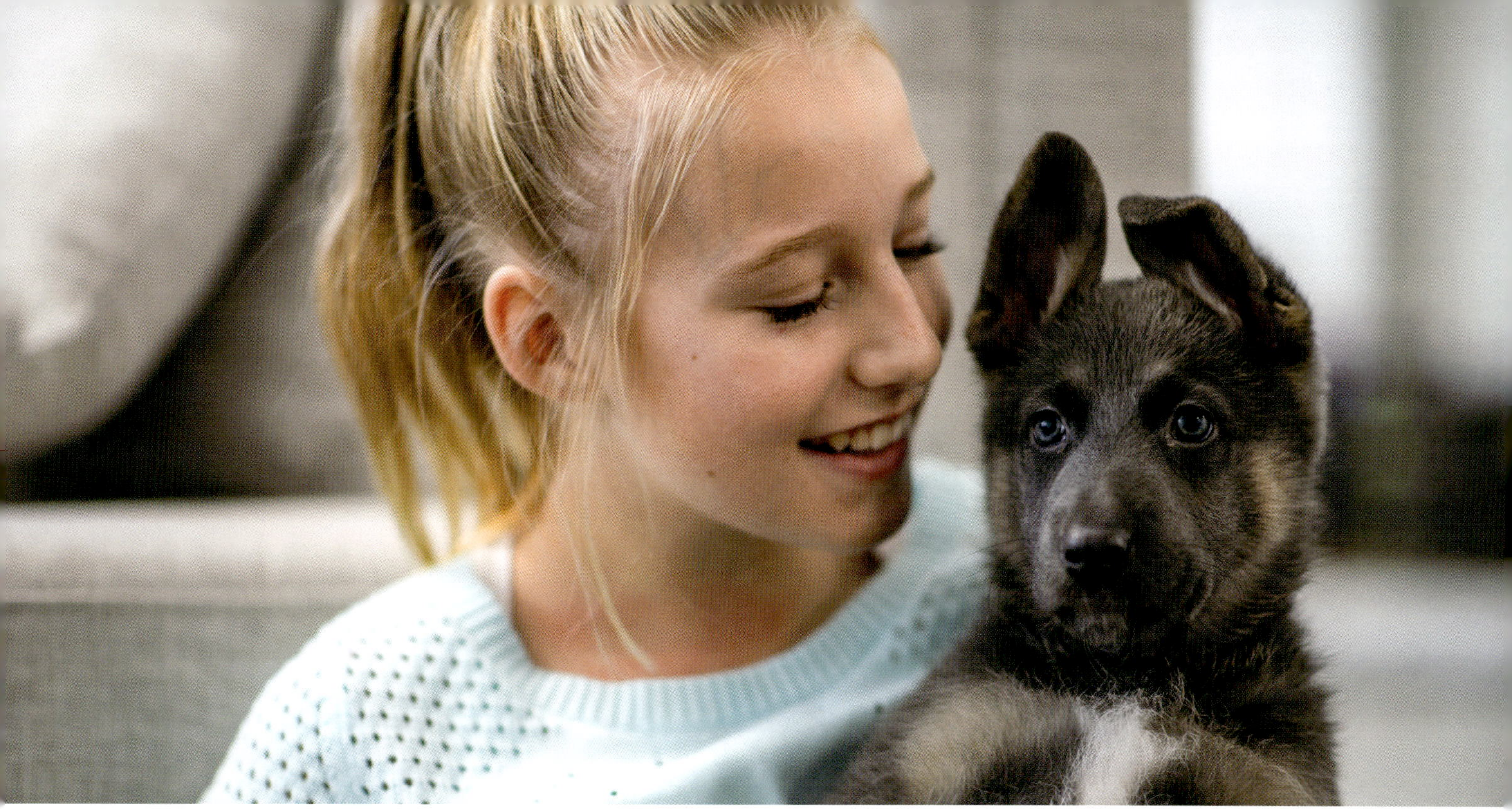

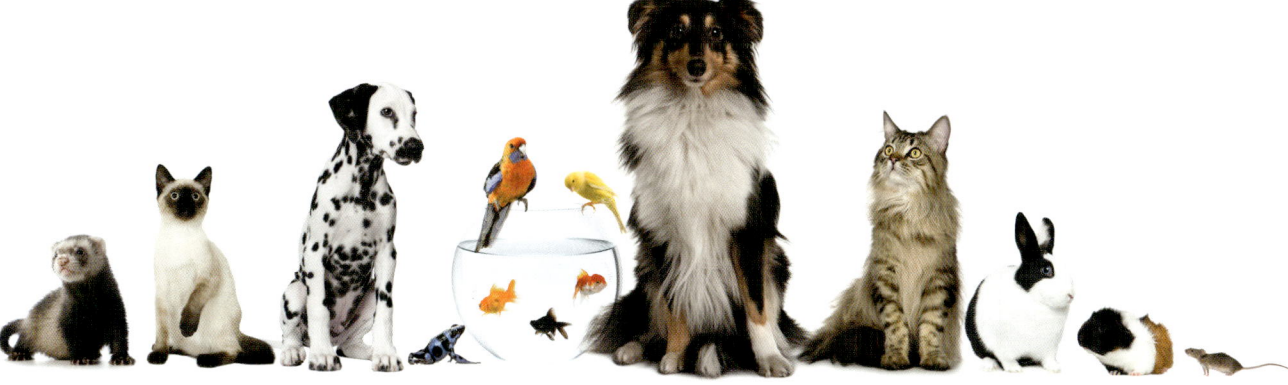

ANIMAL THERAPY

Are you looking for a relationship with a friend who will stick with you through good times and bad? Look no further than your closest furry friend. Domestic animals, such as dogs and cats, offer their owners an unconditional love that doesn't just soothe the mind, but may also heal the body as well. In one study, it was found that a dog's effect on lowering blood pressure is greater than that of a good friend. Why is this the case? It seems the friend was often perceived as judgmental, in contrast to the dog, which obviously wasn't.[100]

Another study found that one year after being hospitalized with chest pains or a heart attack, only six percent of the pet owners had died, compared to 28 percent of the patients who did not own pets. That's over four times as many people. This finding was independent of disease severity, exercise or other known factors.[101]

 **Do you have a pet? How have you experienced their unconditional love?**

But what if you don't have a dog or if you are allergic to certain types of animals? The good news is that even small pets can have a huge impact on your life. In one of the most successful programs of its kind, social worker David Lee of Lima State Hospital for the Criminally Insane in Ohio introduced small animals such as fish and parakeets to prisoners as "mascots." Among the prisoners who received the pets were those who had committed violent crimes. Allowing the criminals to care for the animals almost completely stopped fighting among prisoners, as well as suicide attempts.[102]

INTERPERSONAL

GIVING BACK

Many people who volunteer and serve in their communities claim to receive more back than they give. There are a number of incredible benefits to giving and helping others. For starters, there are the feelings of happiness and goodwill you receive when you give back. According to research, these feelings are even greater when you're in direct contact with the people you are helping. One research study found that 95 percent of those volunteers who had regular personal contact with the individuals whom they helped experienced a feel-good sensation, which has become known as the "helper's high."[103]

Colleges and universities across the United States have begun to incorporate volunteer service into their curricular requirements. While they're hoping to encourage students to become actively involved in helping their communities, short-term studies have also shown that service participation may have positive effects on academics, including knowledge gained, grades earned, degrees sought after and time devoted to academic endeavors. In addition, volunteering for service may influence the development of important life skills in the students. Additional benefits included the perception that their college had provided them with practical experience in the "real world," doubled involvement in volunteer activities after college, a greater sense of empowerment to bring about change in society and development of a meaningful philosophy of life. This study suggests that students who participate in service are more socially responsible and committed to serving their communities for years to come.[104]

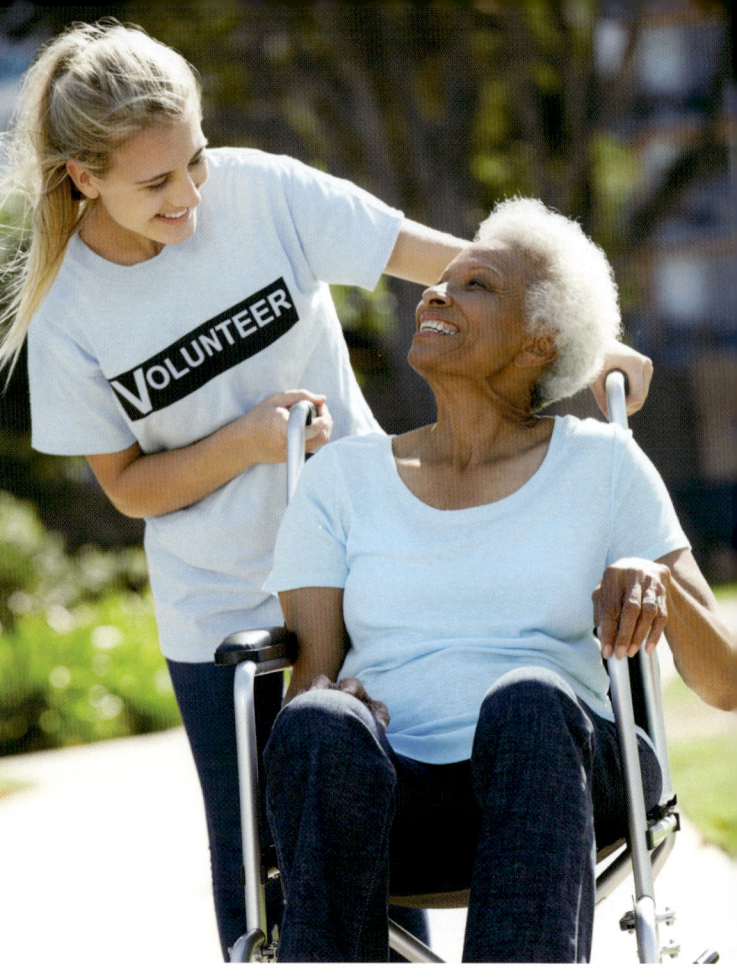

"Life's most urgent question is: What are you doing for others?"

MARTIN LUTHER KING JR.

ENHANCE YOUR VOLUNTEER EXPERIENCE

Use the following tips to get more when you give back:

- Have personal contact with the person you help, especially if they're a stranger.

- Set a goal of two hours of service per week.

- Volunteer at something you are already equipped to do, or something you can be trained to do.

- Choose service opportunities that are especially relevant to your personal interests.

- Find what works for you, and don't give up if you have one or two bad experiences. Be persistent.

INTERPERSONAL

FINAL THOUGHTS

You've probably heard the old saying, "If you want to make friends, be friendly." Most people tend to underestimate the significance of this truth. If you want to have strong, healthy relationships that sustain you through the good times as well as the bad, you must be the kind of person that you want your friends to be.

Shelly Gable, professor of psychology at UCLA, demonstrated through her research that how people talk about the good things that happen to them is more predictive of strong relationships than how people handle the bad things. The people you care about often tell you about their triumphs, victories and many other smaller things that happen to them on a daily basis. How you respond to them can either build up your relationship or undermine it.[105] Through open, positive, supportive communication you can bond with others. These bonds will strengthen when you affirm others by focusing on their positive traits and the positive events in their lives, and by verbally and physically expressing support for them in a sincere, authentic way.

When your friends and family share good news with you, make an effort to respond with genuine support and enthusiasm. Let them know you are truly happy and want to celebrate with them. You may even want to practice being supportive in this way, but in the end, remember, people are looking for authenticity. They desperately want someone they can be real with, someone they can trust to love and accept them the way they truly are. You can be that person for others and experience the joy God intended. It may sound overly simplistic, but following the Golden Rule is still the best way to manage and maintain all of your interpersonal relationships. Jesus said, *"Treat others the same way you want them to treat you"* (Luke 6:31). This is God's prescription for living.

POWER TIPS — IMPROVE YOUR RELATIONSHIPS

Consider these suggestions for improving your social health and your interpersonal relationships:

1. **Invest in friendships.** Take time to meet new people and renew old friendships.

2. **Stay in contact.** Meet often to do things together to enrich your social and emotional life.

3. **Develop a close confidant.** Find someone with whom you can share your most private fears, worries, successes and joys.

4. **Join a group.** Community, church and school organizations provide a way to meet new people and develop caring friends.

5. **Volunteer.** Many churches and organizations need volunteers. It's a great way to stay involved in helping other people, while finding social outlets for yourself.

6. **Look for social opportunities or create them yourself.** Come up with things to do with others. Invite them over, go out to dinner, do an activity together, join a church or school choir or look for someone else who needs a friend.

7. **Interact with others.** Don't isolate yourself completely. People are always more important than things.

REFERENCES

1. *Merriam-Webster*, s.v. "inter," Accessed August 28, 2018, https://www.merriam-webster.com/dictionary/inter.

2. Kaplan, Robert M. and Richard G. Kronick. "Marital Status and Longevity in the United States Population." *Journal of Epidemiology & Community Health* 60, no. 9 (2006): 760-765. http://dx.doi.org/10.1136/jech.2005.037606.

3. Robison, Jon and Karen Blockman Carrier. *The Spirit and Science of Holistic Health: More than Broccoli, Jogging, and Bottled Water More than Yoga, Herbs, and Meditation*. Bloomington: AuthorHouse, 2004.

4. Ornish, Dean. *Love and Survival: The Scientific Basis for the Healing Power of Intimacy*. New York: HarperPerennial, 2011.

5. Positano, Rock. "The Mystery of the Rosetan People." Last modified November 17, 2011. http://www.huffingtonpost.com/drrock-positano/the-mystery-of-the-roseta_b_73260.html.

6. Wolf, Stewart, and John G. Bruhn. The Power of Clan: *The Influence of Human Relationships on Heart Disease*. New Brunswick: Transaction Publishers, 1993.

7. Egolf, Brenda, Judith Lasker, Stewart Wolf, and Louise Potvin. "The Roseto Effect: A 50-year Comparison of Mortality Rates." *American Journal of Public Health* 82, no. 8 (1992): 1089-1092. https://doi.org/10.2105/AJPH.82.8.1089.

8. Cohen, Sheldon, William J. Doyle, David P. Skoner, Bruce S. Rabin, and Jack M. Gwaltney. "Social Ties and Susceptibility to the Common Cold-Reply." *Journal of the American Medical Association* 278, no. 15 (1997): 1232-1232. https://doi.org/10.1001/jama.1997.03550150036020.

9. Kiecolt-Glaser, Janice K., Ronald Glaser, Daniel Williger, Julie Stout, George Messick, Sharon Sheppard, Denise Ricker, Stephen C. Romisher, William Briner, George Bonnell, and Roy Donnerber. "Psychosocial Enhancement of Immunocompetence in a Geriatric Population." *Health Psychology* 4, no. 1 (1985): 25-41. http://dx.doi.org/10.1037/0278-6133.4.1.25.

10. Epplein, Meira, Ying Zheng, Wei Zheng, Zhi Chen, Kai Gu, David Penson, Wei Lu, and Xiao-Ou Shu. "Quality of Life After Breast Cancer Diagnosis and Survival." *Journal of Clinical Oncology* 29, no. 4 (2011): 406-412. https://doi.org/10.1200/JCO.2010.30.6951.

11. Ruberman, William, Eve Weinblatt, Judith D. Goldberg, and Banvir S. Chaudhary. "Psychosocial Influences on Mortality After Myocardial Infarction." *New England Journal of Medicine* 311, no. 9 (1984): 552-559. https://doi.org/10.1056/NEJM198408303110902.

12. World Health Organization. "Depression." Last modified March 22, 2018. http://www.who.int/en/news-room/fact-sheets/detail/depression.

13. McPhillips, Deidre. "U.S. Among Most Depressed Countries in the World" Last modified September 14, 2016. https://www.usnews.com/news/best-countries/articles/2016-09-14/the-10-most-depressed-countries.

14. Camfield, Laura, Kaneta Choudhury, and Joe Devine. "Well-Being, Happiness and Why Relationships Matter: Evidence from Bangladesh." *Journal of Happiness Studies* 10, no. 1 (2009): 71-91. https://doi.org/10.1007/s10902-007-9062-5.

15. Ibid.

16. Ibid.

17. Ibid.

18. Delle Fave, Antonella, Ingrid Brdar, Teresa Freire, Dianne Vella-Brodrick, and Marié P. Wissing. "The Eudaimonic and Hedonic Components of Happiness: Qualitative and Quantitative Findings." *Social Indicators Research* 100, no. 2 (2011): 185-207. https://doi.org/10.1007/s11205-010-9632-5.

19. Burt, Ronald S. "A Note on Strangers, Friends and Happiness." *Social Networks* 9, no. 4 (1987): 311-331. https://doi.org/10.1016/0378-8733(87)90002-5.

20. Myers, David G. and Ed Diener. "Who is Happy?." *Psychological Science* 6, no. 1 (1995): 10-19. https://doi.org/10.1111/j.1467-9280.1995.tb00298.x.

21. Ibid.

22. Levin, Jeffrey S. *God, Faith, and Health: Exploring the Spirituality-Healing Connection*. New York: Wiley, 2001.

23. Berkman, Lisa F. and S. Leonard Syme. "Social Networks, Host Resistance, and Mortality: A Nine-Year Follow-up Study of Alameda County Residents." *American Journal of Epidemiology* 109, no. 2 (1979): 186-204. https://doi.org/10.1093/oxfordjournals.aje.a112674.

24. Aschleman, Kristy A. "Forgiveness as a Resiliency Factor in Divorced or Permanently Separated Families." University of Wisconsin-Madison, 1996.

25. Poloma, Margaret M. and George Gallup. *Varieties of Prayer: A Survey Report*. Philadelphia: Trinity Press International, 1991.

26. Johnson, Ernest H. and Charles D. Spielberger. *Assessment of the Experience, Expression, and Control of Anger in Hypertension Research*. Washington D.C.: Hemisphere Publishing Corp, 1992.

27. McCullough, Michael E., Kenneth I. Pargament, and Carl E. Thoresen, eds. *Forgiveness: Theory, Research, and Practice*. New York: Guilford Press, 2000.

28. Jones, L. Gregory. *Embodying Forgiveness: A Theological Analysis*. Grand Rapids: William B. Eerdmans Publishing, 1995.

29. Lambert, Nathaniel M., Frank D. Fincham, Tyler F. Stillman, Steven M. Graham, and Steven R. H. Beach. "Motivating Change in Relationships: Can Prayer Increase Forgiveness?" *Psychological Science* 21, no. 1 (2010): 126-132. https://doi.org/10.1177/0956797609355634.

30. Zavada, Jack. "Bible Verses About Forgiveness" Thought Co. Last modified July 18, 2018. https://www.thoughtco.com/forgiveness-bible-verses-701330.

31. Demır, Melıkşah and Lesley A. Weitekamp. "I Am So Happy 'Cause Today I Found My Friend: Friendship and Personality as Predictors of Happiness." *Journal of Happiness Studies* 8, no. 2 (2007): 181-211. https://doi.org/10.1007/s10902-006-9012-7.

32. Demır, Melıkşah, Ayça Özen, Aysun Doğan, Nicholas A. Bilyk, and Fanita A. Tyrell. "I Matter to My Friend, Therefore I am Happy: Friendship, Mattering, and Happiness." *Journal of Happiness Studies* 12, no. 6 (2011): 983-1005. https://doi.org/10.1007/s10902-010-9240-8.

33. Bukowski, William M., Brett Laursen, and Betsy Hoza. "The Snowball Effect: Friendship Moderates Escalations in Depressed Affect Among Avoidant and Excluded Children." *Development and Psychopathology* 22, no. 4 (2010): 749-757. https://doi.org/10.1017/S095457941000043X.

34. Emily. "How to Build Lasting Friendships." Life Goals. Last modified May 18, 2010. https://www.lifegoals.org/how-to-build-lasting-friendships/.

35. Ibid.

36. Ibid.

37. Ibid.

38. Ibid.

39. Ibid.

40. Ibid.

41. Ibid.

42. Ibid.

43. Absolute Astronomy. "Peer Pressure." Accessed July 9, 2018. http://www.absoluteastronomy.com/topics/Peer_pressure.

44. Knee, C. Raymond and Clayton Neighbors. "Self Determination, Perception of Peer Pressure, and Drinking Among College Students." *Journal of Applied Social Psychology* 32, no. 3 (2002): 522-543. https://doi.org/10.1111/j.1559-1816.2002.tb00228.x.

45. Brown, B. Bradford, Donna R. Clasen, and Sue A. Eicher. "Perceptions of Peer Pressure, Peer Conformity Dispositions, and Self-Reported Behavior Among Adolescents." *Developmental Psychology* 22, no. 4 (1986): 521-530.

46. Shore, Elsie R., P. Clayton Rivers, and John J. Berman. "Resistance by College Students to Peer Pressure to Drink." *Journal of Studies on Alcohol* 44, no. 2 (1983): 352-361. https://doi.org/10.15288/jsa.1983.44.352.

47. Silva, Nicole. "Higher Education Cliques: Coolness in College." The Quinnipiac Chronicle. Last modified March 9, 2005. http://www.quchronicle.com/2005/03/higher-education-cliques-coolness-in-college/.

48. Barnardos. "Teen Help: Friends, Cliques and Peer Pressure." Accessed July 9, 2018. https://www.barnardos.ie/resources-advice/young-people/teen-help/bullying/friends-cliques-and-peer-pressure.html.

49. Ibid.

50. Statista. "Number of Monthly Active Facebook Users Worldwide as of 2nd Quarter 2018." Accessed September 4, 2018. https://www.statista.com/statistics/264810/number-of-monthly-active-facebook-usersworldwide/.

51. Nielsen. "U.S. Teen Mobile Report Calling Yesterday, Texting Today, Using Apps Tomorrow." Last modified October 14, 2010. http://www.nielsen.com/us/en/insights/news/2010/u-s-teen-mobile-report-calling-yesterday-texting-today-using-apps-tomorrow.html.

52. Kraut, Robert, Michael Patterson, Vicki Lundmark, Sara Kiesler, Tridas Mukophadhyay, and William Scherlis. "Internet Paradox: A Social Technology That Reduces Social Involvement and Psychological Well-Being?" *American Psychologist* 53, no. 9 (1998): 1017-1031. http://dx.doi.org/10.1037/0003-066X.53.9.1017.

53. Ibid.

54. Sigman, Aric. "Well Connected? The Biological Implications of 'Social Networking'." *Biologist* 56, no. 1 (February 2009): 14-20. http://www.aricsigman.com/IMAGES/Sigman_lo.pdf.

INTERPERSONAL

55. Nie, Norman H. and D. Sunshine Hillygus. "The Impact of Internet Use on Sociability: Time-Diary Findings." *IT & Society* 1, no. 1 (2002): 1-20. https://www.researchgate.net/profile/D_Sunshine_Hillygus/publication/247901330_The_Impact_of_Internet_Use_on_Sociability_Time-Diary_Findings/links/0deec5398cdce1b768000000/The-Impact-of-Internet-Use-on-Sociability-Time-Diary-Findings.pdf.

56. Kalpidou, Maria, Dan Costin, and Jessica Morris. "The Relationship Between Facebook and the Well-Being of Undergraduate College Students." *Cyberpsychology, Behavior, and Social Networking* 14, no. 4 (2011): 183-189. https://doi.org/10.1089/cyber.2010.0061.

57. Ibid.

58. Mehdizadeh, Soraya. "Self-Presentation 2.0: Narcissism and Self-Esteem on Facebook." *Cyberpsychology, Behavior, and Social Networking* 13, no. 4 (2010). https://doi.org/10.1089/cyber.2009.0257.

59. Hunter, Brad. "The Subtle Benefits of Face-To-Face Communication." Accessed September 6, 2018. https://web.stanford.edu/class/symbsys205/facetoface.html.

60. Tash, Joe. "Teen 'Sexting' a Serious Problem Police Report at Community Meeting in Carmel Valley." Delmar Times. Last modified November 9, 2013. http://www.delmartimes.net/sddmt-teen-sexting-a-serious-problem-police-report-at-2013nov09-story.html.

61. Ibid.

62. Leinwand, Donna. "Survey: 1 in 5 Teens 'Sext' Despite Risks." USA Today. Accessed July 9, 2018. https://usatoday30.usatoday.com/news/nation/2009-06-23-onlinekids_N.htm.

63. Ibid.

64. Pew Research Center. "Teens And Mobile Phones". Last modified April 20, 2010. http://www.pewinternet.org/2010/04/20/teens-and-mobile-phones-3/.

65. Ellis, Yvonne, Bobbie Daniels, and Andres Jauregui. "The Effect of Multitasking on the Grade Performance of Business Students." *Research in Higher Education Journal* 8 (2010): 1-10.

66. End, Christian M., Shaye Worthman, Mary Bridget Mathews, and Katharina Wetterau. "Costly Cell Phones: The Impact of Cell Phone Rings on Academic Performance." *Teaching of Psychology* 37, no. 1 (2009): 55-57. https://doi.org/10.1080/00986280903425912.

67. Harman, Brittany A. and Toru Sato. "Cell Phone Use and Grade Point Average Among Undergraduate University Students." *College Student Journal* 45, no. 3 (2011). 544-549. https://www.csus.edu/faculty/m/fred.molitor/docs/cell%20phones%20and%20grades.pdf.

68. StopBullying.gov. "What Kids Can Do." Accessed July 9, 2018. https://www.stopbullying.gov/kids/what-you-can-do/.

69. Ibid.

70. StopBullying.gov. "Report Cyberbulling." Accessed July 9, 2018. https://www.stopbullying.gov/cyberbullying/how-to-report/index.html.

71. The Alannah and Madeline Foundation. "Being Smart, Safe, and Responsible: Some Quick Tips for Using Technology." Accessed July 9, 2018. http://www.distance.vic.edu.au/wp-content/uploads/2012/08/eSmart_TipsBrochure.pdf.

72. Ibid.

73. Schaffer, Russell and Carina Wong. "Kaplan Test Prep Survey Finds That College Admissions Officers' Discovery of Online Material Damaging to Applicants Nearly Triples in a Year." Kaplan Test Prep. October 4, 2012. http://press.kaptest.com/press-releases/kaplan-test-prep-survey-finds-that-college-admissions-officers-discovery-of-online-material-damaging-to-applicants-nearly-triples-in-a-year.

74. The Alannah and Madeline Foundation. "Being Smart, Safe, and Responsible: Some Quick Tips for Using Technology." Accessed July 9, 2018. http://www.distance.vic.edu.au/wp-content/uploads/2012/08/eSmart_TipsBrochure.pdf.

75. Ibid.

76. Mehrabian, Albert. "Significance of Posture and Position in the Communication of Attitude and Status Relationships." *Psychological Bulletin* 71, no. 5 (1969): 359-372. http://dx.doi.org/10.1037/h0027349.

77. Ibid.

78. Ibid.

79. Field, Tiffany M., Saul M. Schanberg, Frank Scafidi, Charles R. Bauer, Nitza Vega-Lahr, Robert Garcia, Jerome Nystrom, and Cynthia M. Kuhn. "Tactile/Kinesthetic Stimulation Effects on Preterm Neonates." *Pediatrics* 77, no. 5 (1986): 654-658.

80. McKinney, William T. "Primate Social Isolation: Psychiatric Implications." *Archives of General Psychiatry* 31, no. 3 (1974): 422-426. https://doi.org/10.1001/archpsyc.1974.01760150122018.

81. Fisher, Jeffrey, Marvin Rytting, and Richard Heslin. "Hands Touching Hands: Affective and Evaluative Effects of an Interpersonal Touch." *Sociometry* 39, no. 4 (1976): 416-421. https://pdfs.semanticscholar.org/c052/0ccdee06d0b3bbdab8b7f2d0b0e7ea8839d8.pdf.

82. Grewen, Karen M., Susan S. Girdler, Janet Amico, and Kathleen C. Light. "Effects of Partner Support on Resting Oxytocin, Cortisol, Norepinephrine, and Blood Pressure Before and After Warm Partner Contact." *Psychosomatic Medicine* 67, no. 4 (2005): 531-538. https://doi.org/10.1097/01.psy.0000170341.88395.47.

83. ezTalks. "8 Useful Face to Face Communication Tips." Accessed September 5, 2018. https://www.eztalks.com/unified-communications/face-to-face-communication-tips.html

84. Ibid.

85. Ibid.

86. Ibid.

87. Munroe, Myles. *Waiting and Dating: a Sensible Guide to a Fulfilling Love Relationship.* Shippensburg: Destiny Image Publishers, 2005.

88. Ibid.

89. Ibid.

90. Barna, George. *The Future of the American Family.* Chicago: Moody Press, 1993.

91. Bachman, Jerald G., Lloyd D. Johnston, and Patrick M. O'Malley. *Monitoring the Future: Questionnaire Responses from the Nation's High School Seniors 2012.* Ann Arbor: Institute for Social Research, 2014. http://www.monitoringthefuture.org/datavolumes/2012/2012dv.pdf.

92. Nock, Steven L. "A Comparison of Marriages and Cohabiting Relationships." *Journal of Family Issues* 16, no. 1 (1995): 53-76. https://doi.org/10.1177/019251395016001004.

93. Popenoe, David and Barbara Dafoe Whitehead. *Should We Live Together?* Piscataway: National Marriage Project, 2002.

94. Waite, Linda and Maggie Gallagher. *The Case for Marriage: Why Married People are Happier, Healthier and Better Off Financially.* New York: Broadway Books, 2002.

95. Cloud, Henry and John Sims Townsend. *Boundaries in Dating: Making Dating Work.* Grand Rapids: Zondervan, 2001.

96. Hamilton, B. E., J. A. Martin, and S. J. Ventura. "Births: Preliminary Data for 2012," *National Vital Statistics Reports* 62, no. 3 (2013): 1-20. https://www.ncbi.nlm.nih.gov/pubmed/24321416.

97. Beck, Melinda. "Chlamydia, the Silent STD That Can Cause Infertility." The Wall Street Journal. Last modified June 30, 2009. https://www.wsj.com/articles/SB100014240529702039375045742523622862563486.

98. Rowatt, Wade C. and David P. Schmitt. "Associations Between Religious Orientation and Varieties of Sexual Experience." *Journal for the Scientific Study of Religion* 42, no. 3 (2003): 455-465. https://doi.org/10.1111/1468-5906.00194.

99. Russek, Linda G. and Gary E. Schwartz. "Feeling of Parental Caring Predict Health Status in Midlife: A 35-year Follow-up of the Harvard Mastery of Stress Study." *Journal of Behavioral Medicine* 20, no. 1 (1997): 1-13. https://doi.org/10.1023/A:1025525428213.

100. Friedmann, Erika, Aaron H. Katcher, James J. Lynch, and Sue Ann Thomas. "Animal Companions and One-Year Survival of Patients After Discharge From a Coronary Care Unit." *Public Health Reports* 95, no. 4 (1980): 307-312. https://lemosandcrane.co.uk/resources/Public%20Health%20-%20Animal%20Companions%20and%20One-Year%20Survival%20of%20Patients%20After%20Discharge%20from%20a%20Coronary%20Care%20Unit.pdf.

101. Siegal, J. M. "Stressful Life Events and Use of Physician Services Among the Elderly: The Moderating Role of Pet Ownership." *Journal of Personality and Social Psychology* 58, no. 6 (1990). 1081-1086.

102. Lee, David R. "Pet Therapy: Helping Patients Through Troubled Times." *California Veterinarian* 5 (1983): 24-25.

103. Luks, Allan. "Helper's High: Volunteering Makes People Feel Good, Physically and Emotionally." 22 (1988): 39, 42.

104. Sax, Linda J., Alexander W. Astin, and Juan Avalos. "Long-Term Effects of Volunteerism During the Undergraduate Years." *The Review of Higher Education* 22, no. 2 (1999): 187-202. https://humansciences.okstate.edu/community-engagement/student/research-articles/long-term-effects-of-volunteerism.pdf.

105. Gable, Shelly L., Gian C. Gonzaga, and Amy Strachman. "Will You Be There for Me When Things Go Right? Supportive Responses to Positive Event Disclosures." *Journal of Personality and Social Psychology* 91, no. 5 (2006): 904-917. https://doi.org/10.1037/0022-3514.91.5.904.

INTERPERSONAL

NOTES

INTERPERSONAL

OUTLOOK

Be optimistic, express gratitude

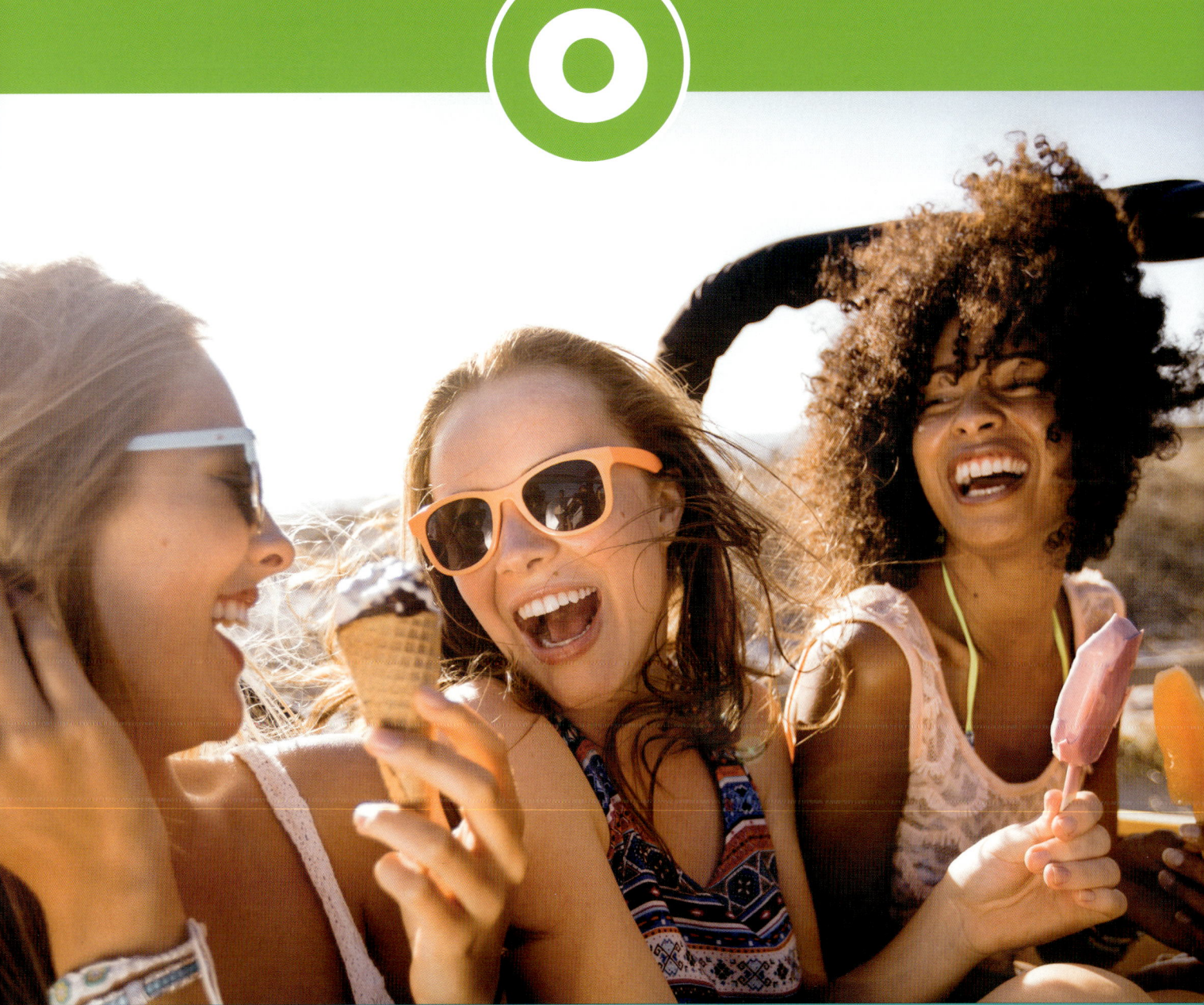

OUTLOOK [out-look] *noun* **1:** the way you view your world. A positive attitude shapes your choices and how you interact with others.

THE BIG PICTURE

It may be hard to imagine, but high school doesn't last forever. Right now you may feel like you'll never be free of term papers, cafeteria food and grade point averages, but just like a pint of Ben and Jerry's *Chunky Monkey®*, all good things must come to an end. The good news is that in a short time you will finally be free. The The challenge is figuring out what to do with the rest of your life. Will you go to a university or a community college? Will you live at home or can you afford to move out? Should you become an international fashion model or take that clandestine black-op with the CIA? You have some big choices to make, and it's not going to get any easier. But you also have an amazing tool at your disposal that, just like the beloved knife carried by the military forces of Switzerland, will help you face any number of sticky situations. You have a positive outlook.

Or do you? No doubt you've come across people in your travels who see the world as dark and foreboding as the land of Mordor. Do you follow in their footsteps, eternally taking a "glass half-empty" approach to life? Do you scan every blue sky, expecting grey clouds to show up at any minute? You were not designed to go through life with a negative point of view. Quite the opposite; you were created for much more.

As the seventh principle of CREATION Life, Outlook refers to your own unique point of view, but it's more than that. How you react to the situations you face shapes your attitude in ways that can either help or harm you. A negative outlook turns off the lights of hope, changes love to hate and makes other people want to be around you less than the guy in gym who doesn't use deodorant. But a positive outlook does just the opposite. It turns on the lights, ignites love and gives you a contagious personality. You become a person others want to be around. "Positive" is what you were made to be.

In this section, you'll see how outlook impacts everything you say and do. You'll focus on how to have a more positive and optimistic attitude toward life and you'll see how negative thinking can be destructive to your health.

OUTLOOK is how you approach the world and your life. In other words, it is your general attitude. Outlook affects how you see the world, what you think of yourself, of the people around you, your family, your schoolmates, your friends — everything.

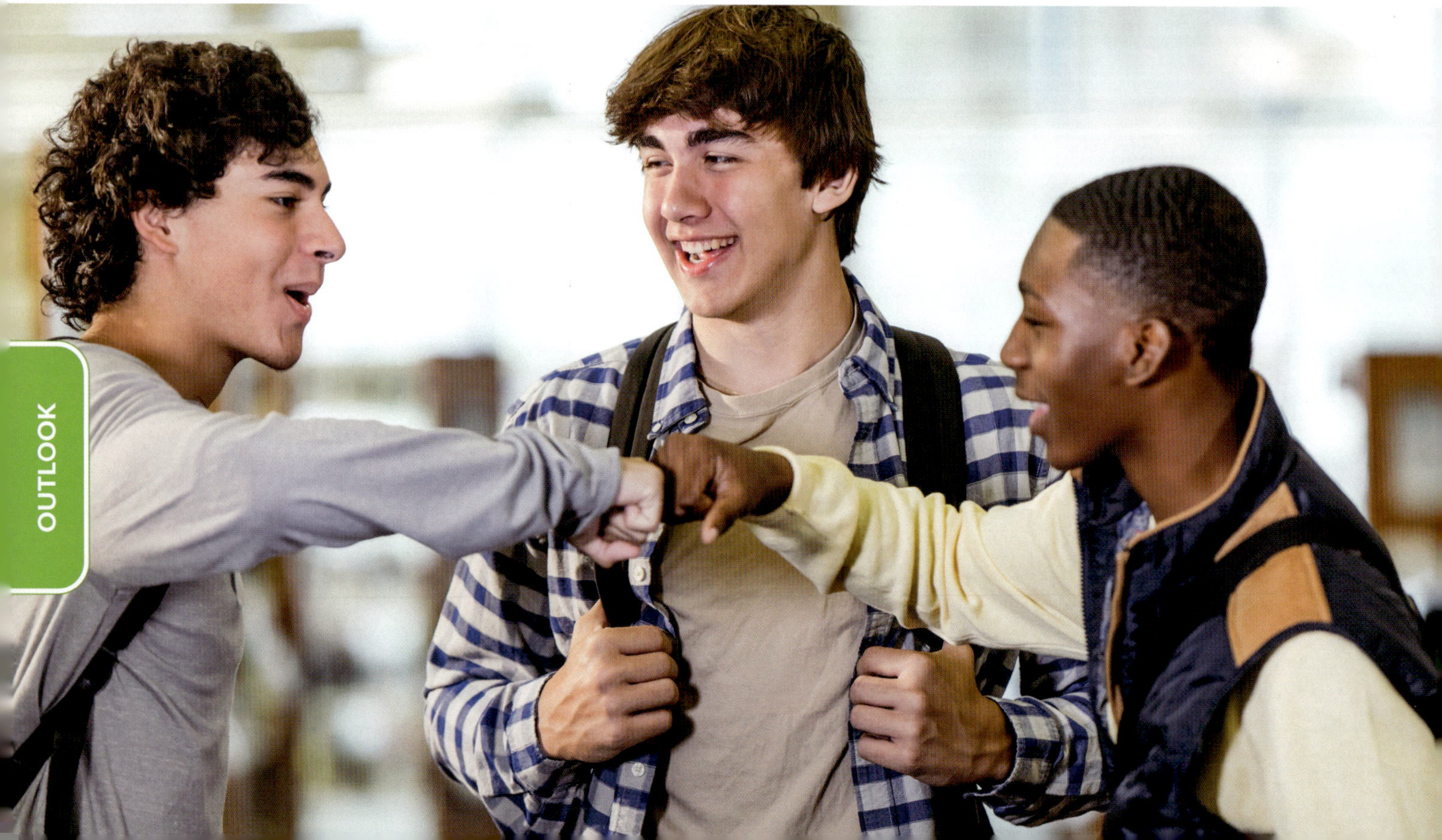

OUTLOOK

THE GIFT OF OUTLOOK

God saw all that He had made, and behold, it was very good. And there was evening and there was morning, the sixth day. GENESIS 1:31

When God made the world, He pronounced that it was all good. God approached His creation with a powerfully positive attitude. As a reflection of His glory, God was pleased with everything He had made. There wasn't a stone or a plant out of place. Like a beautiful symphony written by a master composer, all of creation rang with praises to its divine Creator. It was very good.

God shared this gift of a positive outlook with Adam and Eve when He blessed them. In Genesis 1:28, He gave the couple instructions to *"Be fruitful and multiply, and fill the earth, and subdue it; and rule over the fish of the sea and over the birds of the sky and over every living thing that moves on the earth."* One thing you should notice about these instructions is how overwhelmingly positive they are. In fact, the only prohibition God gave to Adam and Eve was against their eating from the tree of the knowledge of good and evil, and even that was for their own good. It was designed to protect them from the consequences of evil.

Sadly, sin destroyed the paradise Adam and Eve once enjoyed. Humanity lost the perfection and beauty of Eden, but what about the positive outlook? Has that been lost as well?

In the New Testament, the apostle Paul writes these words in the letter to the church in Rome:

And we know that God causes all things to work together for good to those who love God, to those who are called according to His purpose. ROMANS 8:28

> *"You'll never find a rainbow if you're looking down."*
>
> CHARLIE CHAPLIN

Let's be clear — God is not the cause of the struggles and hardships in your life. These are all the consequences of a fallen and imperfect world. But God has allowed these things to occur for a greater purpose. When you love God, you understand that He will never waste a single moment of your life. Sure, humanity may have lost its perfect home in Eden, but you can still have a positive outlook. God wants you to stay positive because He is there with you in the hard times, working out every circumstance for your good. He will turn even your time of deepest grief and mourning into joy and dancing (Psalm 30:11).

TAKE IT FROM JOE

The Bible is full of individuals who remained positive in the face of difficult trials. One of these was Joseph, the son of Jacob. Joseph was betrayed by his brothers, thrown into a pit and sold into slavery. Later, he was accused of a crime he didn't commit and locked in prison. Yet even in the darkest dungeon, Joseph was faithful to God. Joseph had a unique, God-given ability to interpret dreams. This brought him recognition and fame until he got a big promotion as Pharaoh's right-hand man. He literally went from the pit to the palace.

Later, Joseph had the opportunity to get back at his brothers for the wrongs they had done to him. His brothers were afraid for their lives, assuming their days were numbered. But incredibly he didn't hold a grudge. Instead Joseph told them, *"Do not be afraid, for am I in God's place? As for you, you meant evil against me, but God meant it for good"* (Genesis 50:19–20). Joseph's positive outlook allowed him to see God's purpose in everything that happened to him. And Joseph was able to forgive his brothers instead of exacting revenge. Likewise, when you allow God to mold and shape your outlook you will experience the supernatural power to look beyond your circumstances. You will see God's plan at work in all the areas of your life, and you will be able to love and forgive others no matter what difficulties you face.

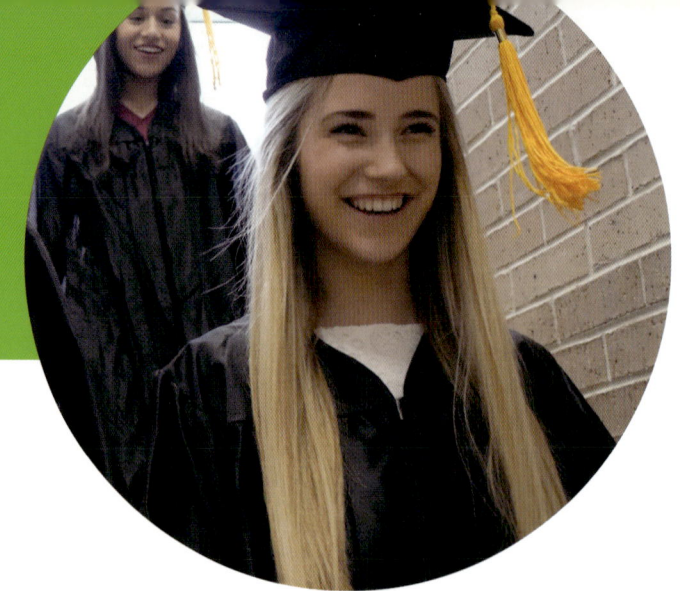

You can do amazing things with the gifts and talents God has given you as long as you keep a positive outlook.

OPTIMISM VS. PESSIMISM

"We're going to lose the game."

"Oh, you're such a pessimist."

"I'm not a pessimist; I'm a realist."

Is always looking on the downside of things a more "realistic" way of thinking? Is it really more likely for things not to go in your favor? Maybe you've heard of Murphy's Law: *Anything that can go wrong, will go wrong.* This particular view of the world doesn't create "realists", it twists people into doubtful cynics, suspicious of any good they encounter. Unable to understand it, they criticize it. They sarcastically mock and question everyone else's motives but not their own. They're not remotely interested in understanding how the world really works. They prefer the feeling of superiority because they're the only ones who have it "figured out."

Do you want to know the truth about pessimism? Always looking for the worst in every situation has long-term effects on the rest of your life. In the book *Learned Optimism,* Dr. Martin Seligman writes about optimism vs. pessimism. Dr. Seligman studied school children, ranking them as either optimists or pessimists. He found that the kids who scored the highest for optimism rarely felt depressed or, if they did get depressed, they recovered rapidly. Not surprisingly, the pessimists were the ones who were most likely to get depressed and stay depressed.

Dr. Seligman also found that college freshmen who rose to the challenges of their first year and did better than expected were optimists when they entered college. Those who did much worse than expected entered their freshman year as pessimists. (The expectations in both groups were based on a student's GPA and how well they had performed on achievement tests such as the SAT).

The research shows that high scores for optimism can actually predict excellence in many areas of your life — from how well you might do in a football game to your ability to achieve in a high-paying sales job. Have you heard of MetLife®? Dr. Seligman's findings have saved that company millions of dollars because now they identify and hire optimists vs. pessimists.

"Over and above their talent-test scores," Dr. Seligman says, "we repeatedly find that pessimists drop below their potential and optimists exceed it. I have come to think that the notion of potential, without the notion of optimism, has very little meaning."[1]

In other words, no matter how gifted or talented you may be right now, if you don't see the world in a positive, optimistic light, you may never live up to your full potential. But there's good news, too. Even if you're not the starting quarterback or first chair in the orchestra, you can still do amazing things with the gifts and talents God has given you as long as you keep a positive outlook.

Optimism is not something you are born with. It's an attitude you can learn, and it starts by properly dealing with disappointment. Seligman states in his book that "becoming an optimist consists not of learning to be more selfish and self-assertive, or presenting yourself to others in overbearing ways, but simply of learning a set of skills about how to talk to yourself when you suffer a personal defeat."[2] Learn to speak encouragingly to yourself instead of beating yourself up over every little setback. You'll feel like you have more control over your life if you adopt the habits of an optimist.

EXPLAIN YOURSELF.

Think about a meaningful event you've experienced in your life. It could be positive, like the time your team won the state championship, or negative, like when a close friend moved away. Somewhere in the back of your mind you explained to yourself why this particular event happened the way it did. Psychologists have identified two "styles" we use to explain events like this to ourselves — pessimistic or optimistic.

For example, let's say your close friend moves away. Naturally, you would be upset and your mind would process the event. If you blame yourself for your friend's move and believe these kinds of negative events will continue indefinitely, you are using a pessimistic explanatory style. You might find yourself saying things like, *This always happens to me.* or *It's all my fault.*

However, if you tell yourself the move has nothing to do with you but is due to events outside your control, you are using an optimistic explanatory style. Optimists believe that such events will end soon, and they refuse to allow them to affect too many aspects of their lives.

So, which style are you?

SMILE FOR YOUR HEALTH

Is smiling good for your health? Research says yes. But not all smiles are created equally. You can probably spot a genuine smile from a fake, "cheeeese" smile a mile away, but what makes them different?

A genuine smile is known as the Duchenne smile, named for the famous French neurologist Duchenne de Boulogne who first discovered it. What makes this smile so special? Well, first of all, two muscle groups create it — one, which turns the corners of the lips up, and another, which squeezes and wrinkles the skin around the eyes. A non-Duchenne smile uses only lip muscles, so an easy way to recognize a true smile is to look for the telltale "crow's feet" wrinkles around the eyes.

Second, research has shown the genuine Duchenne smile to be associated with positive feelings and longevity. "For instance a 30-year-long study published in the *Journal of Personality and Social Psychology* found that women who displayed the Duchenne smile in their college yearbook photos had greater levels of well-being and marital satisfaction three decades later. Another study published in *Psychological Science* went further to make a connection between smiles and longevity. They found that professional baseball players who sported Duchenne smiles in their yearbook photo were only half as likely to die, in any given year, as those who had not."[3]

 Can you think of other examples from the Bible as a reason to have a positive outlook?

You can improve your outlook simply by putting a genuine Duchenne smile on your face and generating positive feelings inside and out.

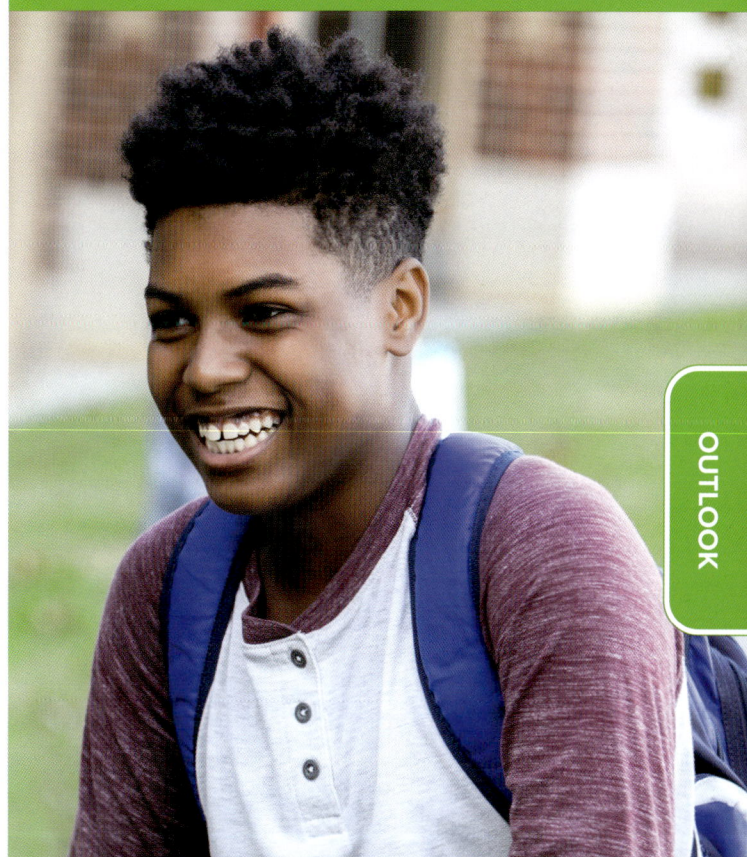

OUTLOOK

A MERRY HEART

A merry heart does good, like medicine,
but a broken spirit dries the bones.

PROVERBS 17:22

Children laugh about 400 times a day. Adults laugh only about 15 times a day. This means that between your childhood and adulthood, you will lose 385 laughs a day. This is a big problem, especially when you consider laughter's incredible power over negative stress.

During negative stress, the body increases the release of several hormones such as epinephrine and cortisol. These are often referred to as stress hormones, which tend to suppress your immune system. When this happens, you can get sick more often. But laughter is considered a healthy stress, also called eustress. This is because it helps reduce the effects negative stress can cause in the body. When you laugh, your body decreases the level of stress hormones present. So, when you find yourself giggling at a joke or funny movie, you're not just enjoying yourself and having a good time. You're actually helping your body to stay healthy.[4]

HAPPINESS

According to 225 studies on the benefits of happiness, happy people:

- Are more productive and creative at work
- Are better leaders and negotiators
- Are more likely to marry and to have fulfilling marriages
- Are less likely to divorce
- Have more friends and social support
- Have stronger immune systems and are physically healthier
- Live longer
- Are more helpful and philanthropic
- Cope better with stress and trauma[5]

To enhance your happiness, try the following:

- **Count your blessings.** Express gratitude for what you have (either privately or to a close friend) or express your appreciation to individuals who you've never properly thanked.

- **Cultivate optimism.** Practice looking at the bright side of things. Try keeping a journal in which you imagine and write about the best possible future for yourself.

- **Avoid overthinking and comparison.** Cut down on how often you dwell on your own problems and compare yourself to others.

- **Practice acts of kindness.** Do good things for others, whether friends or strangers, either directly or anonymously, spontaneously or planned.

- **Nurture relationships.** Choose a relationship in need of strengthening and invest time and energy in cultivating it.

- **Do more engaging activities.** Look for activities at home and school that challenge you.

- **Savor the joys of life.** Pay close attention, take delight and reflect on life's pleasures and wonders through thinking, writing, drawing or sharing with another.

- **Commit to your goals.** Pick one, two or three significant goals that are meaningful to you and devote time and effort to pursuing them.

- **Develop strategies for coping.** Practice ways to endure a recent stress, hardship or trauma.

- **Learn to forgive.** Work on letting go of anger and resentment toward others who have hurt or wronged you.

- **Practice religion and spirituality.** Become more involved in your church or read and ponder spiritually themed books.

- **Take care of your body.** Engage in things such as physical activity, smiling and laughing.[6]

THE TRUTH ABOUT DEPRESSION

According to the World Health Organization, about 300 million people worldwide suffer from depression.[7] That's more than the population of the United States. Speaking of the U.S., depression affects over 21 million people. Lost productive time among U.S. workers due to depression is estimated to be in excess of $51 billion per year.[8]

Depression has a strong link to your health. In one study, researchers looked at the connection between depression and how well patients recovered from surgery. They examined 817 patients who underwent coronary artery bypass surgery. They found that patients with moderate to severe depression prior to or up to six months after their surgery had a higher risk of dying earlier than non-depressed patients. Those who were depressed before surgery but were able to get rid of their depression were at no greater risk of dying early than those who were never depressed.[9]

"Big deal," you might be thinking, "I'm not planning on having coronary artery bypass surgery anytime soon." That may be true, but you still have to ask yourself: *If depression can affect my body's ability to heal when I am older, how is it affecting me right now when my body is still growing and developing?*

You already know that, among high school students, depression is a very serious issue. In fact, it is widely considered to be the most common illness teenagers face. Suicide and drug use are also related to the feelings caused by depression.

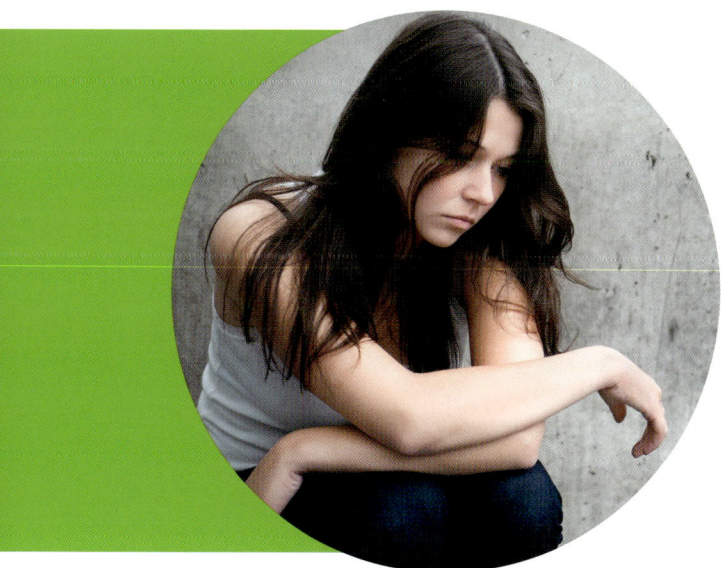

If you are depressed it is crucial for you to remember two important truths:

First, you are not alone. The feelings associated with depression are normal reactions to the disappointments of life. High school is often a confusing time of discovery and challenge. Disappointment may lead you to feel as if you're on a roller coaster of emotion. Remember, what you are feeling is a natural outcome of these up and downs. It doesn't make you strange or worse than anyone else. Everyone experiences these feelings at some point in their life.

Second, if you are depressed there is always hope. Depression is an illness, and many treatments are available from medications to therapy, or a combination of the two. One way to treat depression is through cognitive behavioral therapy. The goal of this kind of treatment is to change the way one thinks by helping them to be more optimistic. This kind of treatment prevents relapses into depression because it teaches skills that can be used again and again without reliance upon medication or doctors. Dr. Seligman sees a great value in cognitive therapy helping depression. "Drugs relieve depression, but only temporarily; unlike cognitive therapy, drugs fail to change the underlying pessimism which is the root of the problem."[10] Seek a treatment that provides you with a way to heal.

If you think you might be experiencing feelings of depression, seek help right away through a family physician, your church, school or counselor. Don't let guilt or shame keep you from getting the help you need. Remember, depression can make you want to be alone and isolate yourself from others. This can actually work against you getting better, so don't withdraw. Reach out.

National Suicide Prevention Lifeline
Call: 800-273-8255

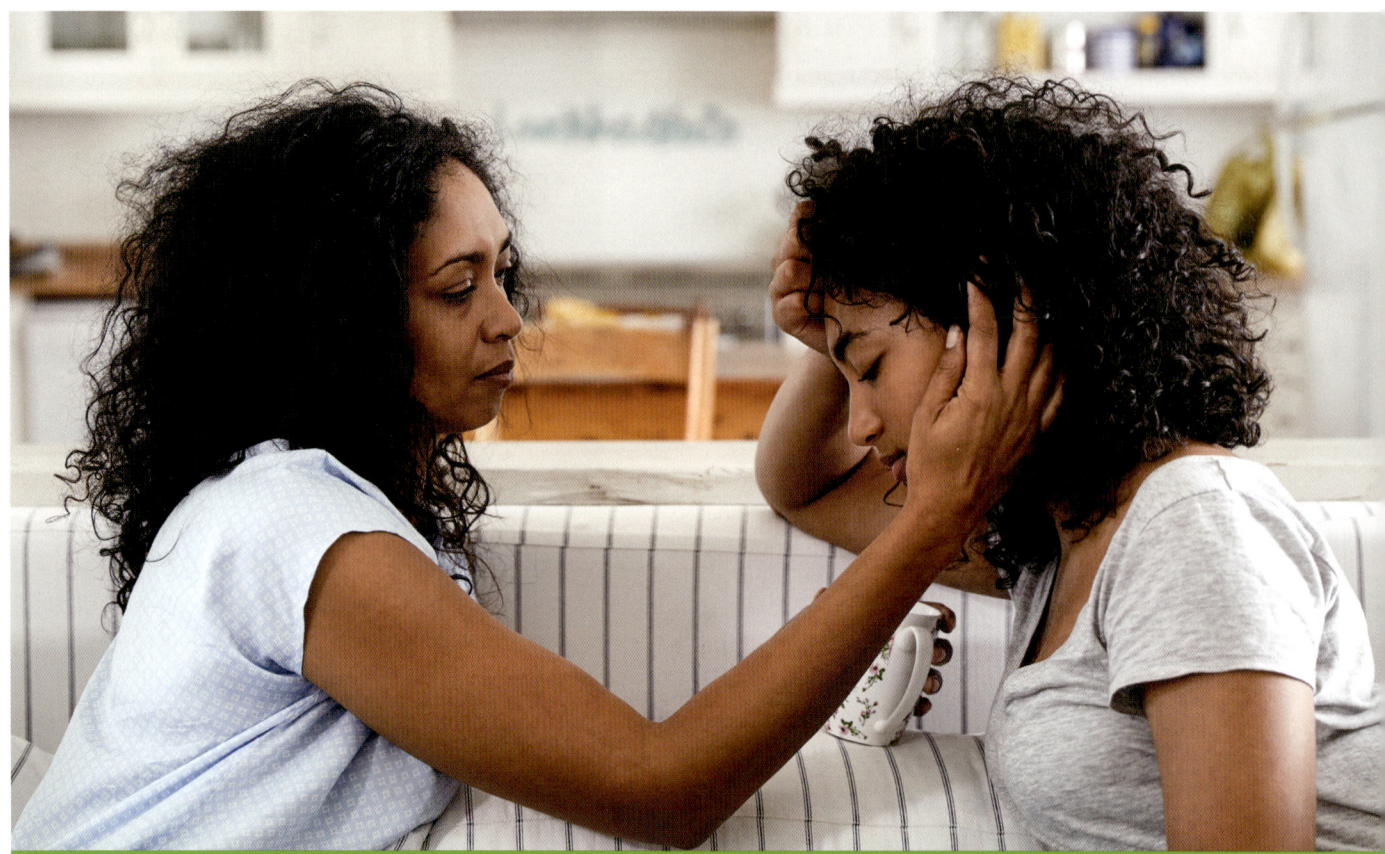

DEALING WITH DEPRESSION

There is no quick fix for breaking the cycle of depression. Being depressed means you are experiencing a variety of emotions including hopelessness, frustration and discouragement. You may also feel numb to doing your schoolwork, participating in extracurricular activities or accomplishing anything with your day. You may want to retreat to your room and seclude yourself from family and friends. Here are some steps you can begin to take to break the cycle of depression in your life.

1. **Build relationships.** Seek out the help of family and friends. Talk about your feelings with others and keep participating in daily activities. Hanging around your friends will help you to feel much better about life.

2. **Help someone else.** One way to counter depression is to reach out and help another person. Try volunteering at your church or through a local ministry such as a shelter or after-school club. By serving others, you will shift the focus from your needs to the needs and concerns of someone else. You'll also exchange negative thoughts for the positive experience of making a difference in someone's life.

3. **Invest in yourself.** The tendency of depressed teens is to stop taking care of themselves. They forget to exercise, eat a balanced diet or get plenty of rest. Make sure you are doing all of these things and more. Spend time outdoors in the sunlight (as you may recall from the section on Environment, sunlight is a great mood enhancer and helps to counteract the effects of seasonal affective disorder or SAD). Find a new hobby or activity in which you can participate. Do something positive for yourself.

TEEN SUICIDE

Suicide is the second leading cause of death among young people ages 15 to 24, according to data taken from the Center for Disease Control and Prevention.[11] The tragedy of teen suicide affects family and friends for years. One reason is because a life has been lost even before it was fully lived. As a teenager, you have incredible potential, and God has so much in store for you in the future. Suicide robs and destroys all of that.

Each case of suicide is unique, and the causes vary from person to person. They may include feelings of stress, confusion, self-doubt and uncertainty about the future. For some, moving to a new community, dealing with divorce or the creation of a new family can also intensify self-doubts.[12] Victims of family violence, bullying or physical or sexual abuse are also at risk.[13] But one thing they all have in common is this — they see suicide as the answer to all their problems.

It never is.

During your life, you are bound to experience some feelings of anxiety, sadness and despair. These are all normal reactions to when you encounter disappointment, loss or rejection. "According to the National Foundation for Suicide Prevention, 90 percent of all people who die by suicide have a diagnosable mental disorder at the time of their death."[14] This means the feelings that lead to suicide are not only common; they are also treatable.

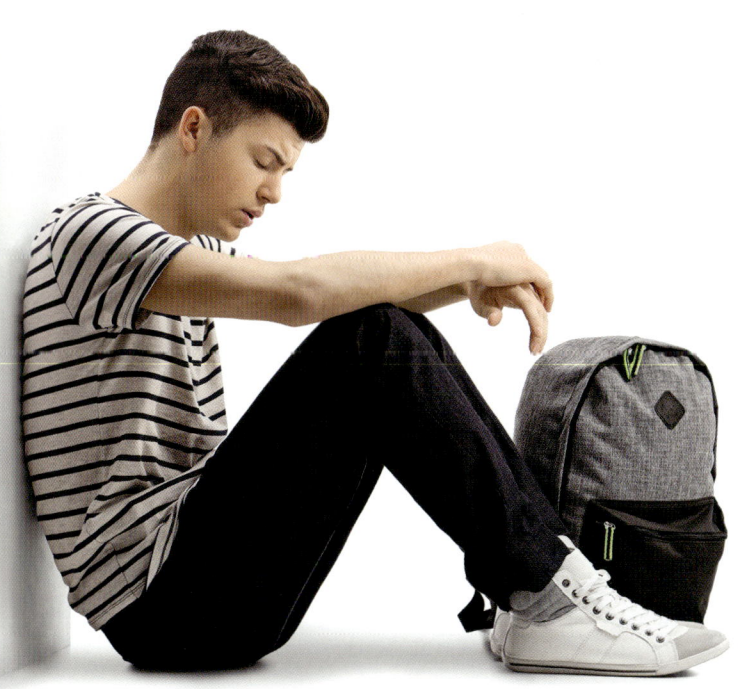

⚠️ DEPRESSION WARNING SIGNS

- Withdrawal from friends and family members
- Trouble in romantic relationships
- Difficulty getting along with others
- Changes in the quality of schoolwork or lower grades
- Rebellious behaviors
- Unusual gift-giving or giving away own possessions
- Appearing bored or distracted
- Writing or drawing pictures about death
- Running away from home
- Changes in eating habits
- Dramatic personality changes
- Changes in appearance (for the worse)
- Sleep disturbances
- Drug or alcohol abuse
- Talk of suicide, even in a joking way
- Having a history of previous suicide attempts[15]

The most important thing you can do is to take suicide seriously. No one can be sure what someone talking of suicide will do, so don't see it as a joking matter. Learn to recognize the signs of suicidal thinking, and if you experience suicidal thoughts, seek help through a doctor or qualified counselor right away.

National Suicide Prevention Lifeline
Call: 800-273-8255

"They say a person needs just three things to be truly happy in this world: someone to love, something to do, and something to hope for."

TOM BODETT

OUTLOOK

> *"The future belongs to those who believe in the beauty of their dreams."*
>
> ELEANOR ROOSEVELT

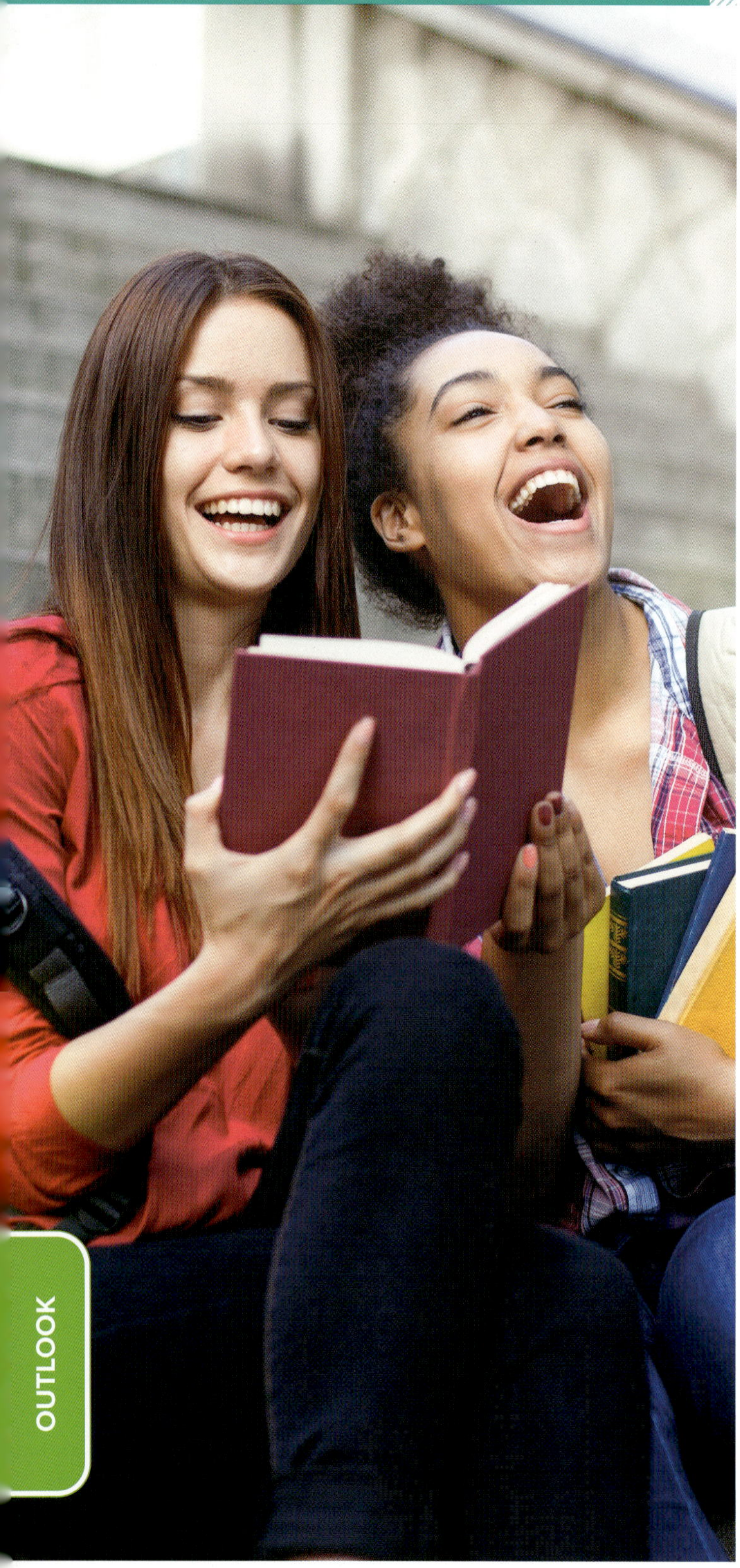

SELF-ESTEEM

God created man in His own image, in the image of God He created him; male and female He created them.

GENESIS 1:27

One problem in high schools today is the ever-increasing number of students with low self-esteem. Excessive feelings of worthlessness or that you can never quite measure up will lead you to crave and seek approval from others. This will damage your relationships and may even lead you to make some dangerous and harmful choices. What is so tragic is that many teens never fully realize just how wonderful and special they truly are. They allow themselves to be defined by what others say rather than by what God says. God created each individual as a unique person with his or her own gifts, talents and abilities. In the book of Psalms, David writes, *"For You formed my inward parts; You wove me in my mother's womb. I will give thanks to You, for I am fearfully and wonderfully made; wonderful are Your works, and my soul knows it very well"* (Psalm 139:13, 14). You are wonderfully made. God crafted you with great precision and care. He formed you in His own image to give Him honor, glory and praise. Do you allow feelings of inadequacy or worthlessness to steal your joy and keep you from being all that God has created you to be? Stop looking at yourself through the eyes of others and begin to view your life through your Father's eyes.

? **Are there areas of life where you feel you aren't measuring up? What would it take for you to see yourself as "fearfully and wonderfully" created by God?**

WHAT IS RUMINATING?

Ruminating involves thinking about something in depth, repeatedly running through what or why something happened. Many times ruminating is focused solely on negative thinking. For example, people who have experienced a messy breakup in the past might analyze their current relationship to excess. In the end, their overthinking could even damage or destroy the current relationship. In one review study, researchers uncovered the very real physical and mental dangers that accompany ruminating. According to their research, "Rumination exacerbates depression, enhances negative thinking, impairs problem solving, interferes with instrumental behavior and erodes social support."[16] "Evidence now suggests that rumination is associated with psychopathologies in addition to depression."[17] These psychopathologies are various types of mental and behavioral disorders that include anxiety, binge-eating, binge-drinking and self-harm.[18]

Negative ruminating is not good for your outlook or your health. Don't allow past mistakes or challenges to negatively affect your future.

BREAK THE CYCLE

Noted psychologist and Yale University Professor, Dr. Susan Nolen-Hoeksema, offers two ways to break the rumination cycle:

1. **Engage in activities that foster positive thoughts.** "You need to engage in activities that can fill your mind with other thoughts, preferably positive thoughts," Nolen-Hoeksema says. That could be anything from a favorite physical activity to a hobby or a prayer. "The main thing is to get your mind off your ruminations for a time so they die out and don't have a grip on your mind."[19]

2. **Problem solve.** "People who ruminate not only replay situations in their head, they also focus on abstract questions, such as, 'Why do these things happen to me?' and 'What's wrong with me that I can't cope?'" Nolen-Hoeksema says. Instead, when you can think clearly, "Identify at least one concrete thing you could do to overcome the problem you are ruminating about." For instance, if you're uneasy about a situation at school, call a close friend to help you think of a solution.[20]

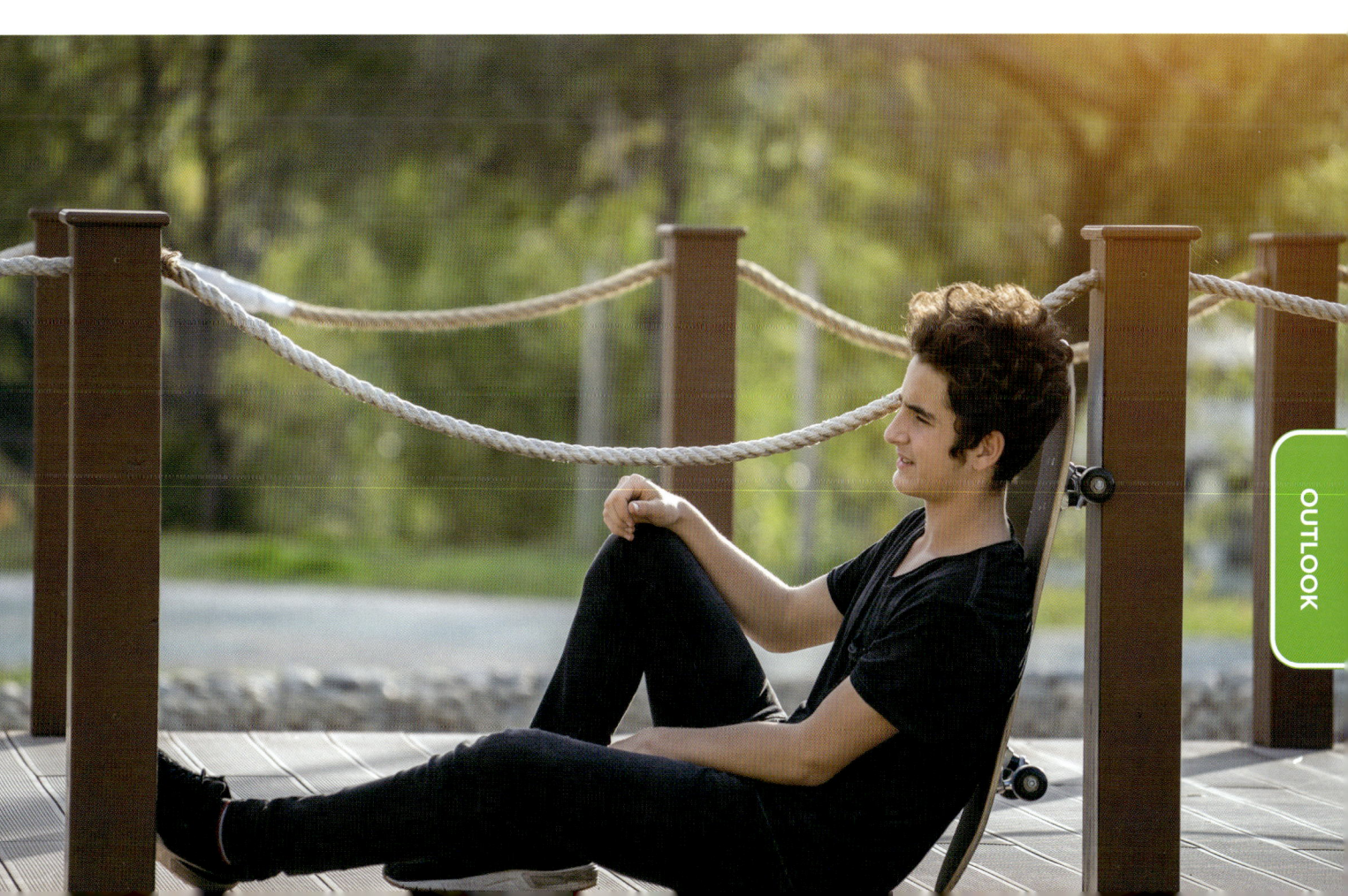

ADJUST YOUR ATTITUDE

The good news is that unlike eye or hair color, pessimism isn't hereditary. With a little practice you can develop your positive thinking skills to become an optimism rock star. Check out the following list to see how boosting the "power of the positive" can impact every aspect of your life:

1. Optimism will help you realize you have healthy choices available. It will help you think of and act on those good healthy choices. When you are optimistic, you will feel in control of your life because you will understand that your choices really do make a difference.

2. Optimism will help you rest easier; a positive view of your future will allow you to relax today and help you sleep well at night.

3. Optimism will help you seek an environment that is healing and restorative. When you are optimistic, you will believe that you can make changes in your room by cleaning the closet, getting organized and keeping it that way.

4. Optimism will help you believe that you have what it takes to be mentally and physically active on a regular basis. When you do have setbacks or "road blocks," your optimistic outlook will help you get back on track.

5. Optimism will help you trust in God and believe that He has your best interests in mind. Optimism will help you trust others, too. It will help you make new friends, give you peace of mind and lower your stress.

6. Optimism will help you have a bright, positive outlook, and this will improve your interpersonal relationships as others are drawn to you. When you have a positive outlook, you will also look for and encourage the positive in others. You will also "stick with" others through challenging times because you believe in them and in the truth that it all will work out for the good.

7. Optimism will help you think positively about your nutrition choices. If you have had challenges with diet in the past, or if you feel like you have never been able to eat the way you want, having an optimistic outlook will help you succeed. It will help you realize that you do have the power to influence your health by choosing the best possible food for your body.

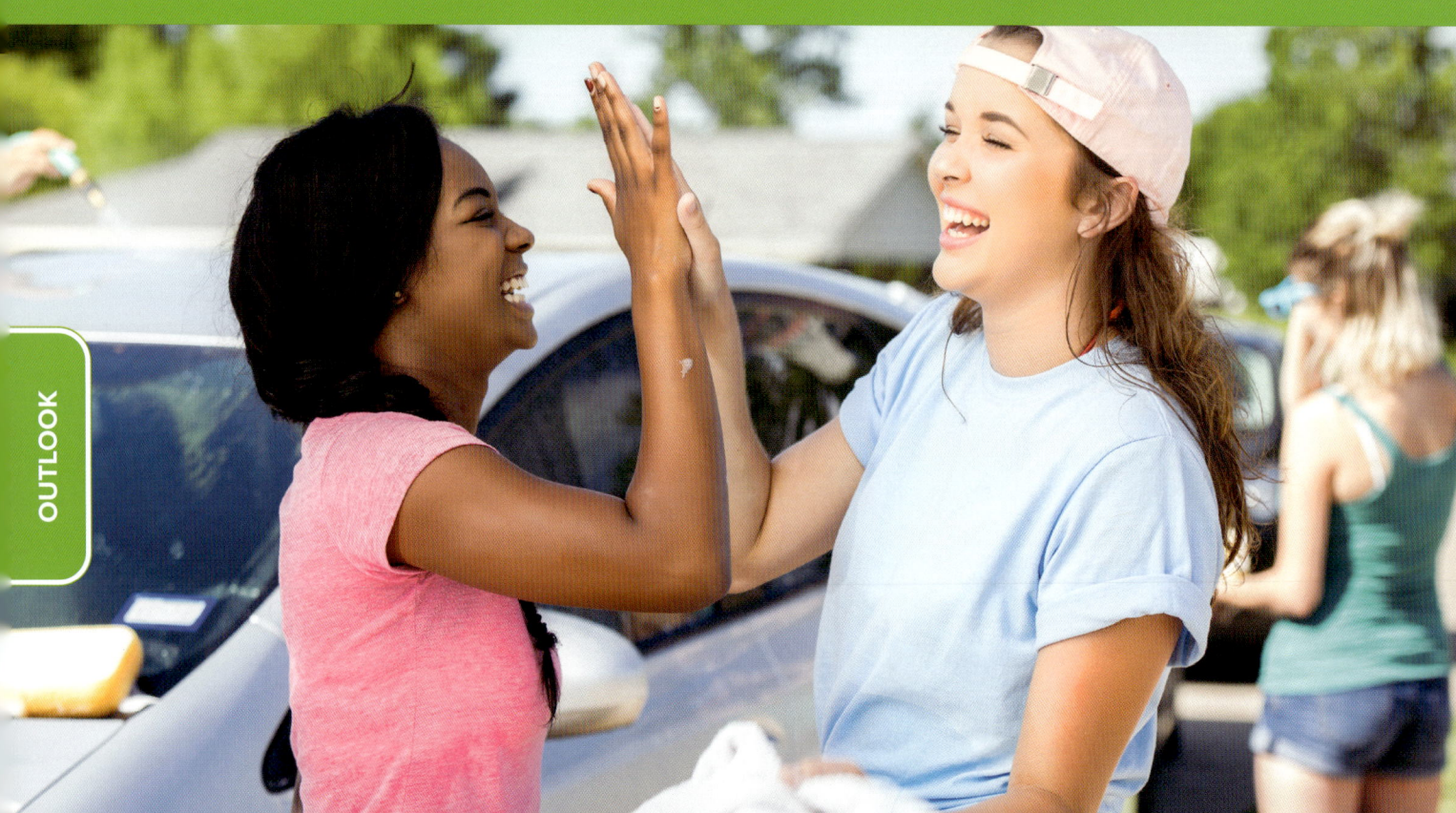

OPPORTUNITYISNOWHERE

In the 1920s, English mountain climber George Mallory was asked by a *New York Times* reporter why, after two failed attempts, he would want to attempt the deadly climb of Mt. Everest a third time. Mallory famously replied, "Because it's there." Where others saw only danger, Mallory saw a challenge. Where others saw only struggle and pain, Mallory saw his chance at greatness.

Look again at the title of this section. What did you see when you first read it? Did you see it as "opportunity is nowhere" or as "opportunity is now here?" Though both readings are possible, what makes the difference is on what you choose to focus. In the same way, the difficult circumstances you face in life can be viewed either as opportunities for failure or success. It just depends how you're looking at them.

The facts show that what you choose to believe about a situation seriously affects your reality. When you have an outlook of hope and positive belief, it's like building a bridge from your thoughts to your success. Take a look at the following scientific study to see what we mean:

Researchers at Rutgers University and Yale Medical School asked more than 2,800 men and women age 65 or older the following question, "Is your health excellent, good, fair or poor?" Seems simple enough, right? What they discovered was that those who felt their health was "poor" were up to six times more likely to die earlier than those who felt their health was "excellent."[21] The results of this study strongly suggest that your point of view may positively or negatively affect your health.

Your opinion about yourself or your circumstances affects more than just your health. Your ability to do well in school, form and maintain relationships and get a good job in the future are all connected to how you perceive the world around you. So take another look:

OPPORTUNITYISNOWHERE

What do you see?

THE PLACEBO EFFECT

What you believe about a situation will either become a drop to failure or a bridge to success. How your mind perceives the world around you is what makes the difference, maybe even when it comes to your health. Perhaps the best-known example of the mind creating powerful, physical changes in the body is found in what science terms "the placebo effect." A placebo is "a treatment or aspect of treatment that does not have a specific action on a patient's symptom of disease." In other words, a placebo is a substance or procedure that doesn't physically change or alter a patient's condition. Placebos are often considered by many to be useless substances or procedures, yet across a broad range of medical conditions and treatments, the placebo effect accounts for 25 to 35 percent of the beneficial effect. And when a procedure or a drug is brand new, the placebo effect is even greater, accounting for up to 70 to 80 percent of the beneficial effect.[22]

Make no mistake, getting proper medical treatment when you are sick is vitally important, but this research shows that what you think about the treatments you receive does play a part in helping your body to heal itself. Even having faith in your doctor may help you have a better outcome. The *Journal of the American Medical Association* looked at 25 plus years of research on pain medications. In the end, the researchers concluded, "The quality of interaction between the patient and the physician can be extremely influential in patient outcomes, and, in some (perhaps many) cases, patient and provider expectations and interactions may be more important than the specific treatments."[23]

NEGATIVE NEWS

If positive thoughts have the power to heal, what do you think negative thoughts might do to you physically, mentally or even spiritually? Think about this in light of the following story:

A young man arrived at a monastery to begin the process of becoming a full-fledged monk. A wiser, older monk told him he would have to take a three-year vow of silence to complete the process; however, at the end of each year he would be permitted to speak a brief sentence consisting of only two words.

At the end of the first year the man walked up to the monk and said his first two words, "Bed hard."

At the end of the second year the man approached the monk and said, "Bad food."

At the end of the third year the man angrily told the older monk, "I quit."

"Well, I'm not surprised," said the monk. "You've done nothing but complain since you got here."

You may think that negativity has little effect on you, but all your thoughts shape who you are inside and out. The following passage takes this a step further to show how your thoughts can even affect the future:

- Watch your thoughts;
  they become your words.

- Watch your words;
  they become your actions.

- Watch your actions;
  they become your habits.

- Watch your habits;
  they become your character.

- Watch your character;
  it becomes your destiny.[24]

Because your thoughts have such a powerful influence on your life, it is vitally important to be careful what you choose to think. It's also important to watch what you consume when it comes to the Internet or media. *Turn on, tune in, drop out* was the counterculture slogan of the 1960s when young people experimented with mind-altering psychedelic drugs in order to reach newer realms of "spiritual discovery." These days you might also apply the slogan to the culture's love of cell phones, social media and video streaming. While all of these can be used to access good content, they can also be misused and abused to open the door to a flood of negativity and discouragement. Maybe you or someone you know has personally experienced the "dark side" of the Internet through cyberbullying, lack of privacy settings or online predators. The dangers are very real, and the pain they cause can last a lifetime. Protect yourself now by *"guarding your heart"* (Proverbs 4:23). In the Bible and other literature, the heart is defined not as the muscle in your chest but the center of your emotions and desires. In essence, it's what makes you unique. You probably think of guarding your heart as keeping out all the bad things in life. Prior to the digital age this was boiled down to an easy-to-follow slogan: *I don't smoke, I don't chew and I don't go out with those who do.* But guarding your heart is more than just keeping things out. It also means keeping things in.

What kind of things? Consider the following verse from the book of Philippians:

"Finally, brothers, whatever is true, whatever is honorable, whatever is just, whatever is pure, whatever is lovely, whatever is commendable, if there is any excellence, if there is anything worthy of praise, think about these things" (Philippians 4:8).

Think about it; if you focus your thoughts on the true and honorable things of life, you will be less swayed by temptation and corruption. Sure, there are a lot of terrible things on the outside just aching to get to your heart, but you don't need to feel overwhelmed because it's not about avoiding the bad; it's about embracing God and making Him the center of your outlook. Focus on His goodness and keep it in the center of your heart.

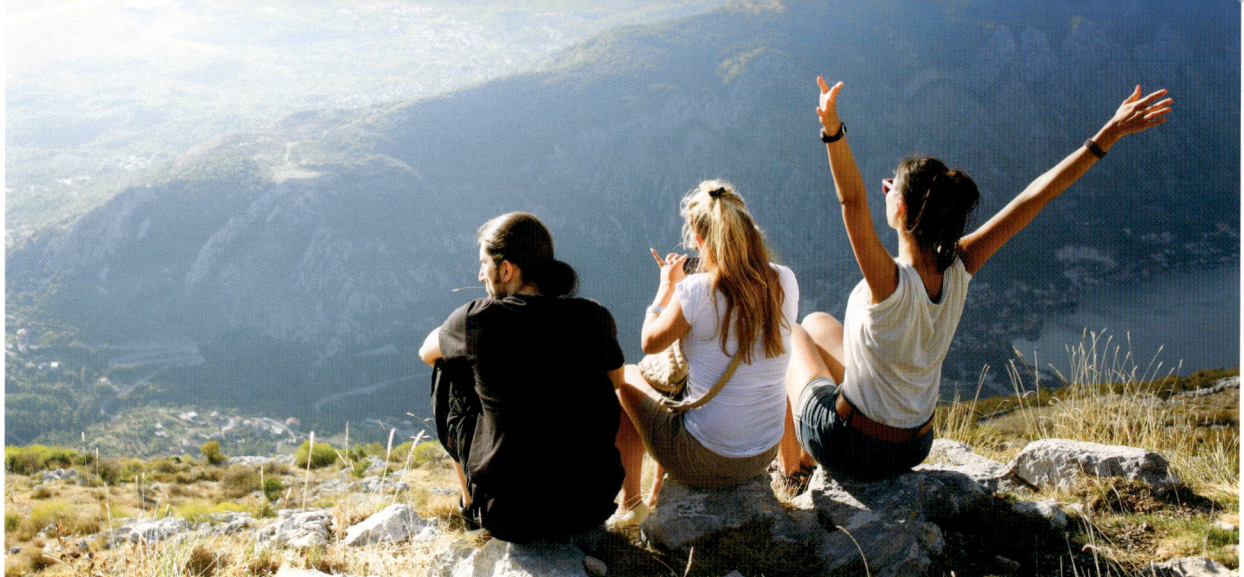

THE BIOLOGY OF HOPE

One morning over breakfast, two oncologists were discussing papers they were going to present that day at the national meeting of the American Society of Clinical Oncology. One of the doctors was very upset because his patients' success rate was far lower than his colleague's patients.

Finally he started complaining bitterly, "You know, Bob, I just don't understand it. We used the same drugs, the same dosage, the same schedule and the same entry criteria. Yet I got a 22 percent response rate, and you got a 74 percent response rate. That is unheard of for metastatic lung cancer. How do you do it?"

The other doctor responded, "We're both using Etoposide, Platinol, Oncovin and Hydroxyurea. You call yours EPOH. I tell my patients I'm giving them HOPE. Sure, I tell them this is experimental, and we go over the long list of side effects together. But I emphasize that we have a chance. As dismal as the statistics are for non-small cell, there are always a few percent who do really well."

When you are hopeful in the face of challenges, you can turn positive thinking into action. Your hope can actually help to heal you. Norman Cousins, a well-known political journalist, author and professor called this phenomenon "the biology of hope."[25] No matter how dark things may look, you can never stop believing in the best. You can never lose your hope.

Remember the optimistic explanatory style? Researcher Toshihiko Maruta and his colleagues found that people with this style were linked with a 50 percent decrease in the risk of mortality or early death.[26] They also found that optimists had a decrease in bodily pain and the role limitations due to emotional and physical problems. In the same study, these optimists also enjoyed an increase in physical function and vitality, general health perception, social functioning and mental health.[27] Hope, or the lack thereof, has been shown to impact other diseases (such as Parkinson's) as well.[28-29]

Hope is one of the most powerful forces you have available to you today.

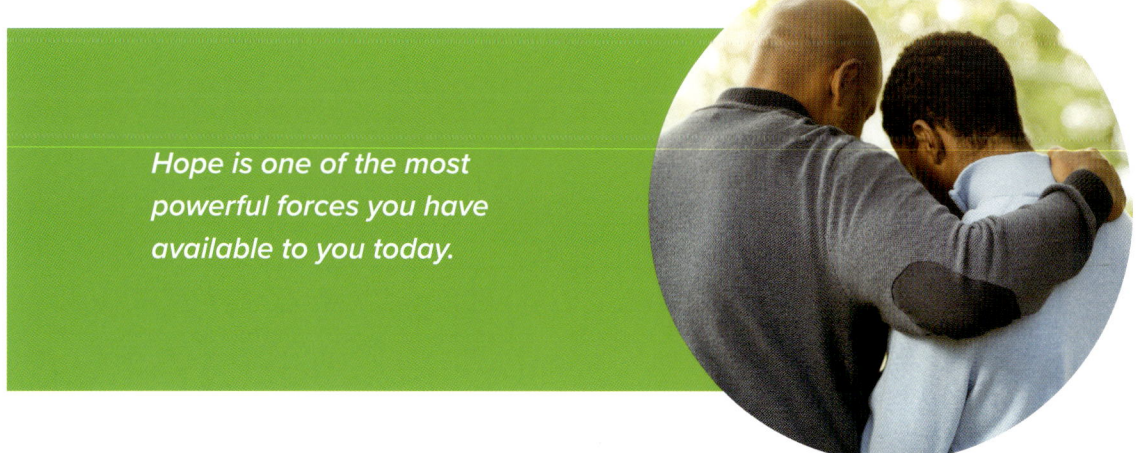

> *"Be of good cheer. Do not think of today's failures, but of the success that may come tomorrow. You have set yourselves a difficult task, but you will succeed if you persevere; and you will find a joy in overcoming obstacles. Remember, no effort that we make to attain something beautiful is ever lost."* HELEN KELLER

20/20 VISION

Do you have big plans for your future? After high school is finally over, do you have your sights set on achieving great and glorious things? If so, then you have vision — this means you aspire to accomplish something positive with your life. Vision is a powerful force in the world. It helps you see the possibilities available to you and motivates you to live up to your full potential.

We tend to think of vision only as it relates to sight. Someone who has perfect eyesight is said to have "20/20 vision." Dewitt Jones, one of America's top professional photographers, traveled the globe for twenty years taking pictures for *National Geographic* Magazine. During this time, he captured extraordinary moments in the lives of people all over the world. Jones called these moments "visions."

I learned a great deal from these visions; about society, about geography, about people. But the vision that most changed my life was not photographic. It was an attitude, a perspective that exists at the core of the *National Geographic*. A vision so simple, yet so profound. A vision I'd like to share with you: Celebrate What's Right with the World. When I was growing up I used to hold that maxim: I won't believe it until I see it, yet the more I shot for the *National Geographic* the more I realized that I had it backwards. That the way it really works is, I won't see it, till I believe it. That's the way life works. Well I believed it, I believed the vision of the *National Geographic* and the more I did the more I'd see it in everything.[30]

Vision is all about how you perceive the world around you. Having a good vision will give meaning and purpose to your life. It helps you see the good in all things, even pop quizzes and breakups. What it all boils down to is this: if you have a good vision, then you have a positive outlook. And a positive outlook is what can make your vision a reality.

OUTLOOK

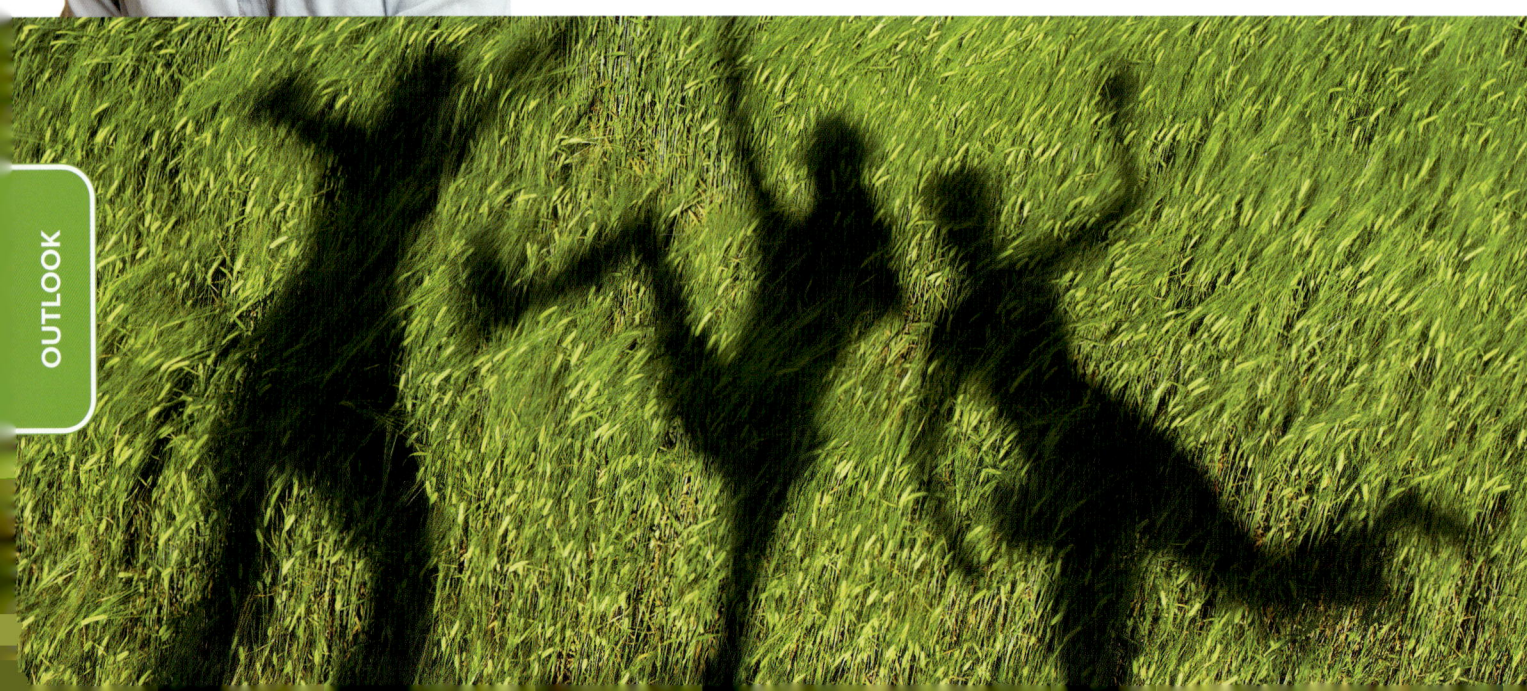

Vision is nothing more than putting your dreams into action. You probably have lots of friends who dream of becoming famous musicians, athletes or YouTube sensations. But how many of them are actually taking the steps necessary to make their dreams a reality? A positive outlook is what you need. You're bound to pass through some dark valleys on the road to fulfilling your dreams. Are you willing to believe in the best and live for your vision? This important truth is seen in the life of Viktor Frankl, a psychiatrist from Vienna who survived the Auschwitz concentration camp. Frankl found that the survivors had something to live for — a golden thread of hope.

"It is a peculiarity of man," Frankl wrote, "that he can only live by looking to the future... And this is his salvation in the most difficult moments of his existence."[31] Optimists have something to live for, and they take positive action to achieve that dream. This makes their life worth living.

Maybe you're living life without a vision. You might even feel unmotivated to do your best in school because you just don't see the point. This characterizes a lot of high school students today. They just don't see the opportunities available to them. They don't believe they have a future.

Eugene Lang, a self-made millionaire, was invited back to speak at his old elementary school in Harlem for the 1981 sixth grade graduating class. As he spoke, he could tell his message just wasn't reaching the 52 students who were gathered together to listen. Lang decided to switch things up. Laying aside his notes, he gave an unplanned talk. He reminded the students of Martin Luther King's "I Have a Dream" speech. He told them that everyone must have a dream if their life is to go anywhere. He emphasized the value of education and of going to college, but then realized that most of the poor students couldn't afford it.

"Don't think for a minute," he said, "that you can't go to college, because you can."

Lang then promised to pay the college tuition for every student in that class who graduated from high school. For the first time, many of the students sensed hope and started developing a vision for their life. One student said, "I had something to look forward to, something waiting for me. It was a golden feeling."[32]

Even as Mr. Lang sat down that day to a cheering audience, he knew that money alone wasn't the answer. By working with teachers and parents, Lang was able to create a support structure in the community that worked with the students to help them establish a vision for their lives.

In the past, only 25 percent of the graduating class of sixth graders would have gone on to high school. And of that 25 percent, almost none would have attended college. But thanks to Mr. Lang and the support of others, 48 of the 52 sixth graders graduated from high school, and 40 went to college.[33]

You may be surprised to learn that being the most intelligent or the highest achieving student in your class is not a guarantee of future success. In the book *The Future-Focused Role Image*, author Benjamin Singer reports that, in his research, IQ and family background are not key indicators of a successful student. The one characteristic that all successful students shared was a profound and positive vision of their future.[34]

So, what is your vision? Take some time this week to write your own personal vision statement. What dream has God given you for your future?

"Only in the darkness can you see the stars."

MARTIN LUTHER KING JR.

OUTLOOK

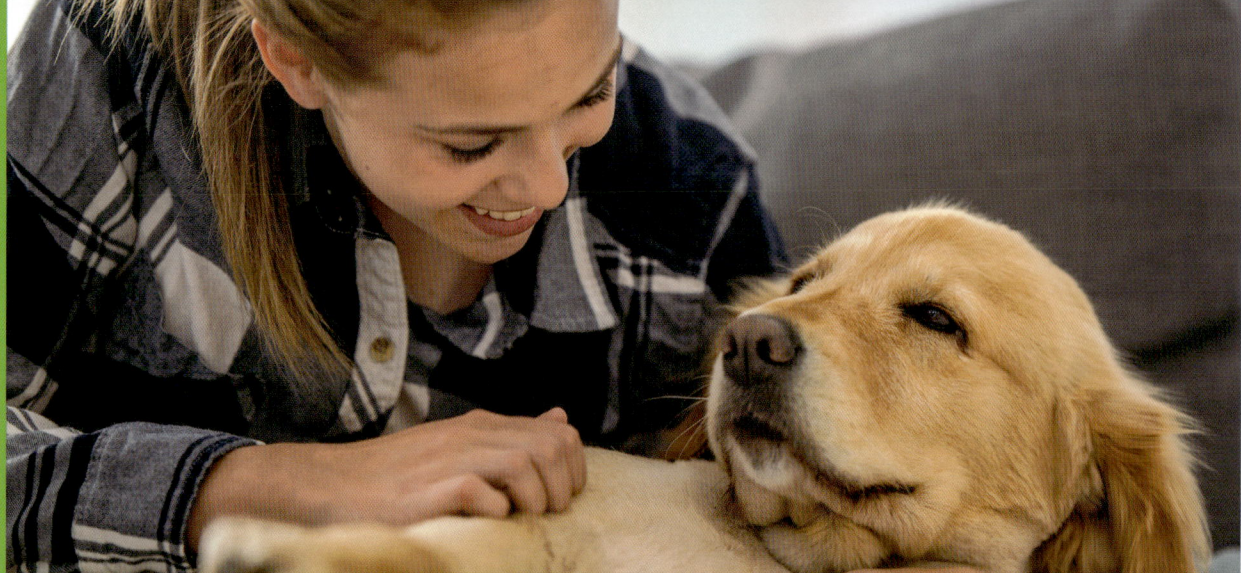

CREATING YOUR VISION

1. **Identify your core values.** These are the fundamental beliefs that you hold most dear. Your core values are the areas of your life where you do not compromise or change.

2. **Decide who you want to be.** You may have your whole life ahead of you, but without a clear vision of the person you want to become, you won't know where to aim.

3. **Set challenging but achievable goals.** You'll need both short- and long-term goals to make your dream a reality.

4. **Write down your vision for the future.** Place where you will see it often. Create an exciting, engaging and specific description of what it will be like when you finally achieve your goal.

5. **Articulate your vision often.** Pray about it, talk about it and rework it as needed, keeping in mind that certain aspects of it should never change while other aspects must change as circumstances demand. Always remain true to your core values and beliefs.

PURPOSE FOR LIVING

You are here for a purpose. It's important because you need to understand why you are here and what you are meant to do with your life.

Perhaps you've known someone living with the debilitating effects of Alzheimer's. This horrible disease affects the memory of a person to the point where they can no longer recognize their own family members. Alzheimer's patients require a safe living environment and around-the-clock care. And even though scientists have yet to uncover what is the cause of this disease, researchers from the Rush Alzheimer's Disease Center have made an incredible discovery. People who have a greater sense of purpose in life are more likely to have slower rates of mental decline. "This is encouraging and suggests that engaging in meaningful and purposeful activities promotes cognitive health in old age," study researcher Dr. Patricia A. Boyle said.

This isn't the first time researchers have discovered a link between having a purpose in life and good health. An article in the journal *Psychosomatic Medicine* showed that having a purpose in life was linked with longevity. And in 2011, *Time* magazine reported on a study suggesting that life fulfillment was linked with a lower risk of Alzheimer's disease.[35]

> *"Don't cry because it's over; smile because it happened."*
>
> DR. SEUSS

GRATITUDE

What are the little things you are grateful for each day? A good conversation? A cool breeze? A favorite intramural game with friends? Showing gratitude is an important part of maintaining a positive outlook regardless of what you have or what you don't have. When you are thankful for the people and things God has given you, you will look at the world through the eyes of an optimist.

Quick. Start making a mental list of the things you are grateful for right now. It might be people or things or whatever. Just start listing them in your head. When you get at least five things, stop and write them down. You may not realize it, but you just counted your blessings. It's really that easy, but don't stop there. Gratitude is even better when it's shared. Let others know about the blessings in your life. If you wrote down a person's name, be sure to tell them as soon as possible how much they mean to you. This is a simple exercise you can do every day. Remember, you're either counting or discounting your blessings.

 **What are some of the incredible blessings God has given to you?**

Gratitude is a powerful weapon against the forces of negativity and depression. Again, photographer Dewitt Jones brings a unique perspective to the subject:

How easy it is to celebrate a birthday, a marriage, a holiday. How hard it is to hold that same perspective in our daily lives. Every day we are inundated with messages that tell us what's wrong with our world. It's not surprising that we lose sight of all the things that are right with it, of all that is truly worth celebrating. As a photographer, I have a choice of what lens I put on my camera, a choice of how I am going to view the world. I choose to celebrate. Why? Because it imbues me with gratitude, because it allows me to see the best in people and situations, because it fills me with energy.[36]

Do you want to experience a higher level of optimism, alertness, enthusiasm, determination, attentiveness and energy? Then get in the habit of regularly listing what you are thankful for. Research has shown that people who express gratitude more often than others have greater amounts of all these qualities, and the benefits don't stop there. They also exercise more regularly, make progress toward their personal goals, enjoy satisfying sleep and feel more connected.[37]

Students who are grateful are more satisfied with their lives than pessimists. They experience less depression and stress, too.

Perhaps you think that grateful, optimistic people are like ostriches with their heads stuck in the sand. After all, aren't they avoiding dealing with all the negativity and discouragement this world affords? Could their positive attitude be just an act? Researchers have learned that grateful people do not deny or ignore the negative aspects of life; they just rise above them. Sure, they experience hard times that knock them down, but they don't stay down. They pick themselves up and look for the next opportunity. Optimistic and grateful people are also more empathetic. They actually care about the health and well-being of others. They are often considered the most helpful and generous by others in their social networks.[38]

LOOKING AHEAD

As you continue your high school journey and move on to your next destination, remember the crucial role your outlook plays in the quality of your life — not just in your mental and physical health, but also in all your future endeavors through college and beyond. Remember, you won't always be able to change the circumstances you face, but you can always change your attitude toward them. God has placed you in control of your outlook, and that makes all the difference in the world.

REFERENCES

1. Seligman, Martin. *Learned Optimism: How to Change Your Mind and Your Life*. New York: Vintage, 2006.

2. Ibid.

3. Nicholson, Christie. "What Makes an Honest Smile Honest?" Podcast. Scientific American. Last modified December 11, 2010. https://www.scientificamerican.com/podcast/episode/what-makes-an-honest-smile-honest-10-12-11/.

4. American Physiological Society. "Anticipating A Laugh Reduces Our Stress Hormones, Study Shows." ScienceDaily. Last modified April 10, 2008. www.sciencedaily.com/releases/2008/04/080407114617.htm.

5. Lyubomirsky, Sonja. "The How of Happiness Boosting Well-Being Through Gratitude, Kindness, and Optimism." Accessed September 4, 2012. http://slideplayer.com/slide/6970869/.

6. Ibid.

7. World Health Organization. "Depression." Last modified March 22, 2018. http://www.who.int/en/news-room/fact-sheets/detail/depression.

8. Mental Health America. "Depression in the Workplace." Accessed June 26, 2018. http://www.mentalhealthamerica.net/conditions/depression-workplace.

9. Blumenthal, James, Heather S. Lett, Michael A. Babyak, William White, Peter K. Smith, Daniel B. Mark, Robert Jones, Joseph P. Mathew, and Mark F. Newman. "Depression as a Risk Factor for Mortality After Coronary Artery Bypass Surgery." *The Lancet* 362, no. 9384 (2003): 604-609. https://doi.org/10.1016/S0140-6736(03)14190-6.

10. Seligman, Martin. *Learned Optimism: How to Change Your Mind and Your Life*. New York: Vintage, 2006.

11. American Psychological Association. "Teen Suicide is Preventable." Accessed July 10, 2018. http://www.apa.org/research/action/suicide.aspx.

12. American Academy of Child and Adolescent Psychiatry. "Teen Suicide." Last Modified October 2013. https://www.aacap.org/App_Themes/AACAP/docs/facts_for_families/10_teen_suicide.pdf.

13. National Institute of Mental Health. "NIMH Answers Questions About Suicide." Accessed September 10, 2018. https://www.nimh.nih.gov/health/publications/nimh-answers-questions-about-suicide/index.shtml.

14. American Foundation for Suicide Prevention. "Suicide Claims More Lives Than War, Murder, and Natural Disasters Combined." Accessed October 2, 2018. https://afsp.donordrive.com/index.cfm?fuseaction=cms.page&id=1226&eventID=5545.

15. Stoppler, Melissa Conrad. "Teen Suicide Warning Signs." MedicineNet.com. Last modified June 13, 2018. https://www.medicinenet.com/teen_suicide_warning_signs/views.htm.

16. Nolen-Hoeksema, Susan, Blair E. Wisco, and Sonja Lyubomirsky. "Rethinking Rumination." *Perspectives on Psychological Science* 3, no. 5 (2008): 400-424. https://doi.org/10.1111/j.1745-6924.2008.00088.x.

17. Ibid.

18. Ibid.

19. Tartakovsky, Margarita. "Why Ruminating is Unhealthy and How to Stop." Psych Central. Last modified January 20, 2011. https://psychcentral.com/blog/why-ruminating-is-unhealthy-and-how-to-stop/.

20. Ibid.

21. Idler, Ellen L. and Stanislav Kasl. "Health Perceptions and Survival: Do Global Evaluations of Health Status Really Predict Mortality?" *Journal of Gerontology* 46, no. 2 (1991): S55-S65. https://doi.org/10.1093/geronj/46.2.S55.

22. Robison, Jonathan and Karen Carrier. *The Spirit and Science of Holistic Health*. Bloomington: AuthorHouse, 2004.

23. Turner, Judith A., Richard A. Deyo, John D. Loeser, M. Von Korff, and W. E. Fordyce. "The Importance of Placebo Effects in Pain Treatment and Research." *Journal of the American Medical Association* 271, no. 20 (1994): 1609-1614. https://doi.org/10.1001/jama.1994.03510440069036.

24. Kinkade, Thomas. *My Father's World*. San Jose: Media Arts Group, 2000.

25. Cousins, Norman. *Head First: The Biology of Hope and the Healing Power of the Human Spirit*. New York: E. P. Dutton, 1989. 99.

26. Maruta, Toshihiko, Robert C. Colligan, Michael Malinchoc, and Kenneth P. Offord. "Optimists vs Pessimists: Survival Rate Among Medical Patients Over a 30-year Period." *Mayo Clinic Proceedings* 75, no. 2 (2000): 140-143. https://doi.org/10.4065/75.2.140.

27. Maruta, Toshihiko, Robert C. Colligan, Michael Malinchoc, and Kenneth P. Offord. "Optimism-Pessimism Assessed in the 1960s and Self-Reported Health Status 30 Years Later." *Mayo Clinic Proceedings* 77, no. 8 (2002): 748-753. https://doi.org/10.4065/77.8.748.

28. Fowler, Susan B. "Hope and a Health-Promoting Lifestyle in Persons with Parkinson's Disease." *The Journal of Neuroscience Nursing: Journal of the American Association of Neuroscience Nurses* 29, no. 2 (1997): 111-116.

29. Everson, Susan A., Debbie E. Goldberg, George A. Kaplan, Richard D. Cohen, Eero Pukkala, Jaakko Tuomilehto, and Jukka T. Salonen. "Hopelessness and Risk of Mortality and Incidence of Myocardial Infarction and Cancer." *Psychosomatic Medicine* 58, no. 2 (1996): 113-121. https://doi.org/10.1097/00006842-199603000-00003.

30. Jones, Dewitt. "Celebrate What's Right With the World with Dewitt Jones." Filmed 2002 at TEDxSouthLakeTahoe, Saint Paul, MN. Video, 18:10. https://youtu.be/gD_1Eh6rqf8

31. Frankl, Viktor E. *Man's Search for Meaning.* Boston: Simon and Schuster, 1985.

32. Geist, William E. "One Man's Gift: College for 52 in Harlem." The New York Times. Accessed September 10, 2018. https://www.nytimes.com/1985/10/19/nyregion/about-new-york-one-man-s-gift-college-for-52-in-harlem.html.

33. Barker, Joel Arthur. *The Power of Vision with Joel Barker Training Manual.* Charthouse International Learning Corporation. St. Paul: Star Thrower Distribution, 1993.

34. Singer, Benjamin D. *Future Focused Role Image.* New York: Vintage Books, 1974.

35. HuffPost. "Having a Purpose in Life Could Protect Brain From Mental Decline, Study Suggests." Last modified May 8, 2012. https://www.huffingtonpost.com/2012/05/08/purpose-in-life-mental-decline-brain_n_1497708.html.

36. Healing Images. "Celebrate What's Right with the World." Accessed September 10, 2018. http://www.healingimages.org/resource/2013/03/08/celebrate-whats-right-world.

37. Emmons, Robert A. and Michael E. McCullough. "Counting Blessings Versus Burdens: An Experimental Investigation of Gratitude and Subjective Well-Being in Daily Life." *Journal of Personality and Social Psychology* 84, no. 2 (2003): 377.

38. McCullough, Michael E., Robert A. Emmons, and Jo-Ann Tsang. "The Grateful Disposition: A Conceptual and Empirical Topography." *Journal of Personality and Social Psychology* 82, no. 1 (2002): 112.

"You cannot have a positive life and a negative mind."

JOYCE MEYER

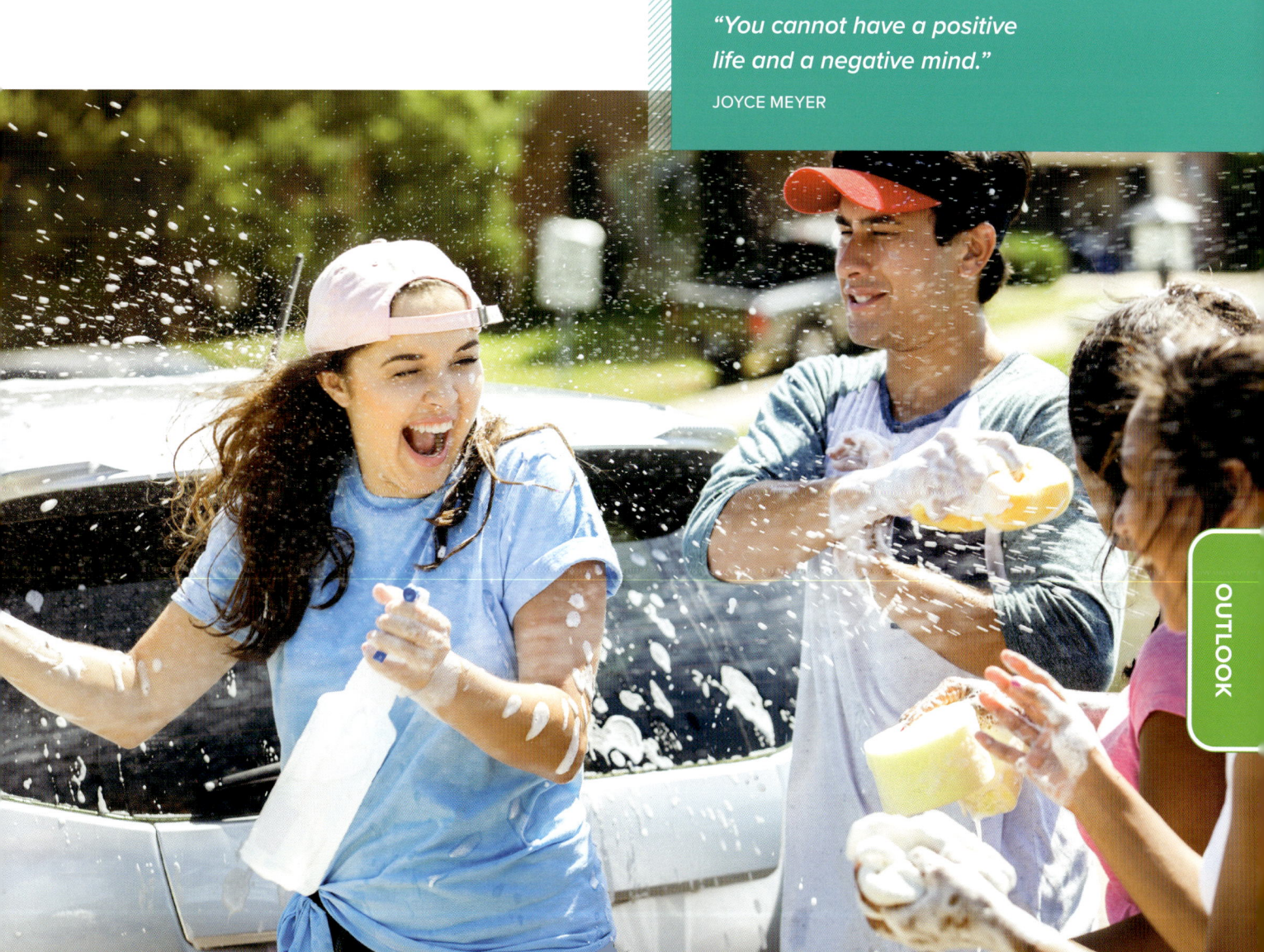

OUTLOOK

NOTES

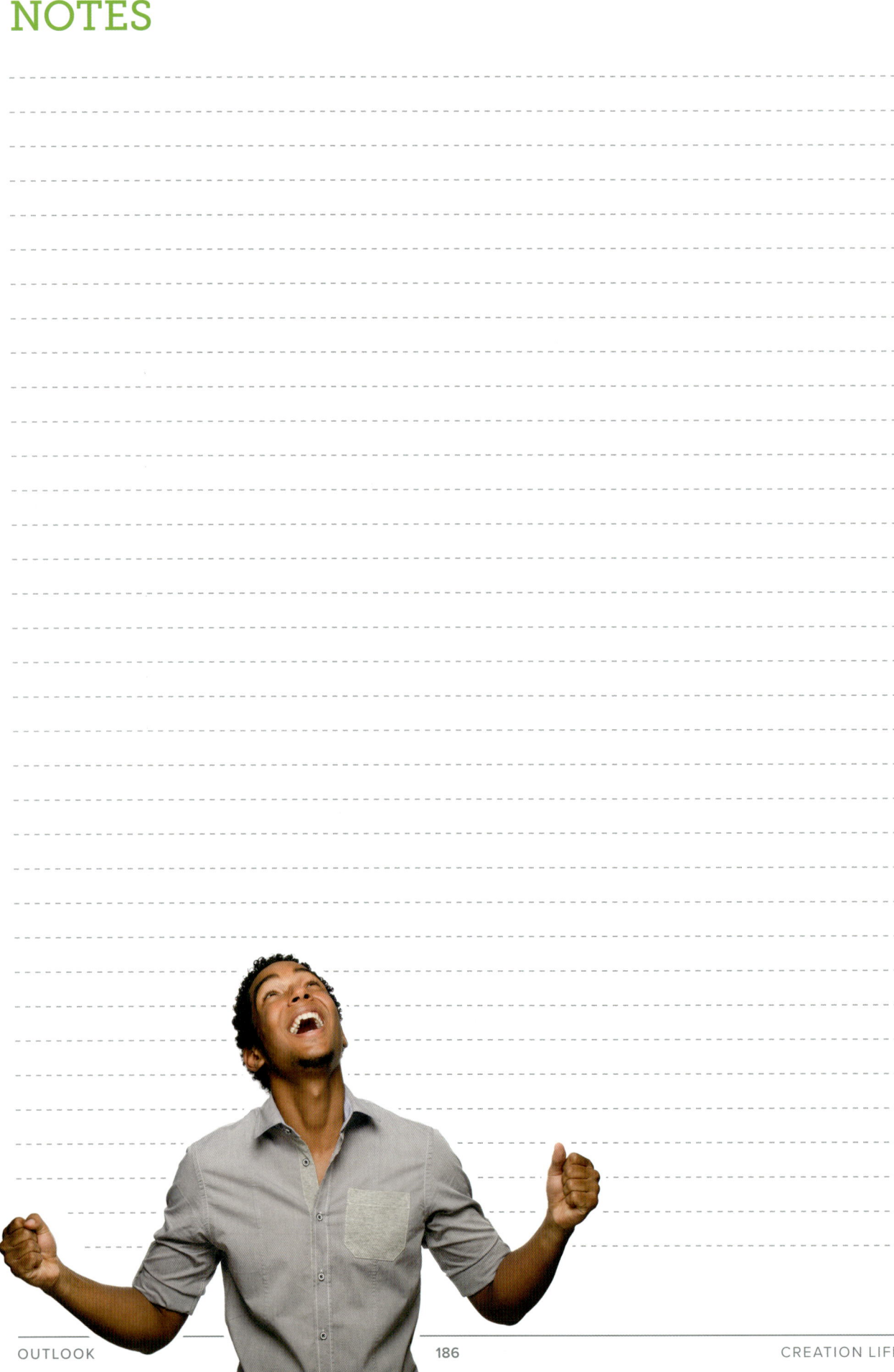

OUTLOOK

NUTRITION

Eat smart

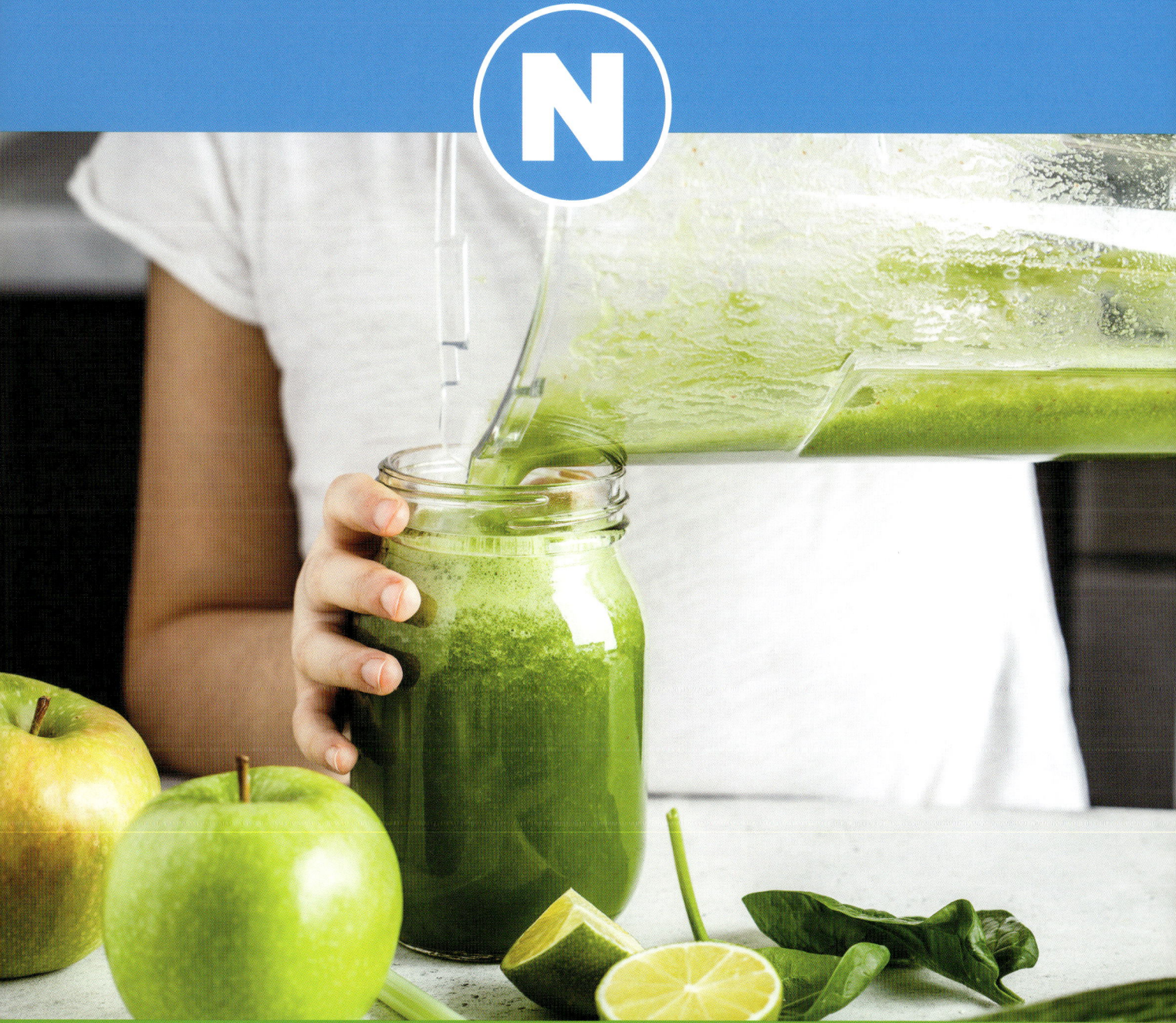

NUTRITION [noo-trish-uhn, nyoo-] *noun* **1:** is nourishment for the body and energy for the mind. Understanding your relationship with food can lead to better choices and improved wellness.

THE BIG PICTURE

So, you finally managed to work up enough nerve to ask that special someone to the spring banquet? You're so excited you decide to get to school extra early, stake out their first class and catch them the minute they arrive. Of course, that means you'll have to skip breakfast but it's a small price to pay, right? Suddenly you see them. The person of your affections is rounding the corner and walking straight towards you. You smile nervously. They smile back. This is it, the moment you've been waiting for. You open your mouth to speak when suddenly your stomach rumbles like Mount Vesuvius. Your "would-be date" can't help but laugh. You're so horrified you dash from the hallway into the nearest restroom to hide. How embarrassing.

All this humiliation could have easily been avoided had you simply eaten a nutritious breakfast. You told yourself you didn't have time and you thought a handful of chips would get you through.

Skipping breakfast is only one of many nutritional blunders teenagers make on a regular basis. In fact, most teenagers pay very little attention to their body's nutritional needs. They simply consume whatever they want whenever they want it, never realizing the impact that poor nutrition has on their lives. What they also fail to understand is how the habits they are forming now will affect them for years to come. As the eighth and final principle of CREATION Life, Nutrition is all about what you choose to put in your body. Making the right food choices is often the difference between health and illness, happiness and depression and in some cases, even life and death.

Food is the body's fuel. Say it's your 16th birthday and your parents are feeling particularly generous. They give you a brand new BMW M3, which can go from a dead stop to 60 miles per hour in under four seconds. You wouldn't dream of filling up the tank with anything less than the highest octane gasoline, would you? Anything less and you'd risk doing serious damage to the engine. Your body operates in much the same way. You need to be filling up with the most nutritious foods available in order to operate at peak performance. Foods overloaded with fat, salt, sugar, preservatives and other undesirable elements may make for a quick, cheap option now, but over time they will wreak havoc on your well-being just like cheap gas in a sports car affects the car's performance.

NUTRITION is the food you eat, but it's also one of the most powerful tools you have available to promote your health. What you put into your body is vitally important to your well-being. The best forms of nutrition come from sticking to a diet as God intended it.

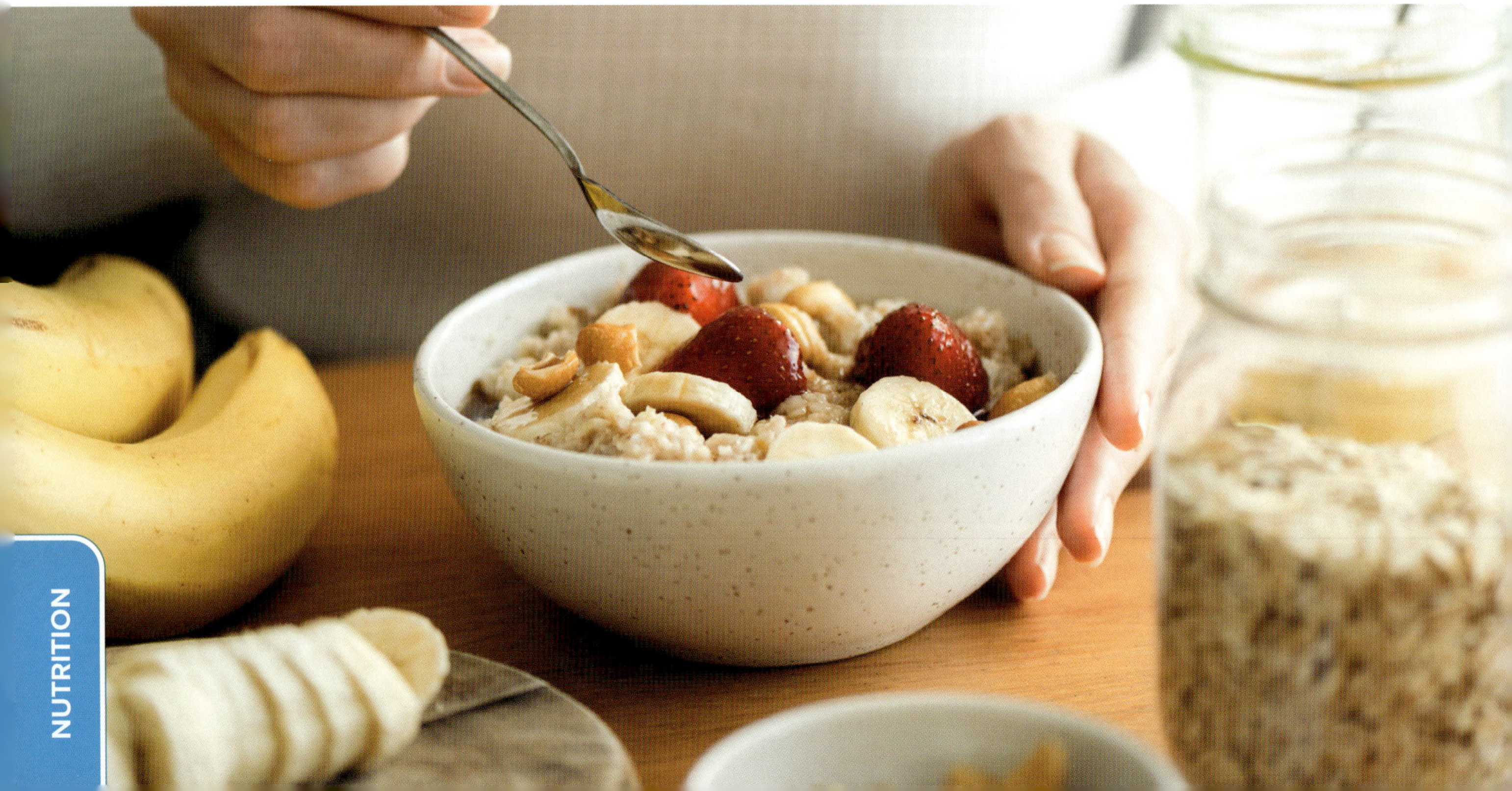

THE GIFT OF NUTRITION

Then God said, "Behold, I have given you every plant yielding seed that is on the surface of all the earth, and every tree which has fruit yielding seed; it shall be food for you... "

GENESIS 1:29

In the Garden of Eden, God gave Adam and Eve the best foods possible. The Creator's original diet was entirely plant-based, full of fruits, grains, seeds and nuts. Scientists are discovering more and more about the amazing benefits of eating these foods. By following God's plan for optimal nutrition, you'll not only experience more happiness and greater energy levels, but you'll also increase your body's disease prevention capabilities and your overall health.[1] In short, God's plan still works for you today.

Want to see a great example of how trusting God's plan for nutrition impacts your health and well-being? Look no further than your Old Testament friend Daniel and his three pals, Shadrach, Meshach and Abednego.

But Daniel made up his mind that he would not defile himself with the king's choice food or with the wine which he drank...

DANIEL 1:8

When Daniel and his friends were young, they were taken from their hometown of Jerusalem to the city of Babylon. The plan was to conform them to the Babylonian culture so they could serve King Nebuchadnezzar. They learned the language and history, and they were offered special foods to eat — the same delicacies served to the king himself. Many people wouldn't think twice about gorging themselves silly on the rich offerings of the king's table, but Daniel knew there was a problem. In the eyes of God, much of the food in question was unclean. To eat it meant Daniel and his friends were going against God's plan, but to not eat it could also be seen as an act of rebellion and cost them their lives.

Perhaps some of Daniel's friends urged him to reconsider. "It's only food," they might have said.

Only food? Didn't they realize what was at stake? God's law was clear about acceptable foods. Daniel wasn't trying to cause trouble in Babylon, but he knew he must remain faithful to God above all others.

"You're living in the past," another might have told him. "We are in Babylon now; we must live as they do."

Did Daniel wonder if there was a grain of truth in this statement? After all, God's city was gone, His temple destroyed. Shouldn't he just learn to make the best of it and live as the Babylonians lived? No. God's law had never changed. The Word of the Lord is forever. Daniel and his friends resolved to stay faithful no matter what the cost.

The name Daniel means "God is my judge," and he certainly lived up to it. Daniel followed God's standard for living right down to the foods he ate. Of course this put him at odds with the status quo, so Daniel put the whole Babylonian system to the test. He proposed a 10-day period in which he and his friends would eat and drink nothing but vegetables and water. At the end of the period their captors would evaluate them.

At the end of the ten days they looked healthier and better nourished than any of the young men who ate the royal food. So the guard took away their choice food and the wine they were to drink and gave them vegetables instead.

DANIEL 1:15–16

After just 10 days, Daniel and his friends were healthier, stronger and in better shape than King Nebuchadnezzar's entire court.

Following God's standard is still the best way to live your life, right down to the foods you put on your plate. Take a page from Daniel and don't be afraid to stand up for what you believe in, even when it puts you against the majority. When you follow God's way, you won't lose.

Have you ever been made fun of for not eating or drinking what everyone else is? Do you ever feel excluded from groups because of your food choices?

REALITY CHECK

You don't have to be a nutritionist to figure out that America has a big weight problem. An abundance of cheap, highly processed food combined with low levels of activity led to an obesity epidemic. In the early 1960s, the obesity level among U.S. adults age 20 and older was 13.4 percent. Today, that number has more than doubled increasing to 35.7 percent.[1] According to data from the 2016 National Survey of Children's Health, about one-third (31.2 percent) of adolescents ages 10 to 17 are considered to be overweight or obese.[2]

"We have an epidemic of obesity in the United States and it's only getting worse," said U.S. Surgeon General Richard Carmona. "We are seeing Generation Y grow into Generation XL, and this weight gain has long-term health consequences."[3]

Being overweight will rob you of your quality and quantity of life. Medical problems that doctors once saw only in adults aged 50 or older are now striking kids your age: diabetes, hypertension, kidney disease and heart disease.[4]

Childhood obesity is destroying lives, draining family resources and pushing America dangerously close to a total healthcare collapse — but you have the power to help reverse the trend. You can work to avert the coming crisis by taking control of your own weight challenges and striving to live a CREATION Life.

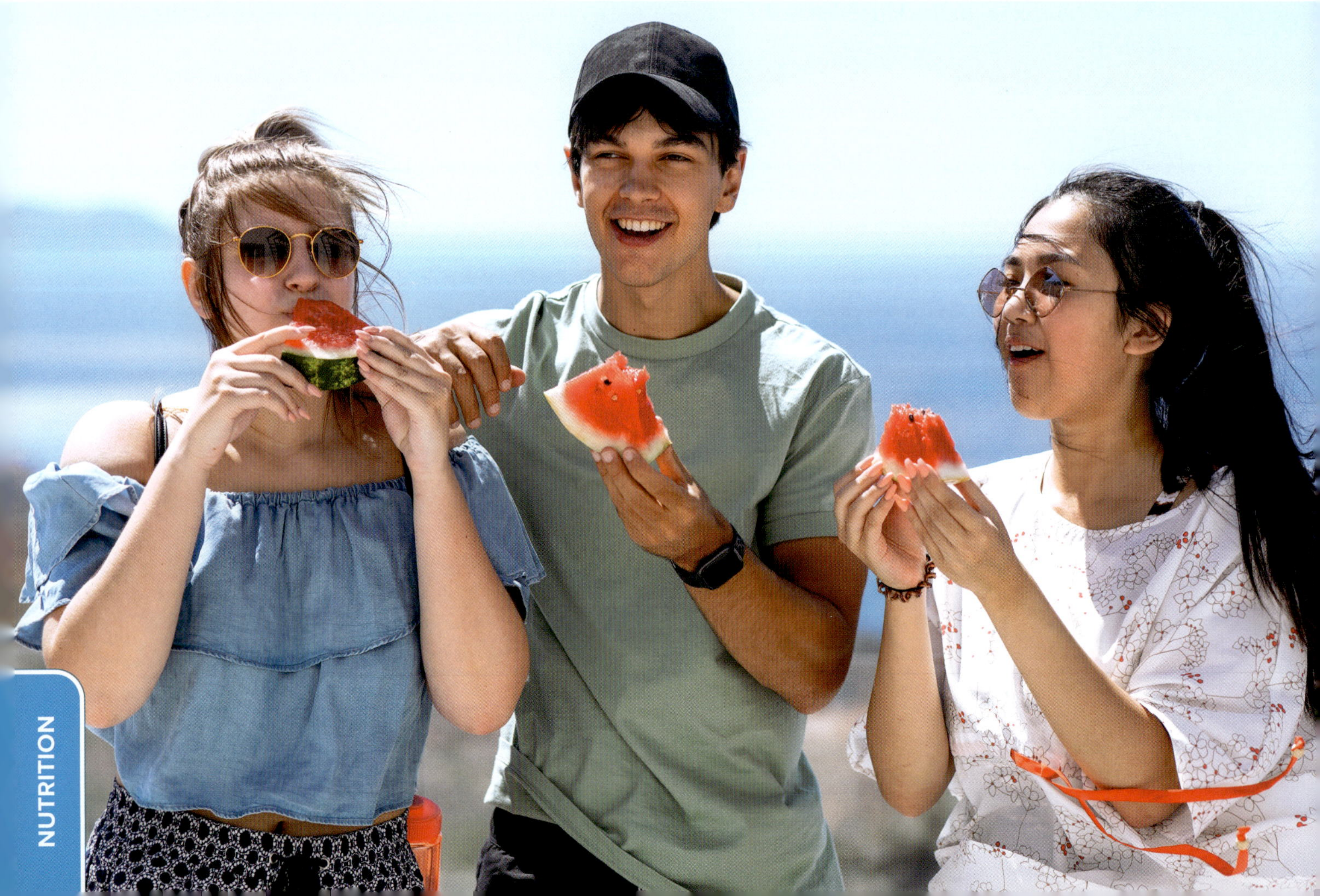

NUTRITION

SMALL POSITIVE STEPS

A student who was seriously overweight desperately wanted to get in shape, but he was too embarrassed to attend a nutrition course offered at his school. So, one day after classes, he secretly went to the teacher and asked if she would be willing to help him individually. She agreed.

For the first week all she asked him to do was to keep track of everything he ate each day. He did, and brought his list to her the next week. She looked it over and then asked him to do the exact same thing the following week, but to add one piece of fruit to his diet every day.

"But what about the three candy bars I eat before lunch?" he said. "What about the milkshake I have after school? What about all the gummy bears, the potato chips and the deep dish pizza?"

She told him not to worry about it. "It will take care of itself," she said.

The next week she asked him to add one vegetable a day. Before this the closest thing he ever got to a vegetable was the ketchup he squirted on his French fries. Each week he continued to add something healthy to his diet. Before he knew it he was eating more than six servings of fruits and vegetables a day. He found he had really grown to like them, too. Now, instead of hitting a vending machine or cruising a drive-thru when school was out, he snacked on healthy foods like carrots, dried fruits and nuts. As his diet changed, so did his weight. In three months he had to buy new pants because his old ones were too big. Little by little, he continued to make progress until one day he looked at himself in the mirror and couldn't believe his eyes. The old, overweight version of himself was a thing of the past. Now, he was lean and healthy, but he hadn't just changed on the outside. He had also gained more confidence and increased his self-esteem.

"Food affects mood, so eat with care."

SEAN COVEY
The 7 Habits of Highly Effective Teens

Many times when people are faced with making a change in their nutrition they go to the extreme. They throw away all the junk food in the house, immediately buy a juicer and start consuming large amounts of kale. In less than a month, they are frustrated, burned out and seriously craving all the yummy goodies they've been missing.

When making a change, focus on the positive. Don't think you have to stop all these bad habits. In the story you just read, the teacher encouraged her student to make small, positive steps. This gave him the ability to make changes that were not only healthy but would also stand the test of time. If you gradually add the positive to your life, pretty soon there won't be any room left for the negative.

Look at the way you currently eat. What is one good thing you could add? Maybe you could try adding a piece of fruit each day. Maybe you could start drinking more water to help your brain and body function better. Maybe you could choose to eat two cruciferous vegetables every week. Cruciferous vegetables such as broccoli, cauliflower, Brussels sprouts, cabbage and kale are super veggies. They contain phytochemicals, vitamins and minerals and fiber that are all important to your health. Consider the results of a study on Chinese women living in Singapore, a city where air pollution from cigarette smoke is often high. This pollution creates extra stress on the cleaning capacity of a person's lungs. The study found that in nonsmokers, eating cruciferous vegetables lowered their risk of lung cancer by 30 percent. In smokers, regularly eating cruciferous vegetables reduced the risk of lung cancer an incredible 69 percent.[6] This study clearly illustrates cruciferous vegetables' amazing ability to help protect your body.

After you have formed a positive and healthy habit, you can add another to your routine. The point is to add something good to your diet and not beat yourself up over the "bad." Dwelling on the good is beneficial for your health and will help you succeed.

What are some small, positive steps you can make this week with your nutrition? Remember, don't focus on eliminating the bad. Think of a simple way you can add something positive to your diet. Here are a few suggestions:

1. Add a side of broccoli or another cruciferous vegetable to one meal each day.

2. Have an apple or another piece of fruit as a midday snack.

3. Try getting some extra water by carrying a water bottle with you to class.

YOU ARE WHAT YOU EAT

Did you know human red blood cells only have a lifespan of 120 days? This means your body is in a constant state of rebuilding and replenishing its supply. There are also thousands of other cells throughout your body that are being regenerated on a daily basis. So, where do you think your body gets its raw material to build these new cells? From your food, of course. Giving your body the best nutrition means you are putting in the highest quality fuel so it will be able to make stronger and healthier cells. It is vitally important to eat a healthy, nutritious diet every day because when it comes down to it, you really are what you eat.

Strive to eat a wide variety of foods and be suspicious of the latest trendy diet fads. Examine new diets carefully before you start following them. One good question to ask is: *How different is this new trend from simply eating a balanced diet?* Remember, advertisers have multimillion-dollar budgets aimed at persuading you to try their latest miracle diet. Eye-catching headlines and doctored before-and-after photos promise incredible results, but you're wise not to believe everything you hear. Stand back and look at the bigger picture. Ask critical questions about the food or dietary practice being promoted. Find out how following this diet will affect your overall health. Get knowledgeable advice from a qualified physician or nutritionist. Seek out other reliable sources that aren't trying to sell you anything.

Remember that for healthy people, dietary changes are best when they are made slowly and after careful consideration. And in order for a change in your diet to last, it must first fit into your balanced lifestyle.

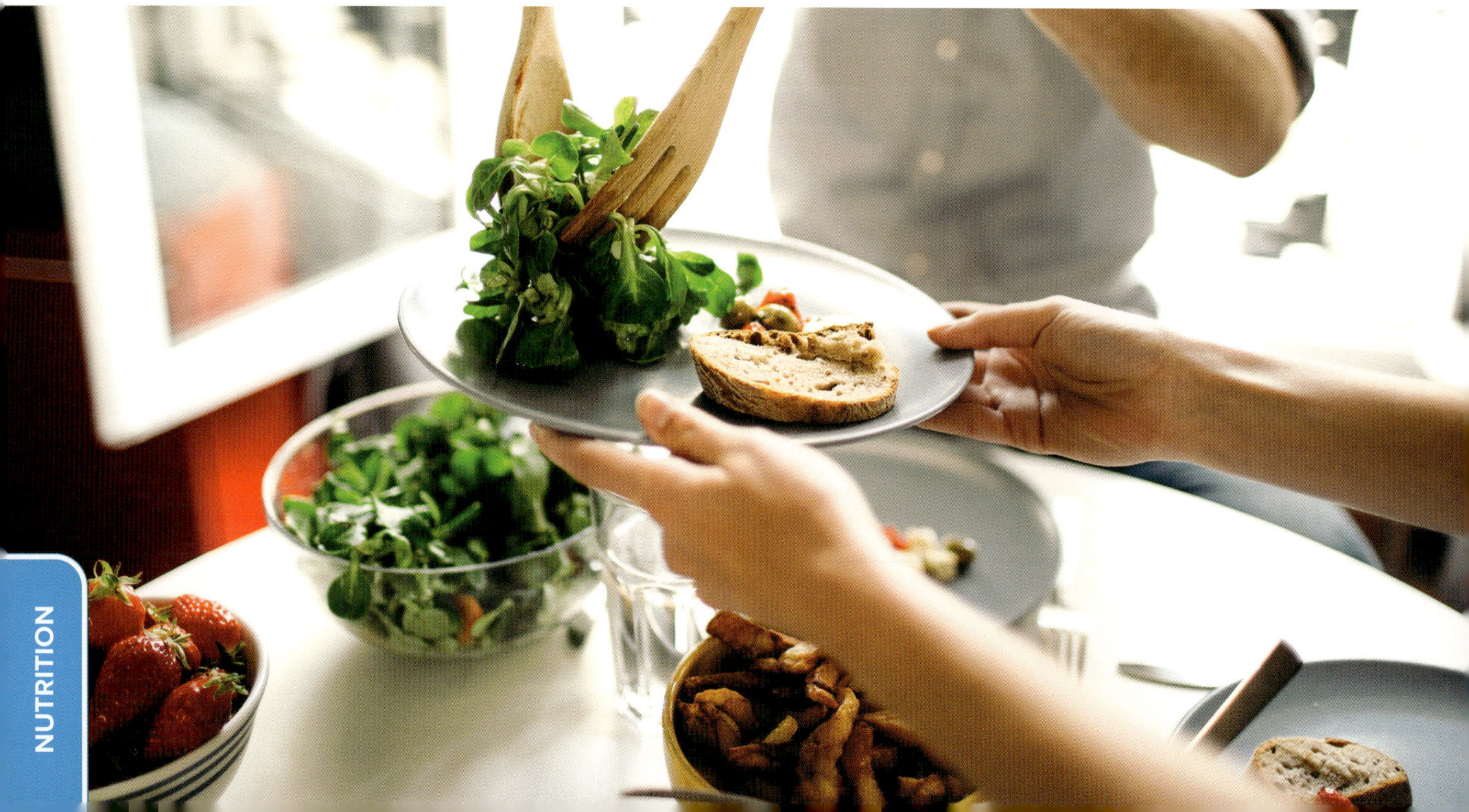

WHAT SHOULD YOU PUT ON YOUR PLATE?

The USDA illustrates a proper balanced diet through MyPlate. As you can see in the illustration, all five food groups that are the building blocks for a healthy diet are represented as a place setting for a meal. This helps you to think about what goes on your plate before you start to eat.

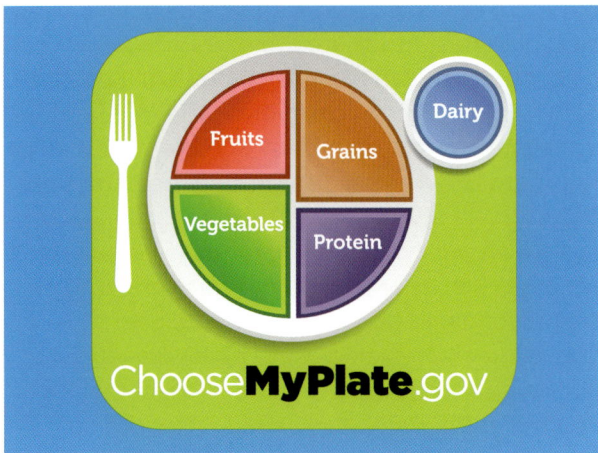

> *"Take care of your body.*
> *It's the only place you have to live."*
>
> JIM ROHN

For using MyPlate, the USDA recommends the following guidelines:

- Make half of your plate fruits and vegetables.

- Make at least half of your grains whole grains.

- Switch to fat-free or one percent milk (almond or soy milk is a great alternative).

- Vary your protein sources.

One very important recommendation is to limit your intake of empty calories, which are calories from added solid fats and/or sugars. While added fat and sugar may make foods a little more desirable, they also make them a lot unhealthier. Foods and beverages that contain the emptiest calories are:

- Cakes, cookies, pastries and donuts (contain both solid fat and added sugars)

- Sodas, energy drinks, sports drinks and fruit drinks (contain added sugars)

- Cheese (contains solid fat)

- Pizza (contains solid fat)

- Ice cream (contains both solid fat and added sugars)

- Meat sausages, hot dogs and ribs (contain solid fat)[7]

You may see some of your favorite foods in the previous list, but this doesn't mean you have to completely wipe eating them from your diet. You can still have a slice of pizza or an ice cream cone. You just need to eat these foods in moderation. "A small amount of empty calories is okay, but most people eat far more than is healthy."[8]

The USDA recommends the following guidelines for empty calorie consumption among teenagers:

- Teen girls 14 to 18 years old should eat no more than 160 empty calories a day as part of a total 1,800 caloric intake.

- Teen boys 14 to 18 years old should eat no more than 265 empty calories a day as part of a total 2,200 caloric intake.

These amounts are for teenagers who get less than 30 minutes of moderate physical activity most days. Physical activity *increases* your calorie needs, so if you are regularly exercising or involved with an extracurricular sports program you will need more overall calories. Just be sure and get those calories from healthy sources.[9]

One quick and easy way to cut empty calories from your diet is to switch to more healthy options. Many low-fat or unsweetened versions of your favorite foods exist. You should also try eating smaller portions of empty calorie foods. That way, you can enjoy more occasional treats without wasting a whole day's allowance on one big indulgence.

BREAKFAST FOR THE BRAIN

Do you know why they call it breakfast? Because your body has been fasting, or going without food all night, and it's hungry. If you are skipping breakfast, you are starting the day at a huge disadvantage, especially when it comes to your brain. Your brain's basic fuel is glucose, and regularly supplying it with a new source of energy is essential. The Pediatrics Department at the University of California at Davis hosted a group of psychologists, neuroscientists, nutritionists and physiologists to review the scientific research on breakfast. The researchers concluded that the "eating of breakfast is important in learning, memory and physical well-being in both children and adults."[10] This means there will never be a time in your life when skipping breakfast is a good idea. In fact, eating a healthy breakfast may be one key to living a long and healthy life. The Alameda County Study found that those who ate breakfast almost every day reported better physical health and tended to live longer than those who skipped breakfast.[11]

Eating a good breakfast is essential for your body and mind to operate at maximum efficiency, especially during the later morning hours. Think about it; how many times have you skipped breakfast only to reach your second or third class feeling groggy or irritable? Breakfast eaters demonstrate more efficient problem solving, increased verbal fluency, an improved attention span, better attitudes and better scholastic scores. In a study directed by Harvard psychologist Michael Murphy, 4,000 elementary school children were reviewed. Half ate breakfast while the other half did not. Across the board, those who ate breakfast exhibited better scores on a series of attention tests. These included a short-term memory test where the children repeated a series of digits, and a verbal fluency test where they were asked to name all of the animals they could think of in 60 seconds.[12]

With so much evidence available, the only question left to ask is, "What's for breakfast?" Not all breakfasts are created alike. Pouring yourself a big bowl of *Chocolate Frosted Sugar Bombs* may sound like a good idea at the time, but there are much better choices available. The best breakfast foods are the ones with a low glycemic load. The glycemic index is a measure of how quickly the carbohydrates in your food are absorbed into your body and converted to fuel. Terrill Bravender, professor of pediatrics at Duke University, explains that when it comes to sustaining your brainpower, foods lower on the scale — such as whole grains — are preferable.[13] As part of a plant-based diet, whole grains, like oatmeal for example, are highly beneficial. However, according to a study published in the *Journal of the American Dietetic Association*, most Americans are simply unaware of this fact. "Whole grain foods are valuable sources of nutrients that are lacking in the American diet, including dietary fiber, B vitamins, vitamin E, selenium, zinc, copper and magnesium. Whole grain foods also contain phytochemicals, such as phenolic compounds that together with vitamins and minerals play important roles in disease prevention."[14] So, even though a bowl of sugary cereal and a bowl of oatmeal may have the same number of carbohydrates, one is healthier than the other. The low glycemic load of oatmeal and its overall health benefits make it a far better choice to start your day.

SIX ESSENTIAL NUTRIENTS

There are six essential nutrients your body needs in order to function: fat, protein, carbohydrates, vitamins, minerals and water. All of these play a different role in helping your body to operate at its maximum potential.

Are you eating a healthy, nutritious breakfast every morning? What are some healthy choices you can start to put on your plate?

FAT

A lot of people think of fat as the mortal enemy of good nutrition, a diabolical Lex Luthor whose delicious schemes keep them from fitting into their skinny jeans. What they fail to realize is that healthy fats are essential in order for you to have a good diet.

Wait a minute. Healthy fats? Isn't that an oxymoron?

Your body needs fat to function. According to the Medline Plus website, fat is a type of nutrient you get from your diet. While it is essential to eat some fat, it is harmful to eat too much. Fat gives your body energy, keeps your skin and hair healthy and helps the absorption of vitamins A, D, E and K, the so-called fat-soluble vitamins.[15] The problem is that not all fats are created equal. Saturated fats and trans fats are considered less healthy types of fats, and both raise the level of "bad" LDL (low density lipoprotein) cholesterol in your blood. However, trans fats also decrease the "good" HDL (high density lipoprotein) cholesterol.[16] Reducing your intake now can make a difference later in minimizing the risks of heart disease and other illnesses.[17-18]

FATS TO AVOID

Saturated fats such as butter and solid vegetable shortening.

Trans fats found in vegetable shortenings, some margarines, crackers, cookies, snack foods and other foods made with or fried in, partially hydrogenated oils.

Try to replace these fats with oils such as canola, olive, safflower, sesame or sunflower. Of course, eating too much of any fat will put on the pounds. Fat has twice as many calories as proteins or carbohydrates.[19]

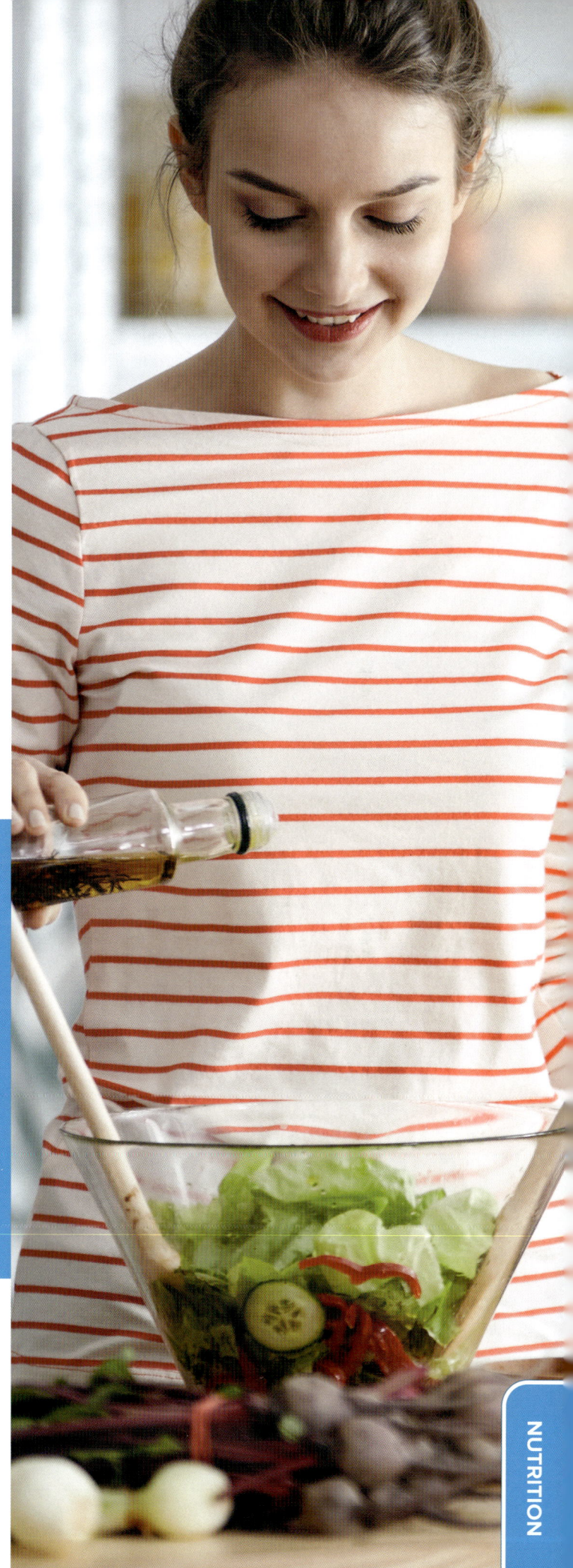

The best place for you to get healthy fats is from natural, plant-based sources. A good rule of thumb to follow is: the closer your food is to nature, the better it is for you. The perfect example is the avocado. Many people only think of avocados when they get a craving for guacamole, but this amazing fruit is bursting with good and nutritious fat that offers you incredible health benefits. Researchers have found that when people on the Standard American Diet were given an avocado-rich diet, their total cholesterol dropped an average of 8.2 percent with no change in their HDL (high-density lipoprotein) cholesterol. HDL is also known as the "good cholesterol," and it plays an important role in preventing heart disease and keeping your body healthy.[20]

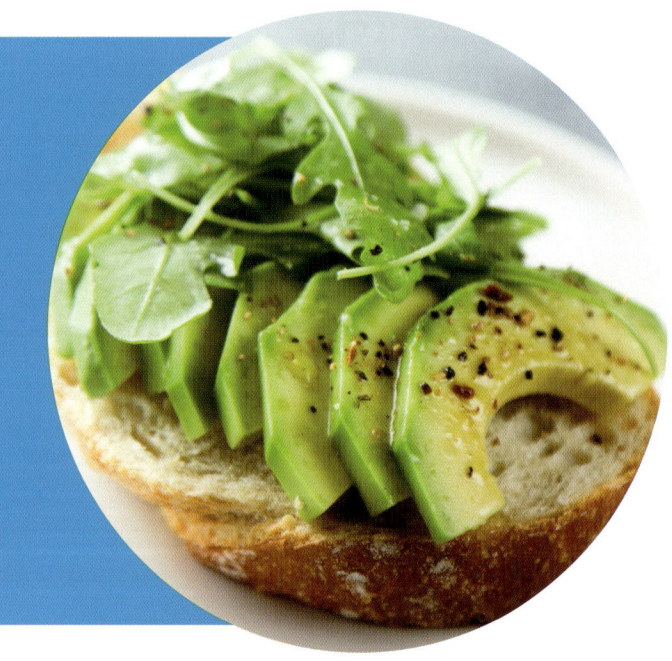

Another good and natural source of healthy fat is nuts. Sometimes these popular snack options get a bad rep for being high in fat, but nuts can actually be a very healthy choice. They not only help you feel full, they also satisfy your hunger and keep cravings under control. Research has shown that adding small amounts of nuts to your diet won't drastically affect your weight. In a review study looking at the association

between nut consumption and energy balance, clinical trials revealed little or no weight change with inclusion of various types of nuts in the diet over six months. Studies indicate this is largely attributed to the high satiety property of nuts. This means people who eat nuts tend to eat less of other foods because they feel full and satisfied. While some people may dispute these findings, there is one thing everyone agrees on: the fat found in nuts is a healthier fat. Like avocados, nuts contain mostly monounsaturated and polyunsaturated fats. These fats are considered more heart friendly. One study found that people who ate nuts five or more times per week cut their risk of having a heart attack by 51 percent. They also had a 48 percent reduction in death from heart attacks compared to those who ate nuts less than once a week.[21]

But nuts are not just good for your heart. They are also excellent "brain food." Researchers have credited nuts with helping to fight Alzheimer's disease and depression. Two studies published in the *Journal of the American Medical Association* suggested that the antioxidant vitamin E and other antioxidants found in nuts might reduce the risk of Alzheimer's.[22-23]

Another crucial area where nuts can make a difference is in hyperactivity, learning disorders and behavior problems. Maybe you know someone who currently struggles with some of these issues or maybe you have personally struggled with these issues in your own life. Well, the problem could have a lot to do with your nutrition. A Purdue University study showed that children who were low in dietary omega-3 essential fatty acids are significantly more likely to be hyperactive, have learning disorders and display behavior problems. Those that had lower total blood omega-3 fatty acids also reported a greater number of behavior problems, temper tantrums, sleep problems, learning issues and health issues.[24] If you suffer from some of these problems you may want to try getting more omega-3 in your diet. Walnuts are excellent sources of omega-3 fatty acids.

UNDERSTANDING FOOD ALLERGIES

For many people, food allergies is a serious concern. Recent studies have found that almost one in 20 young children under the age of five years and almost one in 25 adults are allergic to at least one food. Other studies indicate that food allergies, especially to peanuts, are on the rise. A food allergy is an abnormal response to a food triggered by your body's immune system, and in some cases this response can be life threatening.[25]

According to the National Institute of Allergy and Infectious Diseases, you may experience the following symptoms if you are allergic to a particular food:

- Itching in your mouth
- Swelling of lips and tongue
- GI symptoms, such as vomiting, diarrhea, or abdominal cramps and pain
- Hives
- Eczema
- Tightening of the throat or trouble breathing
- Drop in blood pressure[26]

There is also a chance you could experience a severe form of allergic reaction known as anaphylaxis. "Anaphylaxis includes a wide range of symptoms that can occur in many combinations. Some symptoms are not life-threatening, but the most severe restrict breathing and blood circulation." If not immediately treated, anaphylaxis could lead to death.[27]

In infants and children, the most common foods that cause allergic reactions are:

- Eggs
- Milk
- Peanuts
- Tree nuts, such as walnuts
- Soy (primarily in infants)
- Wheat

In adults, the most common foods that cause allergic reactions are:

- Shellfish, such as shrimp, crayfish, lobster and crab
- Peanuts
- Tree nuts
- Fish, such as salmon[28]

Food allergies can develop at any age. You may outgrow some allergies such as eggs, milk and soy, but people who develop allergies as adults usually have them for life. Children generally do not outgrow their allergy to peanuts.[29]

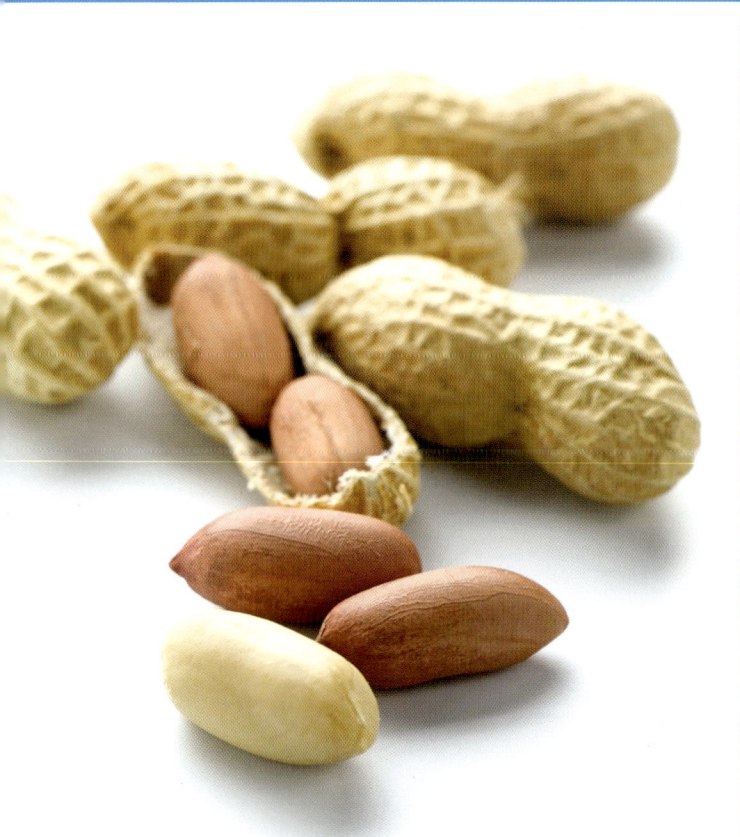

PROTEIN

For many people, it's just not a meal unless a chunk of animal protein is somewhere on the plate. Whether it's roasted, braised, ground into a patty and seared on a grill, meat is a large part of the American diet. According to a report by the U.S. Department of Agriculture, meat consumption in America is at an all-time high. According to their 2018 Red Meat and Poultry Forecasts, the Department of Agriculture projects over 103 billion pounds to be produced nationwide. That is the equivalent to the average American consuming over 220 pounds of meat and poultry in one year.

But according to the Mayo Clinic, eating less meat has many positive health benefits. "A plant-based diet, which emphasizes fruits and vegetables, grains, beans and legumes and nuts, is rich in fiber, vitamins and other nutrients. And people who eat only plant-based foods — aka vegetarians — generally eat fewer calories and less fat, weigh less and have a lower risk of heart disease than nonvegetarians do."[31]

In spite of these positives, many people question the healthiness of a vegetarian lifestyle. In fact, one question vegetarians must routinely field is: "Where do you get your protein?" Carnivores assume that since vegetarians eat no meat, they must be suffering from severe protein deficiencies, but as you'll see, this is not necessarily the case.

Your body does need protein. Protein is in every living cell in your body and you use it to build and maintain bones, muscles and skin.[32] Proteins are made up of amino acids, which are a lot like the building blocks you played with as a kid. Twenty different amino acids join together to make all the types of protein your body needs. However, your body can't make some of these amino acids, so these are known as "essential amino acids."[33] Proteins that come from meat and other animal products are often considered "complete proteins." This means they give your body all of the amino acids it can't make alone, but as you've seen they also provide a number of unhealthy factors as well. Plant proteins are often known as "incomplete proteins," but this term can be confusing and even a bit biased. People tend to think of plant proteins as inferior to the proteins found in meat. However, by combining different plant proteins, you can easily give your body the amino acids it needs.[34]

The Centers for Disease Control and Prevention says, "Most adults in the United States get more than enough protein to meet their needs. It's rare for someone who is healthy and eating a varied diet to not get enough protein." They also recommend the following protein guidelines for teenagers:

- Teen girls 14 to 18 years old should eat 46 grams of protein a day

- Teen boys 14 to 18 years old should eat 52 grams of protein a day

To give you an idea of what this looks like, one cup of dry beans has about 16 grams of protein.[35]

It's not that eating meat is wrong, but a plant-based diet is eating the way God originally intended in the Garden of Eden. If you want to experience the truly abundant life God has for you, consider the benefits of a plant-based, vegetarian diet.

Do you trust God enough to follow His best plan for your life?

Do you believe a plant-based diet will give you the maximum benefits for your health?

If you feel you are eating too much meat or dairy, what are some ways you can begin to change your diet?

"The food you eat can be either the safest and most powerful form of medicine or the slowest form of poison."

ANN WIGMORE

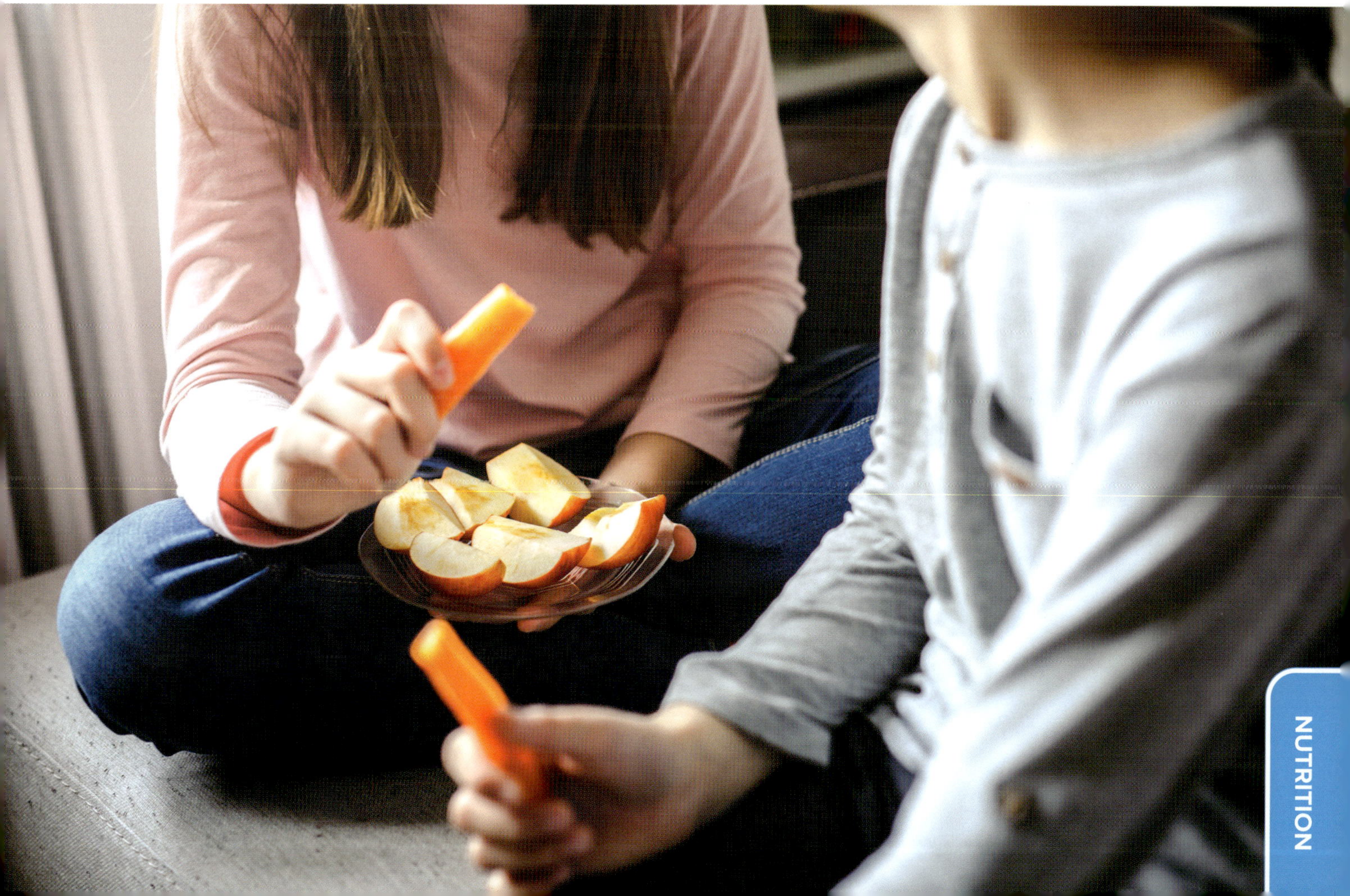

NUTRIENT TIPS FOR VEGETARIANS[36]

Vegetarian diets can meet all the nutritional recommendations. The key is to consume a variety of foods and the right amount of foods to meet your calorie needs. Follow the food group recommendations for your age, sex and activity level to get the right amount of food and the variety of foods needed for nutrient adequacy. Nutrients that vegetarians may need to focus on include protein, iron, calcium, zinc and vitamin B12.[36]

NUTRIENTS TO FOCUS ON FOR VEGETARIANS

- Protein has many important functions in the body and is essential for growth and maintenance. Protein needs can easily be met by eating a variety of plant-based foods. Combining different protein sources in the same meal is not necessary. Sources of protein for vegetarians and vegans include beans, nuts, nut butters, peas and soy products (tofu, tempeh and veggie burgers). Milk products and eggs are also good protein sources for lacto-ovo vegetarians.

- Iron functions primarily as a carrier of oxygen in the blood. Iron sources for vegetarians and vegans include iron-fortified breakfast cereals, spinach, kidney beans, black-eyed peas, lentils, turnip greens, molasses, whole wheat breads, peas and some dried fruits (dried apricots, prunes and raisins).

- Calcium is used for building bones and teeth and in maintaining bone strength. Sources of calcium for vegetarians and vegans include calcium-fortified soymilk, calcium-fortified breakfast cereals and orange juice, tofu made with calcium sulfate and some dark-green leafy vegetables (collard greens, turnip greens, bok choy and mustard greens). The amount of calcium that can be absorbed from these foods varies. Consuming enough plant foods to meet calcium needs may be unrealistic for many. Milk products are excellent calcium sources for lacto vegetarians. Calcium supplements are another potential source.

- Zinc is necessary for many biochemical reactions and also helps the immune system function properly. Sources of zinc for vegetarians and vegans include many types of beans (white beans, kidney beans and chickpeas), zinc-fortified breakfast cereals, wheat germ and pumpkin seeds. Milk products are a zinc source for lacto vegetarians.

- Vitamin B12 is found in animal products and some fortified foods. Sources of vitamin B12 for vegetarians include milk products, eggs and foods that have been fortified with vitamin B12. These include breakfast cereals, soymilk, veggie burgers and nutritional yeast.

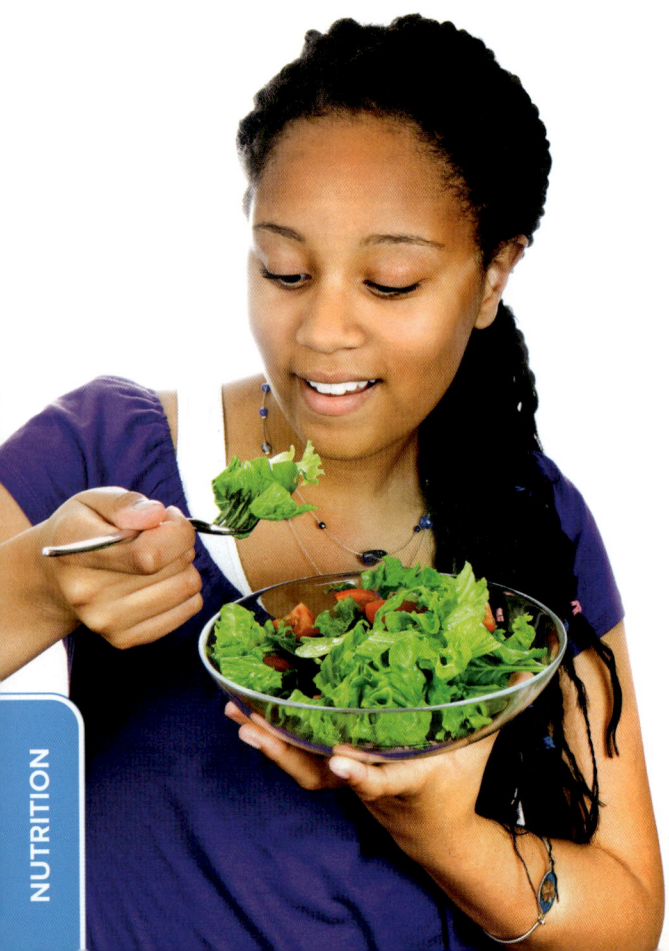

MEAL TIPS FOR VEGETARIANS

- Build meals around protein sources that are naturally low in fat, such as beans, lentils and rice. Don't overload meals with high-fat cheeses to replace the meat.

- Choose calcium-fortified soy milk which provides calcium in amounts similar to milk. It is usually low in fat and does not contain cholesterol.

- Substitute foods that typically contain meat or poultry with plant-based products or vegetables. A variety of vegetarian products look (and taste) like their non-vegetarian counterparts, but are usually lower in saturated fat and contain no cholesterol.

  - Eat soy-based sausage patties or links for breakfast.

  - Try veggie burgers, soy hot dogs, marinated tofu or tempeh and veggie kabobs. A variety of kinds are available, made with soybeans, vegetables and/or rice.

- Add vegetarian meat substitutes to soups and stews to boost protein without adding saturated fat or cholesterol. These include tempeh (cultured soybeans with a chewy texture), tofu or seitan (wheat gluten).

- Make bean burgers, lentil burgers or pita halves with falafel (spicy ground chickpea patties).

- Order vegetarian options at restaurants as a substitute for meat. Most restaurants can accommodate vegetarian modifications to menu items by substituting meatless sauces, omitting meat from stir-fry and adding vegetables or pasta in place of meat.

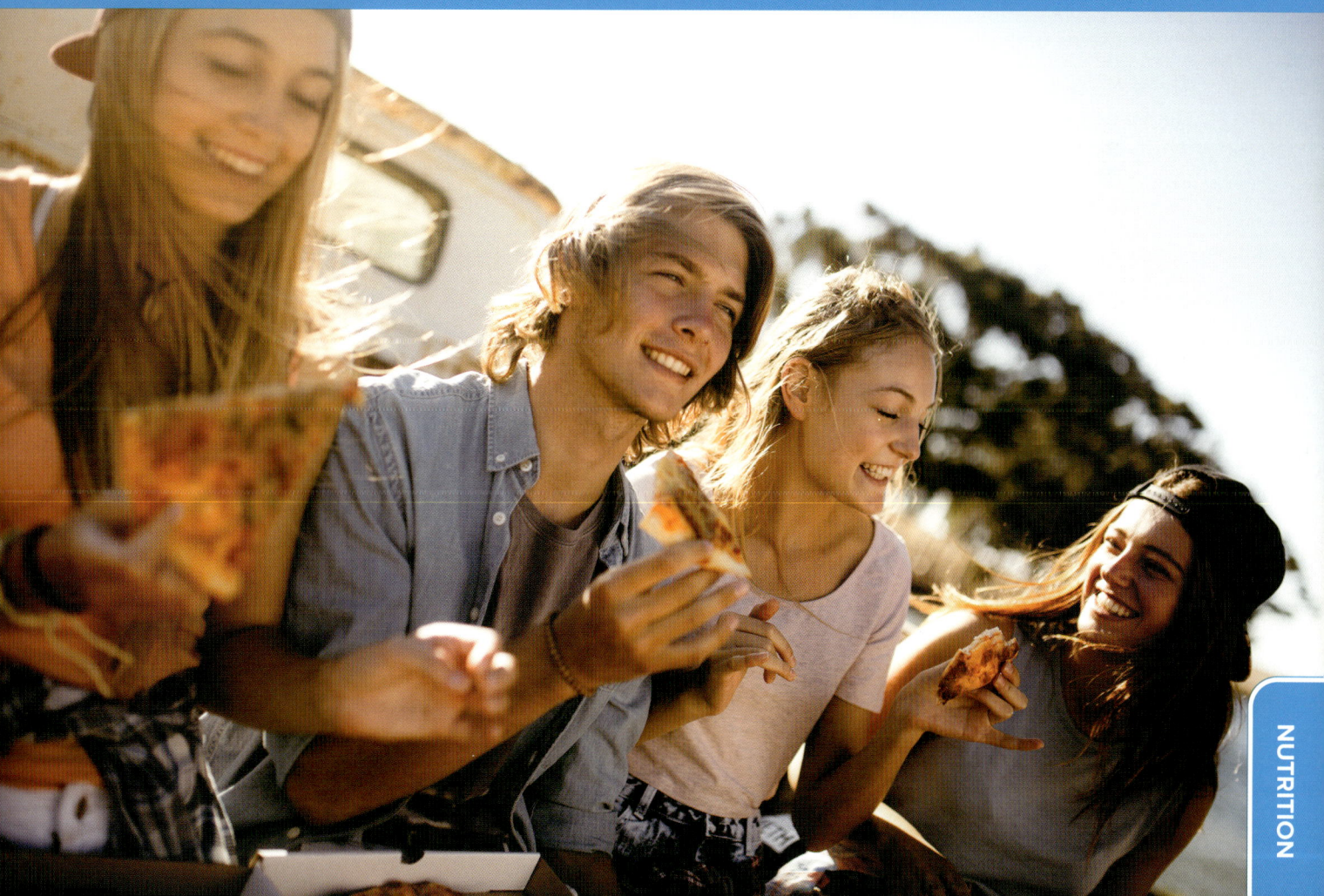

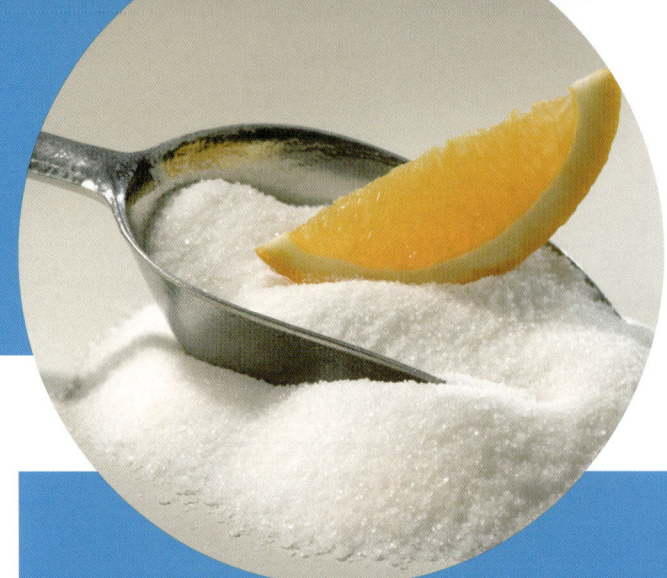

A piece of fruit may contain simple carbs, but it also contains vitamins, minerals and fiber. This makes it a much healthier option.

CARBOHYDRATES

During the early 2000s, carbohydrates got a bad rap. People rejected them in favor of the latest fad — high-protein diets that promised quick weight loss while allowing people to eat all the bacon they wanted. The truth is carbohydrates, or "carbs," aren't bad for you at all. As long as you eat the right kinds of carbs in moderation, they can provide you with some incredible health benefits.

As one of the main types of nutrients, carbs are "the most important source of energy for your body."[37] Your digestive system converts carbs into glucose, also known as blood sugar. This is the energy your cells, tissues and organs require to operate. If you have any extra sugar in your body, it's conveniently stored in your liver and your muscles until you do need it.[38]

There are two kinds of carbs found in foods, simple and complex. Simple carbs are sugars, which are quickly broken down and absorbed into your body. They naturally occur in foods like fruits, vegetables and milk products, but you can find simple carbs in other places as well. Simple carbs also include any refined sugars, which may be added to processed foods such as white bread, baked goods, soda, candy and condiments like ketchup and barbeque sauce[39] You may be wondering why, since they both contain simple carbs, there's so much difference between eating a piece of fruit and a piece of fruit-flavored candy. Well, for starters, the candy is full of empty calories. It provides you with no additional nutrients your body needs. A piece of fruit may contain simple carbs, but it also contains vitamins, minerals and fiber. This makes it a much healthier option.

HIDDEN SUGAR

Are you trying to avoid eating excess sugar? Keep an eye out for these terms on food labels:

- Brown sugar
- Corn sweetener
- Corn syrup
- Dextrose
- Fructose
- Fruit juice concentrates
- Invert sugar
- Lactose
- Maltose
- Glucose
- High-fructose corn syrup
- Malt syrup
- Raw sugar
- Sucrose
- Syrup

Complex carbs, on the other hand, have a different chemical structure than their simpler counterpart. That's why it takes your body longer to digest a complex carb in your digestion. These carbs are found in foods like whole-grain breads and cereals, starchy vegetables and beans. What makes complex carbs such a great source of energy is that many of these foods are also excellent sources of fiber.[40]

Fiber is one of the great benefits of eating a plant-based diet because it satisfies your hunger without adding additional calories. This makes it possible for you to achieve and maintain a healthy weight. Basically, fiber is plant material that is impossible for your stomach to digest. Foods high in complex carbs such as beans, starchy vegetables and whole grains are also high in fiber.[41]

Fiber also has some great health benefits. Diets high in fiber are associated with lower serum cholesterol concentrations, lower risk of coronary heart disease, reduced blood pressure, enhanced weight control, better glycemic control, reduced risk of certain forms of cancer and improved gastrointestinal function.[42] In fact, eating a plant-based diet rich in fiber will give you the lowest risk of cancer possible.[43] Foods high in fiber also provide a slower rise in blood sugar, which means less insulin is required to process a meal.[44] Keeping your insulin levels from spiking is key to feeling less hungry, burning more fat and losing weight. Fiber-rich foods also slow the emptying of food from the stomach, which increases the absorption of simple sugars into the small intestine.[45]

Studies also support the benefits of a plant-based diet full of complex carbs and fiber for children. One study in New York City public schools changed the nutritional content of school lunches to a more wholesome, healthy diet. After just one year, the schools reported a 16 percent increase in academic performance and a 41 percent decrease in the number of learning-disabled children.[46]

You might be surprised to know that fruits and vegetables are also incredible promoters of harmonious living. In a study of 8,000 teenagers at nine juvenile correctional facilities, researchers arranged to have diets high in sugar and other refined carbohydrates replaced with diets high in fruits, vegetables and whole grains. During the year in which the diets were changed, violent and antisocial incidents in the institutions decreased by almost half.[47]

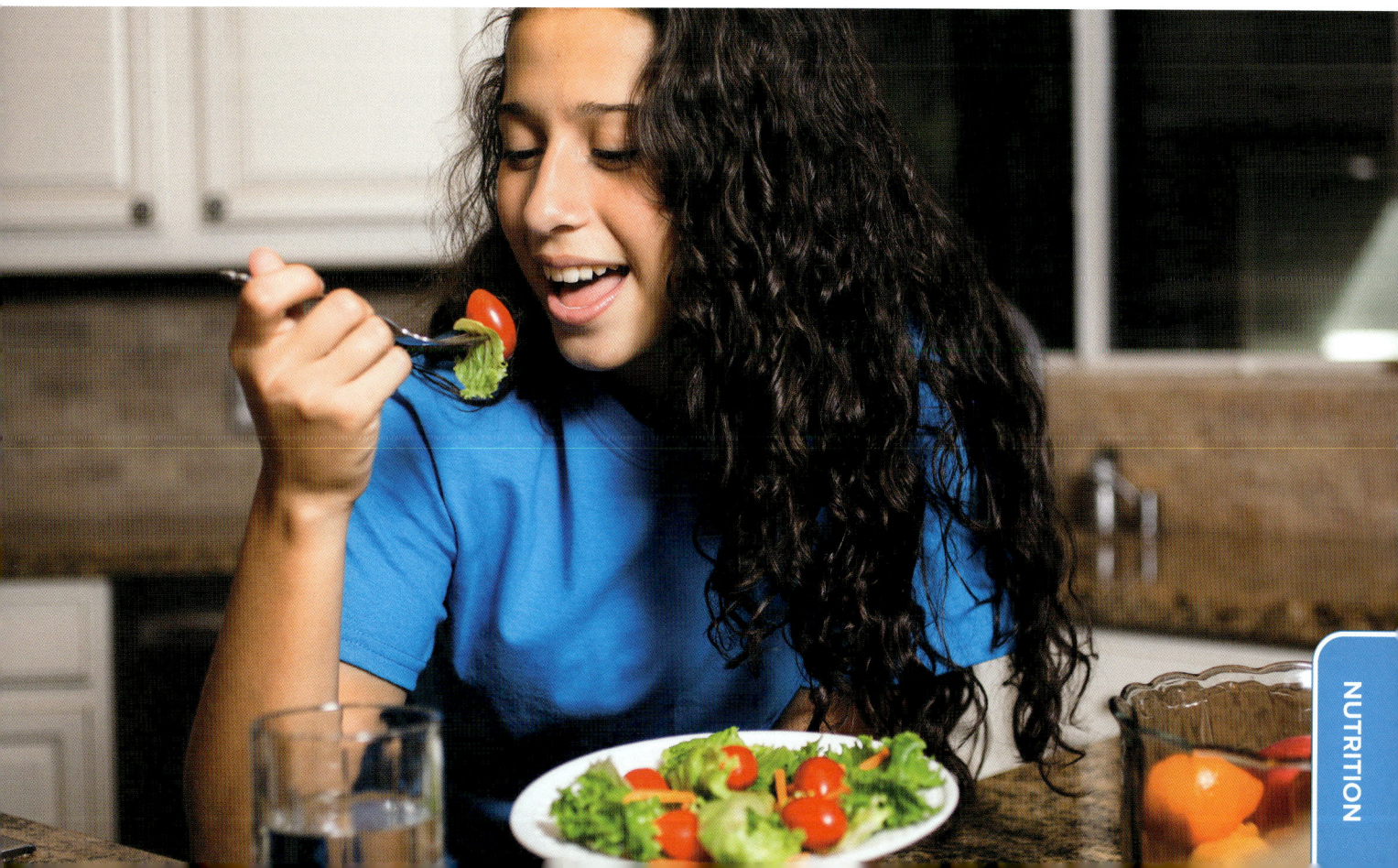

VITAMINS AND MINERALS

Vitamins and minerals are important substances your body needs to grow and develop normally. Each vitamin and mineral has a specific job to do, and when you don't get enough of a certain type, it creates a deficiency. For example, rickets is a disease in children characterized by a softening of the bones. It occurs when children have a Vitamin D deficiency. Usually, you can get all the vitamins and minerals you need from the foods you eat.[48]

These are the 13 vitamins your body needs:

- Vitamin A
- Vitamin C
- Vitamin D
- Vitamin E
- Vitamin K

And the B vitamins, including:

- Thiamine
- Riboflavin
- Niacin
- Pantothenic acid
- Biotin
- Vitamin B6
- Vitamin B12
- Folate

Minerals are divided into two types: macrominerals and trace minerals. You need macrominerals in larger amounts. These include:

- Calcium
- Phosphorus
- Magnesium
- Sodium
- Potassium
- Chloride
- Sulfur

Trace minerals are equally vital, but your body only needs small amounts of them. They include:

- Iron
- Manganese
- Copper
- Iodine
- Zinc
- Cobalt
- Fluoride
- Selenium[49]

Vegetarians may need to take a vitamin B12 supplement because plant-based foods do not typically provide this important nutrient.[50] According to the Office of Dietary Supplements, "Vitamin B12 deficiency causes tiredness, weakness, constipation, loss of appetite, weight loss and megaloblastic anemia. Nerve problems, such as numbness and tingling in the hands and feet, can also occur. Other symptoms of vitamin B12 deficiency include problems with balance, depression, confusion, dementia, poor memory and soreness of the mouth or tongue. Vitamin B12 deficiency can damage the nervous system even in people who don't have anemia, so it is important to treat a deficiency as soon as possible."[51]

If you follow a plant-based diet, make sure you are getting enough vitamin B12. According to the Office of Dietary Supplements:

- Teens 14 to 18 years should get 2.4 micrograms of vitamin B12 a day[52]

Another common deficiency among vegetarians is zinc. As a mineral, zinc is needed by your body to produce proteins and DNA. It's also used by your immune system to fight off bacteria and viruses. Zinc helps wounds to heal and is important for healthy senses of taste and smell.[53] Zinc deficiency causes slow growth in infants and children and delayed sexual development in adolescents. Zinc deficiency also causes hair loss, diarrhea, eye and skin sores and loss of appetite. Weight loss, problems with wound healing, decreased ability to taste food and lower alertness levels can also occur.[54]

While zinc deficiency is rare, vegetarians are more likely to have trouble getting enough in their diets. The foods they eat containing zinc (beans, whole grains, etc.) typically have compounds that keep the zinc from being fully absorbed by the body. Because of this, vegetarians might need to consume as much as 50 percent more zinc than the recommended amounts.[55]

According to the Office of Dietary Supplements, the average daily recommended amount of zinc is:

- Teen girls 14 to 18 years, 9 mcg a day
- Teen boys 14 to 18 years, 11 mcg a day[56]

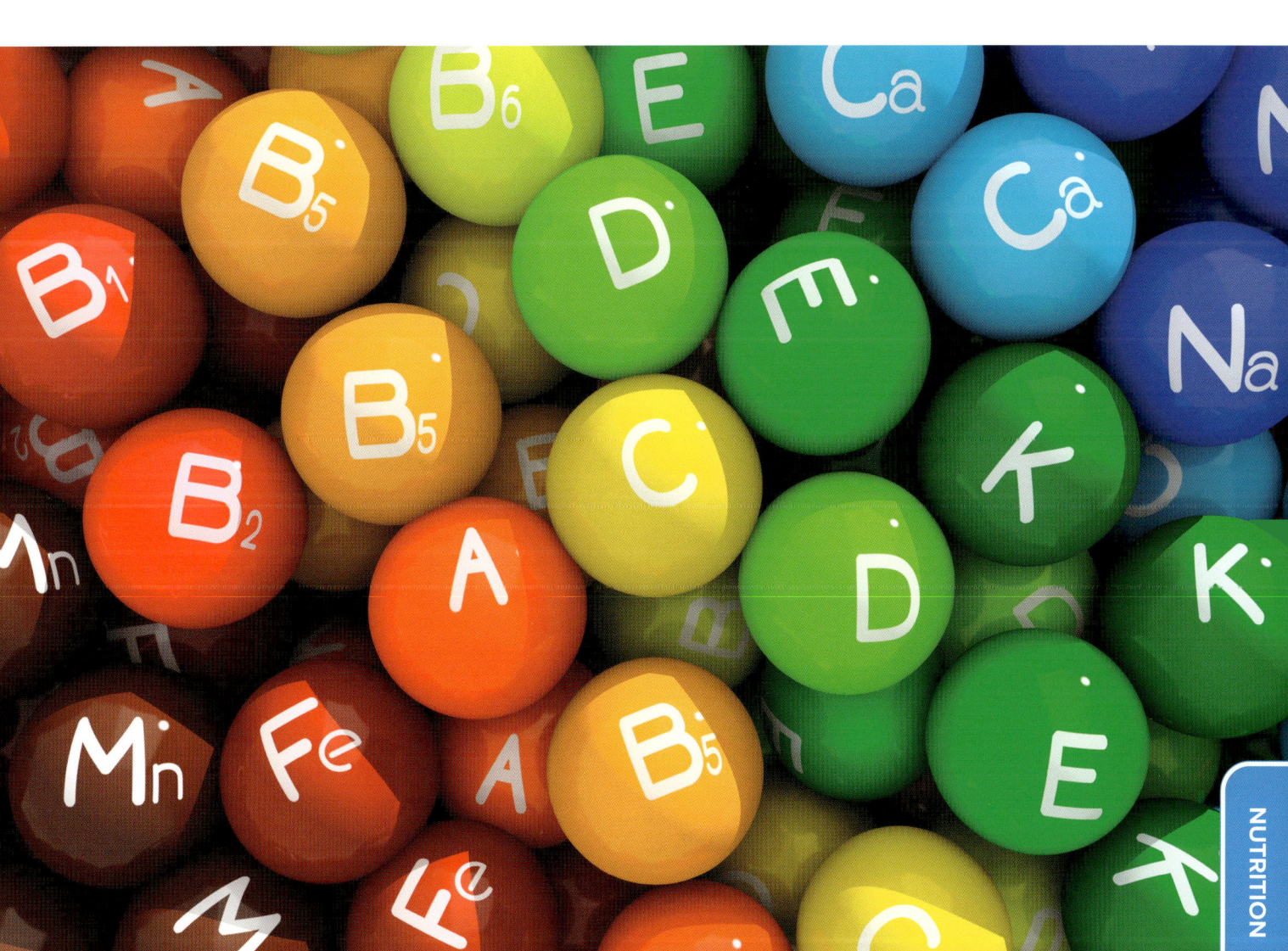

WHAT ABOUT DAIRY?

You are often told to drink milk and eat dairy products in order to get calcium, a valuable mineral your body needs in order to build strong teeth and healthy bones. However, research studies show that dairy foods may have negative effects on your health. You might be familiar with lactose intolerance in humans and the use of antibiotics and hormones in cows, but the problems go beyond that ranging from prostate cancer[57] to diabetes.[58] Cultures that consume the highest amount of milk and dairy products also have the highest rates of osteoporosis and hip fractures.[59] Osteoporosis is a bone disease where a decrease in bone mass and density leads to an increase in fractures. One study, which followed over 75,000 female nurses for 12 years, showed no protective effect of increased milk consumption on fracture risk for the women involved. In fact, the study found increased calcium intake might lead to a higher risk for fractures.[60]

A study published in Osteoporosis International conducted by the University Hospital in Lausanne, Switzerland, found that an overly acidic environment in the body created by too much dairy intake can result in calcium being leached out of the bones and set loose in the bloodstream. Excess calcium may then end up being deposited in joints and other tissues, creating problems that contribute to the development of arthritis.[61] Many doctors, nutritionists and researchers argue that dairy products (primarily cheese, ice cream, butter and milk) contribute significant amounts of fat and cholesterol to a diet, causing the growing rates of obesity, diabetes and heart disease in America. Dr. Dean Ornish is one of many physician-researchers who has shown that diets too high in fat are linked to the development of several chronic diseases, including heart disease, hypertension and high cholesterol.[62]

Lots of non-dairy, plant-based foods naturally contain calcium: leafy greens, broccoli and blackstrap molasses are all excellent sources.

WATER

What's not to love about water? It's wonderfully refreshing, calorie-free and overflowing with health benefits. All this makes perfect sense when you realize your body is mostly made of the stuff. Without food your body could survive for eight weeks, but without water you would only last three to five days. Why is this true? Research shows that all of the body's important chemical reactions take place in water, and it has a vital role in the absorption of nutrients, removal of waste, control of temperature and protection of body tissues, spinal cord and joints.[63] Water's part in many other physical functions is becoming better understood, and the effects of water shortage upon the body is being measured in terms of underperformance, disease and premature death.

If you don't drink enough water, you will soon suffer the effects of dehydration. Mild dehydration begins when you have lost only one or two percent of your total body fluids. In mild dehydration, your skin might appear flushed, dry and loose, with a loss of elasticity.[64-65] This is because your cells are drying up. If you have severely dry skin, it might be a smart move to put down the moisturizer and pick up a glass of water. Loss of skin elasticity is associated with aging as well.[56]

What is one simple thing you can do to improve your mental performance at school? Drink water. Even mild dehydration negatively affects your mental performance in a drastic way. If you are mildly dehydrated, you will experience light-headedness, dizziness, tiredness, irritability and headaches. You will also reduce your alertness and ability to concentrate.[67-69] At dehydration levels of more than two percent, people often report feeling more tired.[70]

For an example of how dehydration can affect your mental performance at school, consider the results of the following study. Researchers looked at the relationship between voluntary dehydration and cognitive performance in elementary school children ages 10 to 12 years in a small desert town in southern Israel. At the beginning of the day, they found no significant differences in mental performance between the hydrated children and dehydrated children. However, by midday the hydrated group performed better in four of five cognitive tests compared to the dehydrated group, especially on a short-term memory task.[71] By staying hydrated when you're at school, you will not only improve your concentration levels, but you will also feel less tired and lethargic. This makes the reusable water bottle the new accessory of choice for school-age children, but staying hydrated has other long-term health benefits as well.

Maintaining good levels of hydration is reported to decrease the risk of fatal coronary heart disease by 46 percent in men and 59 percent in women.[72] Research has also found that drinking water helps you to lose weight regardless of your diet or activity level.[73] By drinking water 15 to 30 minutes before a meal, you will experience a "full" sensation and will consume fewer calories. This is true for both obese[74] and normal weight individuals.[75] A population study of water and food intake in the United States found those who drink water regularly consume nine percent fewer calories than those who do not.[76]

> **?** Are you getting enough water every day? What are some practical ways to get yourself into the habit of drinking more water?

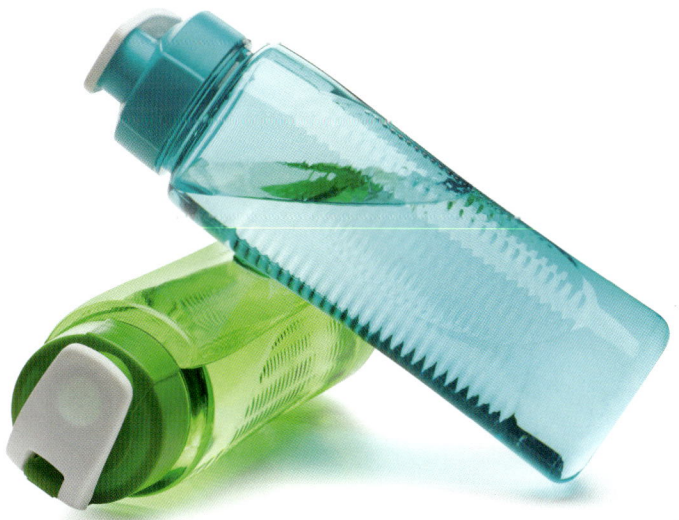

The bottom line is that many people are dehydrated and do not have enough fluid in their systems for the best health. Dehydration makes the blood thicker and more likely to clot, increasing the risk of strokes and heart attacks. One epidemiologic study demonstrated that heart attack risk decreased about 50 percent in people who drank at least five cups of water a day.[77] However, this does not apply to drinking sodas, fruit juice and milk products. Since water is necessary for waste removal through the kidneys, chronic dehydration may cause damage to these vital organs as well.

So, what are you waiting for? Staying well hydrated will not only help your body to function better, it will also keep you mentally alert, help you fight off disease and avoid unwanted weight gain. Of course, like all good things, it is possible to overdo it when it comes to drinking water. If you drink too much, you could wash away your body's sodium, a process called water intoxication. Sodium is a necessary element for your body to function properly. Low levels of sodium can lead to fatigue and even dangerous heart and brain dysfunction, but this is a very rare condition. Most people simply aren't getting enough water. It is recommended that teenagers, 13 or older, drink eight to 10 glasses a day.[78] Of course, if you live in a hot or dry area or if you are doing a lot of heavy work or exercise that causes you to sweat, you should drink even more. Water is absorbed fastest when taken on an empty stomach. Food and sugar slow down the absorption; this means sports drinks, energy drinks or even fruit juices are not as good as water when it comes to quick hydration. Also, if you are exercising at least a couple of hours after a meal, cool water will absorb faster than warm water. Remember, a well-hydrated athlete or worker has much better endurance than a dehydrated one.

How do you know if you're drinking enough water? Look at your urine. It may sound gross, but this is actually one of the best ways to know if you are getting enough water. When your urine is a light straw color, then you are good to go. The darker in color it is, the more water you need to drink.

ALCOHOL

Wine is a mocker and beer a brawler;
whoever is led astray by them is not wise.

PROVERBS 20:1

"Alcohol is the drug of choice among youth," says the National Institute of Alcohol and Alcohol Abuse. "Many young people are experiencing the consequences of drinking too much, at too early an age. As a result, underage drinking is a leading public health problem in this country."[79]

Every year, almost 5,000 young people under the age of 21 die as a result of underage drinking.[80] A mind clouded with alcohol might also make some very unwise or unhealthy choices, which could lead to serious injury or regret.

Because alcohol dulls your senses, it makes it even more difficult to make proper and wise choices. Additionally, research has shown that alcohol is unhealthy to the human body. It hurts the development of your brain, damages your liver and "may upset the critical hormonal balance necessary for normal development of organs, muscles and bones."[81]

Don't be fooled by the empty promises of alcohol. Choose a wise and healthy path by pledging to remain free from the negative effects of alcohol abuse.

"He who cures a disease may be the skillfullest, but he that prevents it is the safest physician."

THOMAS FULLER

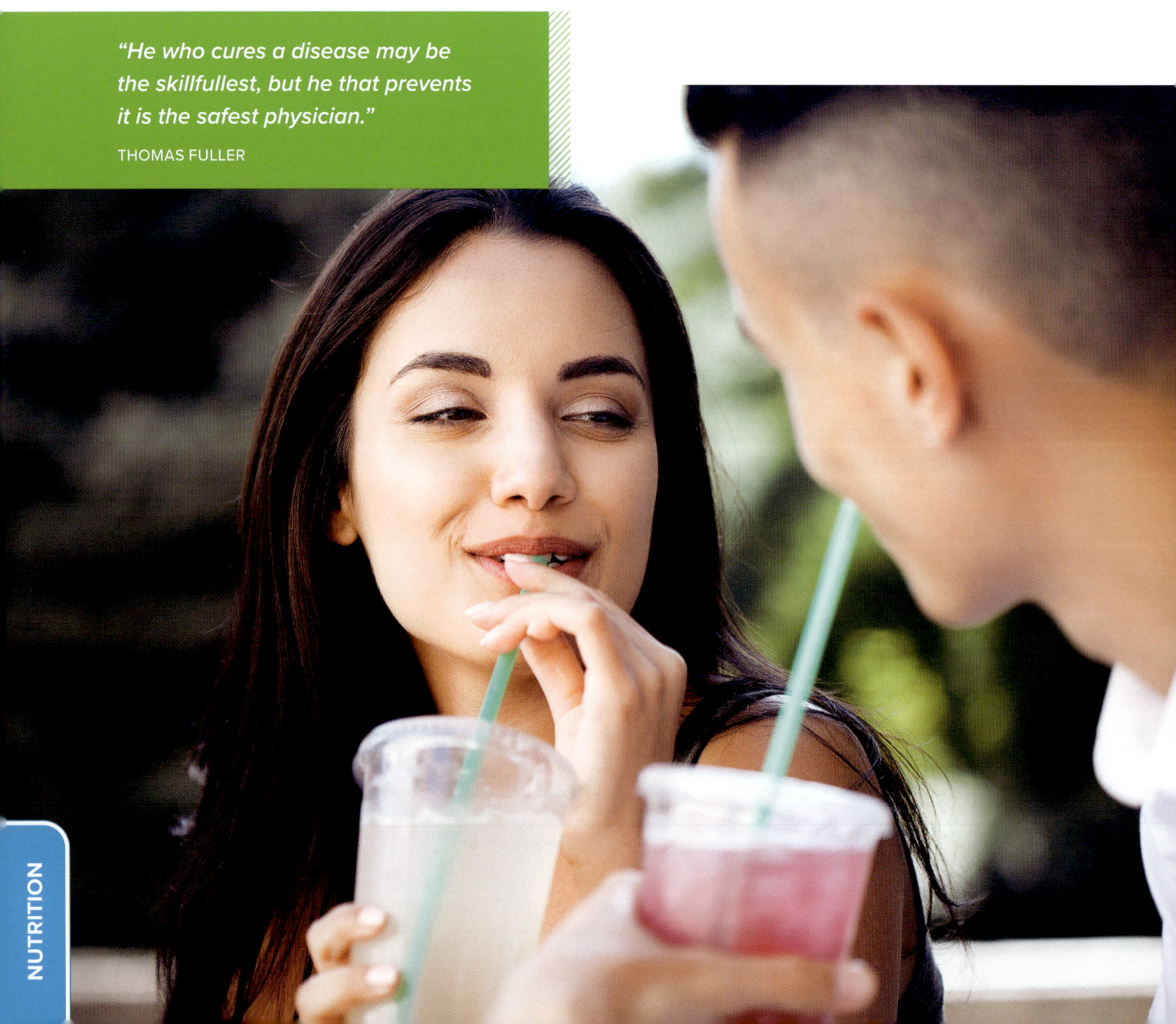

NUTRITION

THE ORIGINAL FAST FOODS

Want a food that's fast, easy to find and readily available at a moment's notice? Look no further than the produce section at your grocery store. Fruits and vegetables are the original fast foods, full of fiber, nutrients and available in their own colorful packaging. In fact, it's these vibrant colors that make fruits and veggies so good for you.

Chemicals called flavonoids create the incredible colors of fruits and vegetables. Flavonoids are found in practically all plants. This is a good thing because science has discovered these chemicals are amazing promoters of health. You can tell what nutrients are in a plant just by looking at the color. For example, purple, red and blue fruits or vegetables are rich in phytochemicals called anthocyanins. Anthocyanins help get rid of free-radical damage in the body and the brain. This makes them powerful disease fighters. Orange, yellow and green vegetables are rich in carotenoids, which help diminish the effects of stress.[82] So, eat your fruits and vegetables in a rainbow of colors every day.

Fruits and vegetables can also be lifesavers. The World Health Organization states that up to 2.7 million lives could be saved annually if people consumed sufficient fruits and vegetables. Low fruit and vegetable intake is among the top 10 risk factors attributable to early mortality, according to evidence presented in the *2002 World Health Report*.[83]

One fruit that has received great attention is the grape. Much of this attention has come from the apparent positive effects that drinking wine has on heart disease. Of course, you're not old enough to buy alcohol yet, and even if you were there are several damaging effects it can have on your body such as addiction, cirrhosis of the liver and an increased risk of cancers. But the good news is that beneficial flavonoids that fight heart disease are found in the grape itself. By drinking grape juice, you can get the same benefits from the grapes and avoid the problems associated with alcohol. A study published in *The Lancet* found that high intakes of flavonoids predicted lower mortality from coronary heart disease and lower incidence of heart attacks.[84]

Maybe you've heard the old saying, "An apple a day keeps the doctor away." Well, recent research shows that this saying is more fact than just wishful thinking. Apples are packed with fiber and flavonoids. These two heavy hitters of nutrition give the humble apple a powerful ability to keep you healthy in all kinds of circumstances. A meta-analysis of over eighty-five studies found that regularly eating apples is the strongest association with a reduced risk of cancer, heart disease, asthma and type 2 diabetes when compared to other fruits and vegetables. Additionally, apple intake was associated with increased lung function and weight loss.[85]

Yet another reason apples are so good for you is they are an excellent source of antioxidants. You may remember that antioxidants remove potentially damaging oxidizing agents from your body and are believed to play a vital role in preventing several life-threatening diseases. When compared to other commonly consumed fruits in the United States, apples were found to have the second highest level of antioxidant activity. Only the humble cranberry has more.[86]

When eating an apple or any fruit with an edible peel, it's always best to eat the whole fruit. You will lose a ton of fiber and valuable nutrients if you peel your fruits.

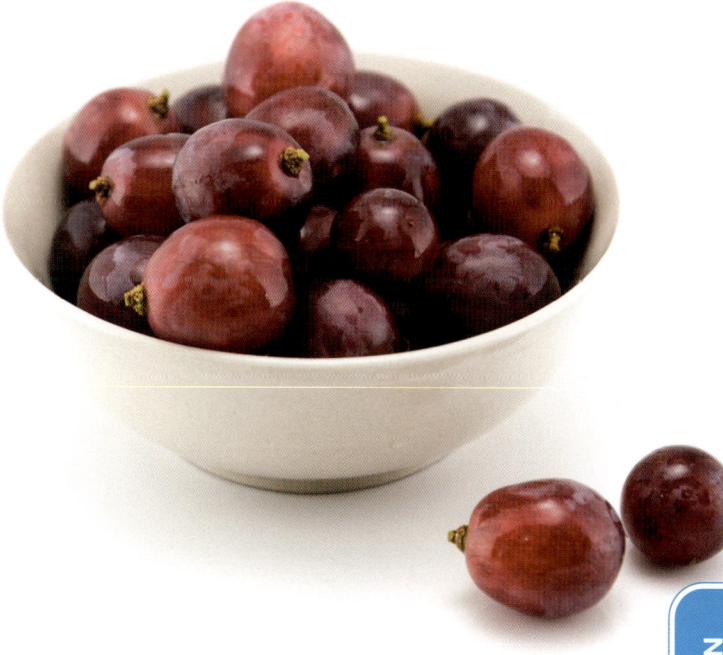

KNOW WHAT YOU'RE EATING

If you are trying to eat healthy, then it's important you learn how to read and understand the nutritional information found on food labels. After all, how can you make a healthy food choice unless you first know what to look for? You can use the Nutrition Facts label located on most foods when you are planning a meal or shopping at the grocery store. Many restaurants also have nutritional information available, which comes in handy the next time you're dining out. By using the label, you'll be able to see the amounts of nutrients you'll be getting in each serving. You'll also be able to compare different food items to see if a better choice is available.

The following guidelines for reading the Nutrition Facts Label are provided by the USDA and the U.S. Department of Health and Human Services:

Check the number and size of servings.

- The Nutrition Facts label information is based on one serving, but many packages contain more. Look at the serving size and how many servings you are actually consuming. If you double the servings you eat, you double the calories and nutrients, including the percent daily value (DVs).

- When you compare calories and nutrients between brands, check to see if the serving size is the same.

Pay attention to calories.

- This is where you'll find the number of calories per serving and the calories from fat in each serving.

- Fat-free doesn't mean calorie-free. Lower fat items may have as many calories as full-fat versions.

- If the label lists that one serving equals three cookies and 100 calories, and you eat six cookies, you've eaten two servings, or twice the number of calories and fat.

Look for foods that are rich in vitamin A, vitamin C, calcium and liron.

- Use the label not only to limit fat and sodium, but also to increase nutrients that promote good health and may protect you from disease.

- Some Americans don't get enough vitamins A and C, potassium, calcium and iron, so choose the brand with the higher percent DV for these nutrients.

- Get the most nutrition for your calories — compare the calories to the nutrients you would be getting to make a healthier food choice.

Know your fats and reduce sodium for your health.

- To help reduce your risk of heart disease, use the label to select foods that are lowest in saturated fat, trans fat and cholesterol.

- Trans fat doesn't have a percent DV, but consume as little as possible because it increases your risk of heart disease.

- The percent DV for total fat includes all different kinds of fats.

- To help lower blood cholesterol, replace saturated and trans fats with monounsaturated and polyunsaturated fats found in fish, nuts and liquid vegetable oils.

- Limit sodium to help reduce your risk of high blood pressure.

Reach for healthy, wholesome carbohydrates.

- Fiber and sugars are types of carbo-hydrates. Healthy sources, like fruits, vegetables, beans and whole grains, can reduce the risk of heart disease and improve digestive functioning.

- Whole grain foods can't always be identified by color or name, such as multigrain or wheat. Look for the "whole" grain listed first in the ingredient list, such as whole wheat, brown rice or whole oats.

- There isn't a percent DV for sugar, but you can compare the sugar content in grams among products.

- Limit foods with added sugars (sucrose, glucose, fructose, corn syrup) that add calories but not other nutrients, such as vitamins and minerals. Make sure that added sugars are not one of the first few items in the ingredients list.

Choose proteins that are lower in fat.

- Most Americans get plenty of protein, but not always from the healthiest sources.

- When choosing a food for its protein content, make choices that are lean, low-fat or fat-free.

Know your daily percent value.

- The percent DV is a general guide to help you link nutrients in a serving of food to their contribution to your total daily diet. It can help you determine if a food is high or low in a nutrient — five percent or less is low, 20 percent or more is high. You can use the percent DV to make dietary trade-offs with other foods throughout the day. The * is a reminder that the percent DV is based on a 2,000-calorie diet. You may need more or less, but the percent DV is still a helpful gauge.[87]

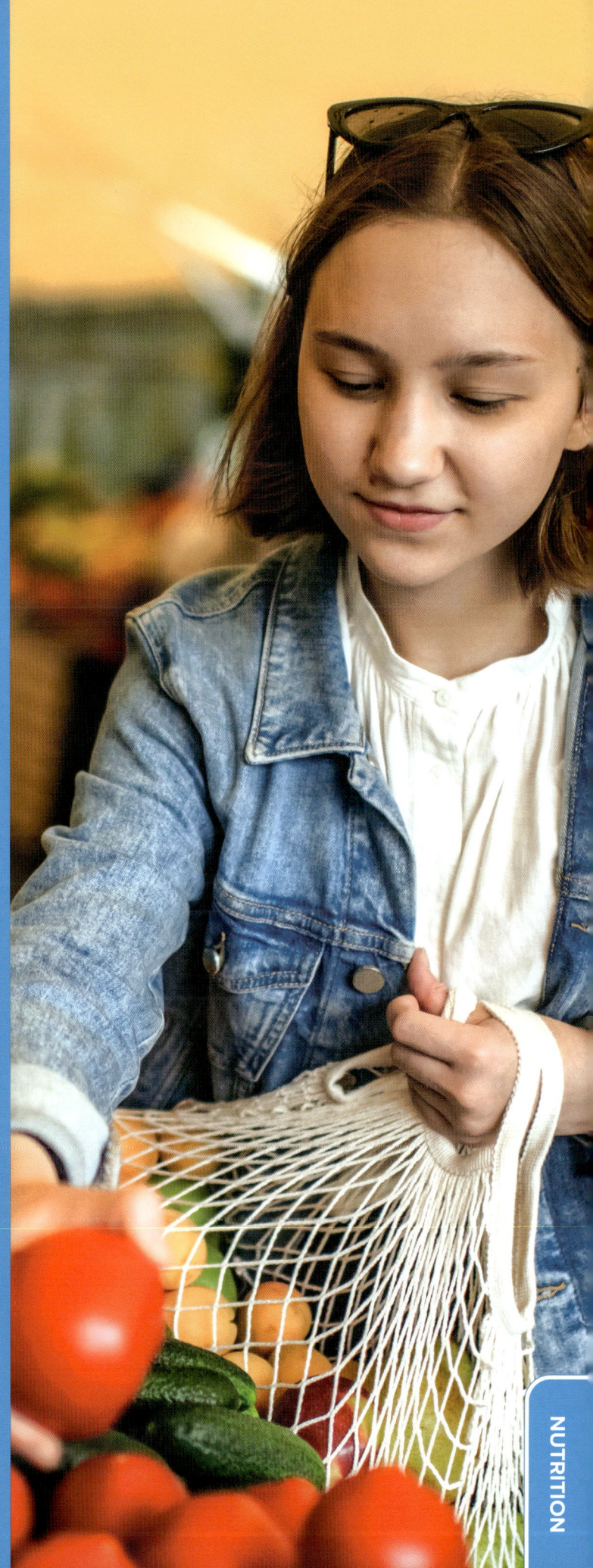

NUTRITION

SEEDS

Want a food that's small, light and bursting with great health benefits? Consider the tiny seed. Like nuts, most people limit seeds to snack status or to sprinkle on top of nutritionally void baked goods, but making these nutritional wonders a regular part of your diet will benefit you in many incredible ways. For starters, seeds are like eggs in the plant world. Inside each one are the essential nutrients needed to nourish a new baby pant.

For example, sesame seeds are a fantastic source of bone-building calcium. In fact, one-quarter cup of unhulled sesame seeds has more calcium than a cup of milk. This is great news if you are lactose intolerant or if you are trying to cut dairy from your diet due to other health concerns.

Flax seeds are another nutritional powerhouse. They are chock full of omega-3 fatty acids, antioxidants and fiber — all of which your body needs. Here's the thing, though: you have to grind up flax seeds in order to get the most benefits from eating them. If you eat them whole, the seeds will simply pass through your intestinal tract without releasing the beneficial nutrients contained within.[88] However, once they are ground, flax seeds have the potential to help with a number of problems such as heart disease,[89] cancer,[90] high cholesterol,[91-92] blood pressure,[93] diabetes,[94] ADHD,[95] memory loss,[96] weight problems,[97] acne[98] and even PMS.[99] Flax seed oil also contains the same essential fatty acids as ground flax seeds and has been shown to bring significant improvements to people suffering from symptoms caused by depression.[100]

Try adding freshly ground flax seed to your diet. You can sprinkle it on cereal, put it in baked goods or add it to your morning smoothie. A coffee or spice grinder is a great and inexpensive tool to grind whole flax seeds. Be sure to keep ground flax seed refrigerated and sealed in a dark, airtight container or else it could become rancid. You can store it even longer in the freezer. It is also recommended you limit your intake to no more than one or two tablespoons of ground flax seed per day. Flax seeds naturally contain small amounts of cyanide, but don't worry; many other foods such as almonds, spinach and lima beans all contain small amounts of naturally occurring cyanide. Eating one to two tablespoons of ground flax seed a day will not cause any problems and will still provide your body with all the necessary fiber and fatty acids it needs.

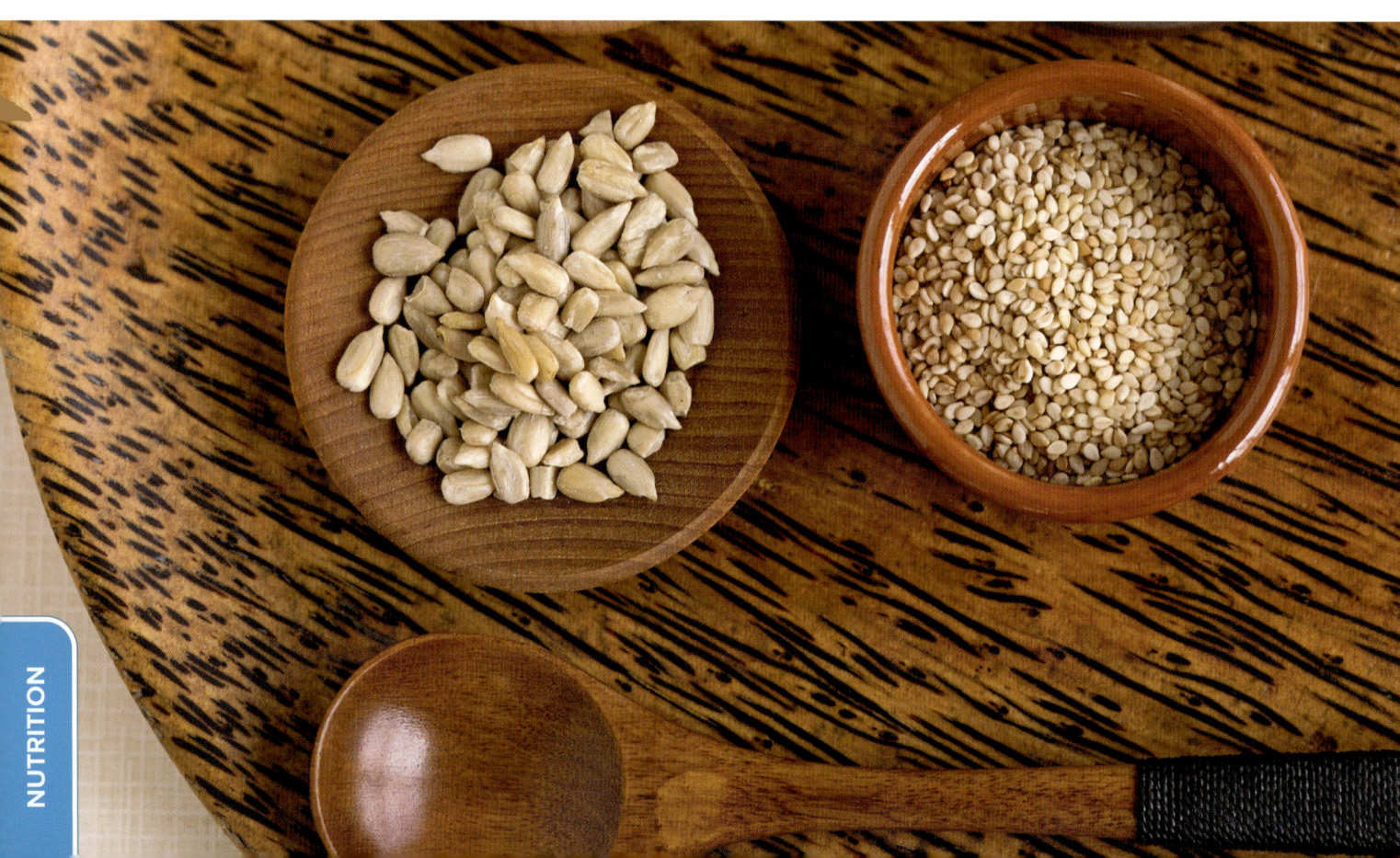

BEANS AND WHOLE GRAINS

Okay, let's face it; beans have a certain... how should we say this... bad reputation. People have long associated eating beans with intestinal gas, or as it's more technically known — flatus. The results of this can either be very embarrassing or absolutely hilarious depending on your maturity level. It's a shame beans have been reduced to middle school jokes and lowbrow humor because when you get down to it, they are actually a very nutritious food packed with some key health benefits.

Beans, or "legumes" as they are often called, are low in calories and fat and are a great source of fiber and folate. Folate is a B vitamin your body uses for a number of things including cell production. Since your body doesn't naturally produce folate, you have to get it from your diet. Beans also contain large amounts of complex carbohydrates and are a wonderful source of protein. In fact, beans typically have the same amounts of protein per serving as most meats minus the saturated fats and cholesterol. This is what makes beans an excellent addition to many meatless dishes such as vegetarian chili.

Beans come in all colors, shapes, sizes and flavors, and they can help you eat less throughout the day. Adding a few beans at breakfast means you won't be so hungry at lunch. Beans are great at helping your body maintain a steady supply of energy throughout the day. Eating beans can also reduce your risk of heart disease, strokes and cancer.[101-102] One study found that eating more pinto beans lowered LDL, or "bad" cholesterol levels, which should reduce the risk of heart disease.[103] Another study found that drinking soy milk more than once a day decreased the risk of prostate cancer by an amazing 70 percent.[104] Beans also make an ideal food for diabetics because their low glycemic index value means they won't cause a sudden increase in blood sugar levels.

BETTER BEANS

Despite all these nutritional benefits, some people still turn up their noses at beans just because of the gas they produce. To understand why this happens, you have to know something about your digestive system. As your body breaks down the foods you eat into usable energy, gases are often released. It's a natural part of digestion. You also swallow air that can build up in your intestines. At some point, all this gas and air has to go somewhere, so if you find you have a problem digesting beans, consider these options:

- Canned beans are quick, easy and often treated in such a way to minimize the problem of gas. You can easily add canned beans to soups, salads or use them in a variety of other recipes.

- Preparing your own beans at home can also minimize the gas-forming elements. Bring a pot of beans to boil and then let them sit overnight. The next morning, pour off the water and replace it with fresh water. The majority of gas-causing substances will float off with the original water. Return the beans to a simmer and complete the cooking process.

- Several natural products are available that can minimize the problem of excessive gas. These are naturally derived enzymes that help your body break down the complex sugars in beans into more digestible simple sugars. You can find them at almost any supermarket or drugstore.

20 POWER TIPS FOR NUTRITION

1. **Focus on the positive.** Add wholesome, healthy foods to what you already eat, and pretty soon your unhealthy choices will disappear. Make a choice to think about your food positively and you will succeed at having a healthy, nutritious diet.

2. **Don't think of mealtime as a chore.** God has given you many different foods to experience and savor. Meals can be a great source of joy in your life when you follow God's standard for living.

3. **Don't eat when you aren't hungry.** Pay attention to God-given internal signals to determine when and how much to eat.

4. **Eat a plant-based diet.** God's diet given in the Garden of Eden gives you the most nutrient-rich foods with the most benefits to your health and well-being.

5. **Experiment and have fun.** Enjoy something new on a regular basis, or try something you like prepared a different way. Don't be afraid to experiment with recipes and tweak them to your specifications.

6. **Color your diet.** Different colors on your plate means different nutrients are present. Make it a goal to eat more than five colorful fruits and vegetables a day.

7. **Reach for whole foods and remember.** Important nutrients and fiber are found in the skins of many foods. Whole grains are one of the foundational whole-food choices.

8. **Pay attention to the fats you are consuming.** Replace bad fats with fats such as those found in nuts, seeds and avocados. Include healthy oils such as olive oil, and avoid partially hydrogenated oils (trans fats) and saturated fats. Remember that moderation is the key. Even good fats have lots of calories and if taken in large amounts can lead to weight gain.

9. **Experiment with natural sweeteners.** Sugar adds extra calories and has a negative effect on your brain function and immune system. Limit the amount of sugar in your diet. For example, dried fruit sprinkled on top of your morning oatmeal makes a much more nutritious choice than sugar. Read labels and educate yourself on what sweeteners are in your food.

10. **Don't get caught up in the latest craze or diet fad.** Choose to eat sensibly and responsibly.

11. **Eat nuts and seeds daily.** Their powerful nutrients fight disease.

12. **Don't be afraid to try new things.** You can learn to like healthier foods; you just need to give yourself time to adjust. Try adding spinach or another leafy green to a morning fruit smoothie for a nutritional punch.

13. **Turn a dull meal into an exciting one with herbs and spices.** Try experimenting with them in recipes for wonderful flavor options and nutrients.

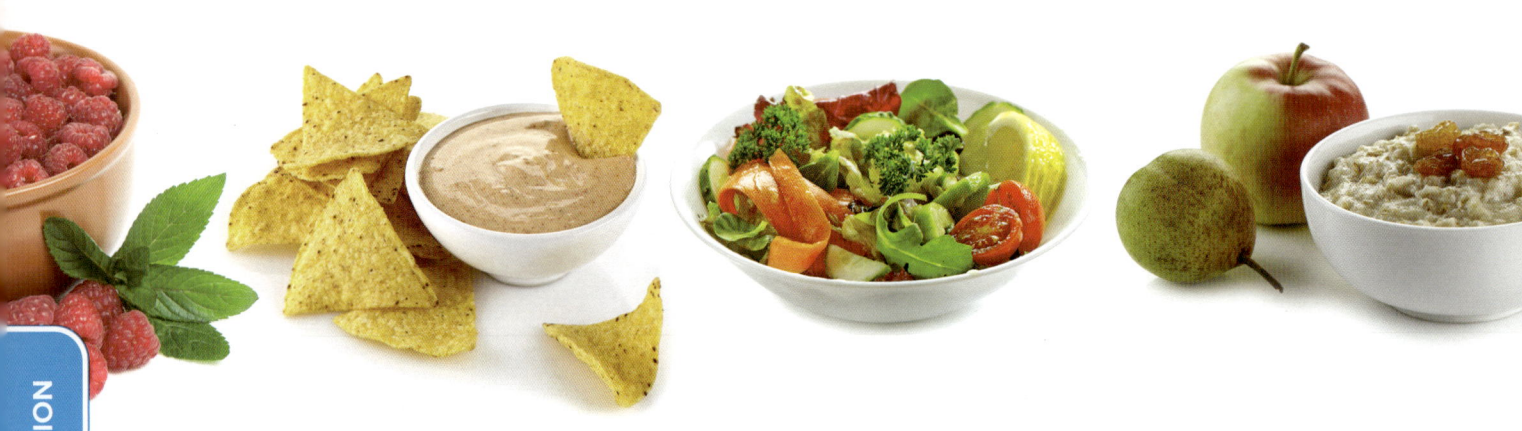

14. **Get back to the basics.** Foods with less processing and fewer ingredients are generally the healthiest for you. It is a good rule of thumb that the fewer the ingredients on the label, the better for you the product is likely to be.

15. **Buy produce grown locally.** Fresh fruits and vegetables have more nutritional content.

16. **Drink pure water.** The health benefits are many.

17. **Start each day with a powerful breakfast.** Eat a well-balanced, healthy breakfast for benefits that will last the whole day.

18. **Plan your meals ahead of time.** This not only saves you time; it reduces the stress of waiting till the last minute.

19. **Make dining out healthy.** Substitute salad or steamed vegetables for french fries or heavy side dishes.

20. **Consider applesauce.** Substitute applesauce for the oil in baked goods for a healthier option.

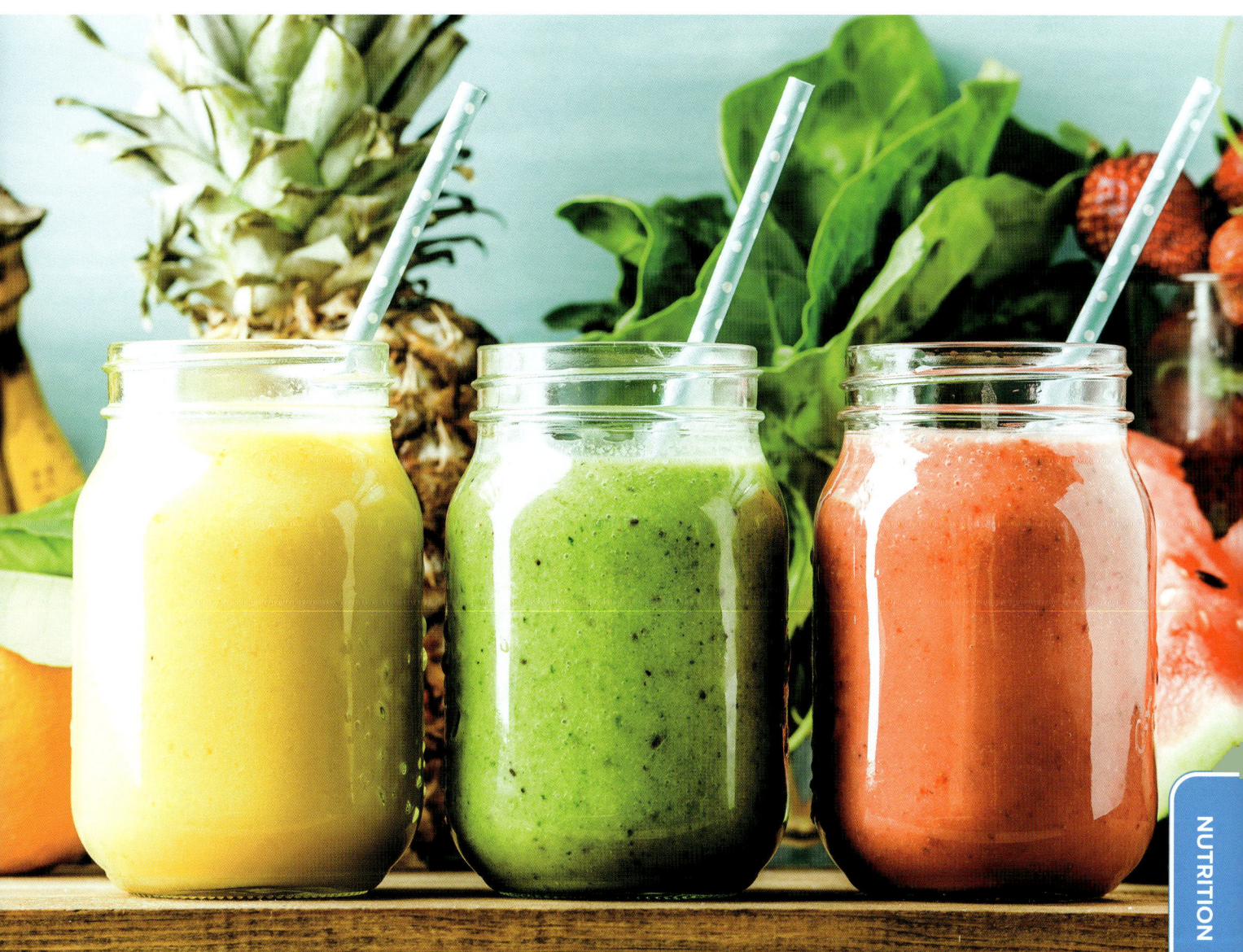

REFERENCES

1. Willett, Walter C. "Diet and Health: What Should We Eat?" *Science* 264, no. 5158 (1994): 532-537. https://doi.org/10.1126/science.8160011.

2. Data Resource Center for Child & Adolescent Health. "2016 National Survey of Children's Health." Accessed July 12, 2018. http://www.childhealthdata.org/browse/survey/results?q=4568&r=1.

3. Larimore, Walt. "The Obesity Crisis: It's a Killer Epidemic." All Pro Dad. Accessed September 17, 2018. https://www.allprodad.com/the-obesity-crisis-its-a-killer-epidemic/.

4. National Kidney Foundation. "High Blood Pressure and Kidney in Children." Accessed October 2, 2018. https://www.kidney.org/atoz/content/hbpchildren.

5. Larimore, Walter L., Sherri Flynt, and Steve Halliday. *Super Sized Kids: How to Rescue Your Child From the Obesity Threat.* New York: Center Street Publishing, 2005.

6. Zhao, Bin, Adeline Seow, Edmund J. D. Lee, Wee-Teng Poh, Ming Teh, Philip Eng, Yee-Tang Wang, Wan-Cheng Tan, Mimi C. Yu, and Hin-Peng Lee. "Dietary Isothiocyanates, Glutathione S-transferase -M1, -T1 Polymorphisms and Lung Cancer Risk among Chinese Women in Singapore." *Cancer Epidemiology, Biomarkers & Prevention: A Publication of the American Association for Cancer Research, Cosponsored by the American Society of Preventive Oncology* 10, no. 10 (2001): 1063-1067. http://cebp.aacrjournals.org/content/10/10/1063.

7. Choose My Plate. "What Are Empty Calories?" Accessed July 10, 2018. http://district.schoolnutritionandfitness.com/simplifiedculinaryservices/files/Wellness/What_Are_Empty_Calories_ChooseMyplate.pdf.

8. Ibid.

9. Beck, Jen. "How Many Empty Calories Can Be Part of a Healthy Diet?" Complete Health Revolution. August 29, 2015. https://www.completehealthrevolution.com/how-many-empty-calories-can-be-part-of-a-healthy-diet/.

10. UC Davis Health. "Researchers Find Breakfast Critical to Performance." Last modified September 19, 1995. https://www.ucdmc.ucdavis.edu/publish/news/newsroom/3052.

11. Belloc, Nedra B. and Lester Breslow. "Relationship of Physical Health Status and Health Practices." *Preventive Medicine* 1, no. 3 (1972): 409-421. https://doi.org/10.1016/0091-7435(72)90014-X.

12. Aubrey, Allison. "A Better Breakfast Can Boost a Child's Brainpower." NPR. September 4, 2006. http://www.npr.org/templates/story/story.php?storyId=5738848.

13. Ibid.

14. Slavin, Joanne L., David Jacobs, Len Marquart, and Kathy Wiemer. "The Role of Whole Grains in Disease Prevention." *Journal of the American Dietetic Association* 101, no. 7 (2001): 780-785. https://doi.org/10.1016/S0002-8223(01)00194-8.

15. MedlinePlus. "Dietary Fats Explained." Accessed July 10, 2018. https://medlineplus.gov/ency/patientinstructions/000104.htm.

16. Healthy Kids. "Facts About Fats." Accessed September 21, 2018. https://www.healthykids.nsw.gov.au/recipes/facts-about-fats.

17. Hu, Frank B., Eric B. Rimm, Meir J. Stampfer, Alberto Ascherio, Donna Spiegelman, and Walter C. Willett. "Prospective Study of Major Dietary Patterns and Risk of Coronary Heart Disease in Men." *The American Journal of Clinical Nutrition* 72, no. 4 (2000): 912-921. https://doi.org/10.1093/ajcn/72.4.912.

18. Kaartinen, K., K. Lammi, M. Hypen, M. Nenonen, O. Hänninen, and A. L. Rauma. "Vegan Diet Alleviates Fibromyalgia Symptoms." *Scandinavian Journal of Rheumatology* 29, no. 5 (2000): 308-313. https://doi.org/10.1080/030097400447697.

19. MedlinePlus. "Dietary Facts." Accessed July 10, 2018. http://www.nlm.nih.gov/medlineplus/dietaryfats.html.

20. Colquhoun D. M., D. Moores, S. M. Somerset, and J. A. Humphries. "Comparison of the Effects on Lipoproteins and Apolipoproteins of a Diet High in Monounsaturated Fatty Acids, Enriched with Avocado, and a High-Carbohydrate Diet." *The American Journal of Clinical Nutrition* 56, no. 4 (1992): 671-677. https://doi.org/10.1093/ajcn/56.4.671.

21. Fraser, Gary. E., J. Sabate, W. L. Beeson, and T. M. Strahan. "A Possible Protective Effect of Nut Consumption on Risk of Coronary Heart Disease: the Adventist Health Study." *Archives of Internal Medicine* 152, no. 7 (1992): 1416-1424. https://doi.org/10.1001/archinte.1992.00400190054010.

22. Morris, M. C., D. A. Evans, J. L. Bienias, C. C. Tangney, D. A. Bennett, N. Aggarwal, R. S. Wilson, and P. A. Scheer. "Dietary Intake of Antioxidant Nutrients and the Risk of Incident Alzheimer Disease in a Biracial Community Study." *Journal of the American Medical Association* 287, no. 24 (2002): 3230-3237. http://doi.org/10.1001/jama.287.24.3230.

23. Engelhart, Marianne J., M. I. Geerlings, A. Ruitenberg, et al. "Dietary Intake of Antioxidants and Risk of Alzheimer Disease." *Journal of the American Medical Association* 287, no. 24 (2002): 3223-3229. https://doi.org/10.1001/jama.287.24.3223.

24. Burgess, John R., Laura Stevens, Wen Zhang, and Louise Peck. "Long-Chain Polyunsaturated Fatty Acids in Children with Attention-Deficit Hyperactivity Disorder." *The American Journal of Clinical Nutrition* 71, no. 1 (2000): 327S-330S. https://doi.org/10.1093/ajcn/71.1.327S.

25. ENT Associates. "What is Food Allergy?" Accessed July 11, 2018. http://entflorida.com/what-is-food-allergy/.

26. Ibid.

27. Ibid.

28. Ibid.

29. Ibid.

30. Haley, Mildred and Kim A. Ha. *Livestock, Dairy, and Poultry Outlook*. Ithica: 2018. Accessed September 17, 2018. https://www.ers.usda.gov/webdocs/publications/88516/ldp-m-286.pdf?v=43206.

31. Mayo Clinic. "Meatless Meals: The Benefits of Eating Less Meat." Accessed July 10, 2018. http://www.mayoclinic.com/health/meatless-meals/my00752.

32. MedlinePlus. "Dietary Proteins." Last modified January 31, 2018. https://medlineplus.gov/dietaryproteins.html.

33. Centers for Disease Control and Prevention. "Protein." Last modified October 2, 2013. http://comenius.susqu.edu/biol/010/tobin-janzen/nutrition%20for%20everyone_%20basics_%20protein%20_%20dnpao%20_%20cdc.pdf.

34. MedlinePlus. "Dietary Proteins." Last modified January 31, 2018. https://medlineplus.gov/dietaryproteins.html.

35. Centers for Disease Control and Prevention. "Protein." Last modified October 2, 2013. http://comenius.susqu.edu/biol/010/tobin-janzen/nutrition%20for%20everyone_%20basics_%20protein%20_%20dnpao%20_%20cdc.pdf.

36. Choose My Plate. "10 Tips: Healthy Eating for Vegetarians." Last modified July 25, 2017. http://www.choosemyplate.gov/healthy-eating-tips/tips-for-vegetarian.html.

37. MedlinePlus. "Carbohydrates." Accessed July 10, 2018. https://medlineplus.gov/carbohydrates.html.

38. Ibid.

39. Ibid.

40. Ibid.

41. MedlinePlus. "Carbohydrates: MedlinePlus Medical Encyclopedia." https://medlineplus.gov/ency/article/002469.htm.

42. Schneeman, Barbara O. "Dietary Fiber and Gastrointestinal Function." *Nutrition Reviews* 45, no. 7 (1987): 129-132. https://doi.org/10.1111/j.1753-4887.1987.tb06343.x.

43. Colditz, G. A., K. A. Atwood, K. Emmons, R. R. Monson, W. C. Willett, D. Trichopoulos, and D. J. Hunter. "Harvard Report on Cancer Prevention Volume 4: Harvard Cancer Risk Index." *Cancer Causes & Control* 11, no. 6 (2000): 477-488. https://doi.org/10.1023/A:1008984432272.

44. Tabatabai, A. and S. Li. "Dietary Fiber and Type 2 Diabetes." *Clinical Excellence for Nurse Practitioners: The International Journal of NPACE* 4, no. 5 (2000): 272-276. https://doi.org/10.1111/j.1753-4887.1987.tb06343.x.

45. Colditz, G. A., K. A. Atwood, K. Emmons, R. R. Monson, W. C. Willett, D. Trichopoulos, and D. J. Hunter. "Harvard Report on Cancer Prevention Volume 4: Harvard Cancer Risk Index." *Cancer Causes & Control* 11, no. 6 (2000): 477-488. https://doi.org/10.1023/A:1008984432272.

46. Tabatabai, A. and S. Li. "Dietary Fiber and Type 2 Diabetes." Clinical Excellence for Nurse Practitioners: The International Journal of NPACE 4, no. 5 (2000): 272-276. https://doi.org/10.1111/j.1753-4887.1987.tb06343.x.

47. B. Schneeman, "Dietary Fiber and Gastrointestinal Function," *Nutrition Research* 18, no. 4 (1998): 625–632.

48. MedlinePlus. "Vitamins." Accessed September 13, 2013. https://medlineplus.gov/vitamins.html.

49. MedlinePlus. "Minerals." Accessed September 13, 2013. https://medlineplus.gov/minerals.html.

50. Food Revolution Network. "5 Key Supplements for Vegans and Vegetarians to Thrive on A Plant-Based Diet." Last modified December 1, 2017. https://foodrevolution.org/blog/supplements-vegetarians-vegans-plant-based/#vitamin-b12.

51. Office of Dietary Supplements. "Vitamin B12." Accessed September 13, 2013. http://ods.od.nih.gov/factsheets/VitaminB12-QuickFacts/.

52. Ibid.

53. Office of Dietary Supplements. "Zinc." Accessed September 16, 2013. http://ods.od.nih.gov/factsheets/Zinc-QuickFacts/.

54. Ibid.

55. Ibid.

56. Ibid.

57. Tseng, Marilyn, Rosalind A. Breslow, Barry I. Graubard, and Regina G. Ziegler. "Dairy, Calcium, and Vitamin D Intakes and Prostate Cancer Risk in the National Health and Nutrition Examination Epidemiologic Follow-up Study Cohort." *The American Journal of Clinical Nutrition* 81, no. 5 (2005): 1147-1154. https://doi.org/10.1093/ajcn/81.5.1147.

58. Luopajärvi, Kristiina, Erkki Savilahti, Suvi M. Virtanen, Jorma Ilonen, Mikael Knip, Hans K. Åkerblom, and Outi Vaarala. "Enhanced Levels of Cow's Milk Antibodies in Infancy in Children Who Develop Type 1 Diabetes Later in Childhood." *Pediatric Diabetes* 9, no. 5 (2008): 434-441. https://doi.org/10.1111/j.1399-5448.2008.00413.x.

59. Goldschmidt, Vivian. "Debunking The Milk Myth: Why Milk is Bad for You And Your Bones." Accessed November 25, 2013. http://saveourbones.com/osteoporosis-milk-myth/.

60. Feskanich, Diane, Walter C. Willett, Meir J. Stampfer, and Graham A. Colditz. "Milk, Dietary Calcium, and Bone Fractures in Women: a 12-Year Prospective Study." *American Journal of Public Health* 87, no. 6 (1997): 992-997. https://doi.org/10.2105/AJPH.87.6.992.

61. Pineda, Sofia. "7 Ways Milk and Dairy Products Are Making You Sick." Forks Over Knives. Last modified March 19, 2016. https://www.forksoverknives.com/7-ways-milk-and-dairy-products-are-making-you-sick/.

62. Ornish, Dean. "The Myth of High-Protein Diets." The New York Times. Last modified March 23, 2015. https://www.nytimes.com/2015/03/23/opinion/the-myth-of-high-protein-diets.html?smprod=nytcore-iphone&smid=nytcore-iphone-share.

63. Laskey, Jen. "The Health Benefits of Water." Everyday Health. Last modified February 16, 2015. https://www.everydayhealth.com/water-health/water-body-health.aspx.

64. Eastwood, Martin A., *Principles of Human Nutrition.* London: Blackwell Publishing, 2003.

65. Kleiner, Susan M. "Water: An Essential But Overlooked Nutrient." *Journal of the American Dietetic Association* 99, no. 2 (1999): 200-206. https://doi.org/10.1016/S0002-8223(99)00048-6.

66. Eisenbeiss, C., J. Welzel, W. Eichler, and K. Klotz. "Influence of Body Water Distribution on Skin Thickness: Measurements Using High-Frequency Ultrasound." British Journal of Dermatology 144, no. 5 (2001): 947-951. https://doi.org/10.1046/j.1365-2133.2001.04180.x.

67. Kleiner, Susan M. "Water: An Essential But Overlooked Nutrient." *Journal of the American Dietetic Association* 99, no. 2 (1999): 200-206. https://doi.org/10.1016/S0002-8223(99)00048-6.

68. Rogers, Peter J., A. Kainth, and H. J. Smit. "A Drink of Water Can Improve or Impair Mental Performance Depending on Small Differences in Thirst." *Appetite* 36, no. 1 (2001): 57-58. https://doi.org/10.1006/appe.2000.0374.

69. Maughan, R. J. "Impact of Mild Dehydration on Wellness and on Exercise Performance." *European Journal of Clinical Nutrition* 57, suppl. 2 (2003): S19–23.

70. Cian, Corinne, N. Koulmann, P. A. Barraud, C. Raphel, C. Jimenez, and B. Melin. "Influences of Variations in Body Hydration on Cognitive Function: Effect of Hyperhydration, Heat Stress, and Exercise-Induced Dehydration." *Journal of Psychophysiology* 14, no. 1 (2000): 29. http://dx.doi.org/10.1027//0269-8803.14.1.29.

71. Bar-David, Y. A. I. R., Jacob Urkin, and Ely Kozminsky. "The Effect of Voluntary Dehydration on Cognitive Functions of Elementary School Children." *Acta Padiatrica* 94 (2005): 1667-1673. https://doi.org/10.1080/08035250500254670.

72. Chan, Jacqueline, Synnove F. Knutsen, Glen G. Blix, Jerry W. Lee, and Gary E. Fraser. "Water, Other fluids, and Fatal Coronary Heart Disease: The Adventist Health Study." *American Journal of Epidemiology* 155, no. 9 (2002): 827-833. https://doi.org/10.1093/aje/155.9.827.

73. Stookey, Jodi D., Florence Constant, Barry M. Popkin, and Christopher D. Gardner. "Drinking Water is Associated with Weight Loss in Overweight Dieting Women Independent of Diet and Activity." *Obesity* 16, no. 11 (2008): 2481-2488. https://doi.org/10.1038/oby.2008.409.

74. Davy, Brenda M., Elizabeth A. Dennis, A. Laura Dengo, Kelly L. Wilson, and Kevin P. Davy. "Water Consumption Reduces Energy Intake at a Breakfast Meal in Obese Older Adults." *Journal of the American Dietetic Association* 108, no. 7 (2008): 1236-1239. https://doi.org/10.1016/j.jada.2008.04.013.

75. Lappalainen, R., L. Mennen, and H. Mykkänen. "Drinking Water with a Meal: A Simple Method of Coping with Feelings of Hunger, Satiety and Desire to Eat." *European Journal of Clinical Nutrition* 47, no. 11 (1993): 815-819.

76. Popkin, Barry M., Denis V. Barclay, and Samara J. Nielsen. "Water and Food Consumption Patterns of U.S. Adults from 1999 to 2001." *Obesity* 13, no. 12 (2005): 2146-2152. https://doi.org/10.1038/oby.2005.266.

77. Chan, Jacqueline, Synnove F. Knutsen, Glen G. Blix, Jerry W. Lee, and Gary E. Fraser. "Water, Other fluids, and Fatal Coronary Heart Disease: The Adventist Health Study." *American Journal of Epidemiology* 155, no. 9 (2002): 827-833. https://doi.org/10.1093/aje/155.9.827.

78. Healthy Kids. "Choose Water as a Drink." Accessed September 5, 2013, http://www.healthykids.nsw.gov.au/kids-teens/choose-water-asa-drink-kids.aspx.

79. National Institute for Alcohol and Alcohol Abuse. "Underage Drinking." Accessed September 16, 2013, http://pubs.niaaa.nih.gov/publications/AA67/AA67.htm.

80. Ibid.

81. Ibid.

82. Hasegawa, Tohru. "Anti-stress Effect of Beta-Carotene." *Annals of the New York Academy of Sciences* 691, no. 1 (1993): 281–283. https://doi.org/10.1111/j.1749-6632.1993.tb26196.x.

83. World Health Organization. *The World Health Report 2002: Reducing Risks, Promoting Healthy Life.* Switzerland: World Health Organization, 2002.

84. Hertog, Michael G. L., Edith J. M. Feskens, Daan Kromhout, P. C. H. Hollman, and M. B. Katan. "Dietary Antioxidant Flavonoids and Risk of Coronary Heart Disease: The Zutphen Elderly Study." *The Lancet* 342, no. 8878 (1993): 1007-1011. https://doi.org/10.1016/0140-6736(93)92876-U.

85. Boyer, Jeanelle and Rui H. Liu. "Apple Phytochemicals and Their Health Benefits." *Nutrition Journal*, no. 3 (2004): 5. https://doi.org/10.1186/1475-2891-3-5.

86. Sun, Jie, Yi-Fang Chu, Xianzhong Wu, and Rui Hai Liu. "Antioxidant and Antiproliferative Activities of Common Fruits." *Journal of Agricultural and Food Chemistry* 50, no. 25 (2002): 7449-7454. https://doi.org/10.1021/jf0207530.

87. Food and Drug Administration. "Nutrition Facts Label." Accessed September 12, 2013. https://choosemyplate-prod.azureedge.net/sites/default/files/sites/default/files/images/NutritionFactsLabel.pdf.

88. Austria, J. Alejandro, Melanie N. Richard, Mirna N. Chahine, Andrea L. Edel, Linda J. Malcolmson, Chantal MC Dupasquier, and Grant N. Pierce. "Bioavailability of Alpha-Linolenic Acid in Subjects After Ingestion of Three Different Forms of Flaxseed." *Journal of the American College of Nutrition* 27, no. 2 (2008): 214-221. https://doi.org/10.1080/07315724.2008.10719693.

89. Houston, Mark and William Sparks. 2008. "Latest Findings on Essential Fatty Acids and Cardiovascular Health." *The Original Internist*, no. 2 (2008): 65-68.

90. Donaldson, Michael S. "Nutrition and Cancer: A Review of the Evidence for an Anti-Cancer Diet." *Nutrition Journal* 3, no. 19 (2004): 3-5. https://doi.org/10.1186/1475-2891-3-19.

91. Marlett, Judith A., Michael I. McBurney, and Joanne L. Slavin. "Position of the American Dietetic Association: Health Implications of Dietary Fiber." *Journal of the Academy of Nutrition and Dietetics* 102, no. 7 (2002): 993-1000. https://doi.org/10.1016/S0002-8223(02)90228-2.

92. Cunnane, Stephen C., Mazen J. Hamadeh, Andrea C. Liede, Lilian U. Thompson, T. M. Wolever, and D. J. Jenkins. "Nutritional Attributes of Traditional Flaxseed in Healthy Young Adults." *The American Journal of Clinical Nutrition* 61, no. 1 (1995): 62-68. https://doi.org/10.1093/ajcn/61.1.62.

93. Miura, Katsuyuki, Jeremiah Stamler, Hideaki Nakagawa, Paul Elliott, Hirotsugu Ueshima, Queenie Chan, Ian J. Brown et al. "Relationship of dietary Linoleic Acid to Blood Pressure: The International Study of Macro-Micronutrients and Blood Pressure Study." *Hypertension* 52, no. 2 (2008): 408-414. https://doi.org/10.1161/hypertensionaha.108.112383.

94. Dahl, Wendy J., Erin A. Lockert, Allison L. Cammer, and Susan J. Whiting. "Effects of Flax Fiber on Laxation and Glycemic Response in Healthy Volunteers." *Journal of Medicinal Food* 8, no. 4 (2005): 508-511. https://doi.org/10.1089/jmf.2005.8.508.

95. Burgess, John R., Laura Stevens, Wen Zhang, and Louise Peck. "Long-Chain Polyunsaturated Fatty Acids in Children with Attention-Deficit Hyperactivity Disorder." *The American Journal of Clinical Nutrition* 71, no. 1 (2000): 327S-330S. https://doi.org/10.1093/ajcn/71.1.327S.

96. Das, Undurti N. "Long-Chain Polyunsaturated Fatty Acids in Memory Formation and Consolidation: Further Evidence and Discussion." *Nutrition* 19, no. 11 (2003): 988-993. https://doi.org/10.1016/S0899-9007(03)00174-6.

97. Marlett, Judith A., Michael I. McBurney, and Joanne L. Slavin. "Position of the American Dietetic Association: Health Implications of Dietary Fiber." *Journal of the Academy of Nutrition and Dietetics* 102, no. 7 (2002): 993-1000. https://doi.org/10.1016/S0002-8223(02)90228-2.

98. Horrobin, David F. "Essential Fatty Acids in Clinical Dermatology." *Journal of the American Academy of Dermatology* 20, no. 6 (1989): 1045-1053. https://doi.org/10.1016/S0190-9622(89)70130-4.

99. Phipps, W. R., M. C. Martini, J. W. Lampe, J. L. Slavin, and M. S. Kurzer. "Effect of Flax Seed Ingestion on the Menstrual Cycle." *The Journal of Clinical Endocrinology and Metabolism* 77, no. 5 (1993): 1215-1219.

100. Stoll, Andrew L., Carol A. Locke, L. B. Marangell, and W. E. Severus. "Omega-3 Fatty acids and Bipolar Disorder: A Review." *Prostaglandins, Leukotrienes and Essential Fatty Acids* 60, no. 5-6 (1999): 329-337. https://doi.org/10.1016/S0952-3278(99)80008-8.

101. Bazzano, Lydia A., Jiang He, Lorraine G. Ogden, Catherine Loria, Suma Vupputuri, Leann Myers, and Paul K. Whelton. "Legume Consumption and Risk of Coronary Heart Disease in U.S. Men and Women: NHANES I Epidemiologic Follow-up Study." *Archives of Internal Medicine* 161, no. 21 (2001): 2573-2578.

102. Kolonel, Laurence N., Jean H. Hankin, Alice S. Whittemore, Anna H. Wu, Richard P. Gallagher, Lynne R. Wilkens, Esther M. John, Geoffrey R. Howe, Darlene M. Dreon, Dee W. West, and Ralph S. Paffenbarger Jr.. "Vegetables, Fruits, Legumes and Prostate Cancer: A Multiethnic Case-Control Study." *Cancer Epidemiology and Prevention Biomarkers* 9, no. 8 (2000): 795-804.

103. Winham, Donna M., Andrea M. Hutchins, and Carol S. Johnston. "Pinto Bean Consumption Reduces Biomarkers for Heart Disease Risk." *Journal of the American College of Nutrition* 26, no. 3 (2007): 243-249.

104. Jacobsen, Bjarne K., Synnøve F. Knutsen, and Gary E. Fraser. "Does High Soy Milk Intake Reduce Prostate Cancer Incidence? The Adventist Health Study (United States)." *Cancer Causes & Control* 9, no. 6 (1998): 553-557. https://doi.org/10.1023/A:1008819500080.

NOTES